T0172759

Molecular Mechanisms of Skin Aging and Age-Related Diseases

Molecular Mechanisms of Skin Aging and Age-Related Diseases

Editor

Taihao Quan
Department of Dermatology
University of Michigan Medical School
Ann Arbor, Michigan
USA

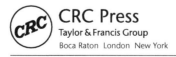

CRC Press
Taylor & Francis Group
Boca Raton London New York

CRC Press is an imprint of the
Taylor & Francis Group, an **informa** business

A SCIENCE PUBLISHERS BOOK

CRC Press
Taylor & Francis Group
6000 Broken Sound Parkway NW, Suite 300
Boca Raton, FL 33487-2742

First issued in paperback 2021

© 2016 by Taylor & Francis Group, LLC
CRC Press is an imprint of Taylor & Francis Group, an Informa business

No claim to original U.S. Government works

ISBN-13: 978-0-367-78300-6 (pbk)
ISBN-13: 978-1-4987-0464-9 (hbk)

This book contains information obtained from authentic and highly regarded sources. Reasonable efforts have been made to publish reliable data and information, but the author and publisher cannot assume responsibility for the validity of all materials or the consequences of their use. The authors and publishers have attempted to trace the copyright holders of all material reproduced in this publication and apologize to copyright holders if permission to publish in this form has not been obtained. If any copyright material has not been acknowledged please write and let us know so we may rectify in any future reprint.

Except as permitted under U.S. Copyright Law, no part of this book may be reprinted, reproduced, transmitted, or utilized in any form by any electronic, mechanical, or other means, now known or hereafter invented, including photocopying, microfilming, and recording, or in any information storage or retrieval system, without written permission from the publishers.

For permission to photocopy or use material electronically from this work, please access www.copyright. com (http://www.copyright.com/) or contact the Copyright Clearance Center, Inc. (CCC), 222 Rosewood Drive, Danvers, MA 01923, 978-750-8400. CCC is a not-for-profit organization that provides licenses and registration for a variety of users. For organizations that have been granted a photocopy license by the CCC, a separate system of payment has been arranged.

Trademark Notice: Product or corporate names may be trademarks or registered trademarks, and are used only for identification and explanation without intent to infringe.

Library of Congress Cataloging-in-Publication Data

Names: Quan, Taihao, editor.
Title: Molecular mechanisms of skin aging and age-related diseases / [edited by] Taihao Quan.
Description: Boca Raton : Taylor & Francis, 2016. | Includes bibliographical references and index.
Identifiers: LCCN 2016002046 | ISBN 9781498704649 (hardcover : alk. paper)
Subjects: | MESH: Skin Aging--physiology | Skin Aging--pathology | Skin Diseases | Aged
Classification: LCC RL96 | NLM WR 102 | DDC 616.5/07--dc23
LC record available at http://lccn.loc.gov/2016002046

Visit the Taylor & Francis Web site at
http://www.taylorandfrancis.com

and the CRC Press Web site at
http://www.crcpress.com

Preface

Human skin is the most voluminous connective tissue and the most abundant type of tissue in the human body. Human skin, like all other organs, undergoes natural aging as a consequence of the passage of time. In addition, human skin, unlike other organs, continuously experience harmful stress and damage from environmental sources such as solar UV irradiation.

Skin is directly accessible and change of skin appearance is among the most visible signs of aging. The directly observable prominent features of human skin aging, i.e. accumulation of tissue damage as well as decline of tissue mass and function with age are a universal characteristic of the aging process in other vital human organs. Therefore, human skin provides a unique source to unravel the progress of human aging at molecular levels, which may have direct relevance to aging in other human tissues. This book presents the most recent progress and understanding on the molecular mechanisms of human skin aging and age-related disorders. It provides a useful resource for researchers, dermatologists, students, teachers and also cosmetic industry interested in the field.

Chapter 1: The prominent molecular feature of aging skin is altered dermal connective tissue characterized by fragmentation and declined synthesis of collagen, the major structural protein in skin. Aberrant homeostasis of dermal connective tissue collagen, which is caused by impaired dermal fibroblast function, is primary responsible for the human skin aging. This chapter reviews molecular mechanisms of human skin connective tissue aging emphasizing three aspects: 1) impaired transforming growth factor-β signaling, 2) elevated matrix-degrading metalloproteinases (MMPs) and 3) age-associated dermal ECM microenvironment and age-related skin diseases.

Chapter 2: The in dermis represents the thickest compartment of the skin and play an important role in maintaining skin structure and function. Dermal (myo) fibroblasts are largely responsible for synthesis and maintenance of the dermal connective tissue. This chapter reviews the biology of dermal (myo) fibroblasts and their critical roles in maintenance of dermal connective tissue homeostasis, skin dermal aging process and age-related skin diseases.

Chapter 3: The epidermis serves as a barrier to protect the body against microbial pathogens, oxidant stress/UV light from the sun and chemical compounds. The two primary barrier functions of skin, permeability and antimicrobial barriers, are provided by lipids and proteins delivered to the extracellular spaces of the stratum corneum. Aged epidermis shows various changes in skin epidermal barrier impairment. This chapter discusses the molecular basis of epidermal barrier function and changes of skin barrier with aging as well as therapeutic strategies in aging skin barrier.

Chapter 4: While skin dryness causes fine epidermal wrinkles, deep wrinkles are caused by dermal connective tissue damage by degradation of collagen, the major structural protein in skin. In this chapter, the author discusses most recent molecular basis of age-related skin wrinkling with emphasize on the roles of proinflammatory cytokines and matrix-degrading metalloproteinases. The author proposed a new concept that skin dryness accelerates dermal wrinkling by promoting collagen degradation. This novel concept provides exciting therapeutic strategies that prevention of skin dryness could delay and/or rejuvenate the dermal wrinkles in aged human skin.

Chapter 5: Emerging evidence indicates that members of the CCN (CYR61/ CTGF/NOV) family proteins mediate aberrant collagen homeostasis in dermal fibroblasts and contributes to human skin connective tissue aging. Altered expression of CCN family members is associated with several pathological states, including tissue fibrosis, inflammation and cancer. This chapter describes the role of CCN proteins in skin connective tissue aging and in age-related skin diseases.

Chapter 6: Communications between cells and extracellular matrix microenvironment is critical and necessary for the maintenance of proper homeostasis of the skin. This chapter discusses the intercellular interactions in human skin and other squamous epithelia and focuses predominantly on the role of fibroblasts in wound healing and cancer development.

Chapter 7: In this chapter, the author discusses mitochondrial DNA common deletion in human skin connective tissue aging. Impairment of dermal fibroblast morphology with aging brings about numerous alterations including increased mitochondrial oxidative stress, which promotes mtDNA common deletion. Increased mtDNA common deletion could further induce oxidative stress through a positive feedback mechanism, forming a critical mechanism of human skin aging. This mechanism extends current understanding of the oxidative theory of aging by recognizing that age-related impairment of dermal fibroblast morphology induces mtDNA common deletion through mitochondrial ROS/oxidative stress.

Chapter 8: Topical application is fundamental in dermatologic therapy. Nanomaterials are very useful for drugdelivery in skin topical treatment. These nanoplatforms have been shown to have great benefit for use as wound healing, antimicrobial therapies, anti-inflammatory therapeutics, antineoplastic agents and cosmetics. This chapter discusses an overview of nanotechnology and the use of nanotechnology in dermatologic disorders (nanodermatology).

Chapter 9: As we grow older, chronic diseases will become more prevalent, including diseases of the skin. Clinicians often see more elderly patients presenting with age-related dermatological conditions, such as xerosis and pruritus. Geriatric dermatology is associated with significant morbidity and financial burden on our health care system. This chapter reviews the most common skin disorders seen in elderly.

Chapter 10: Physical appearance is important to many individuals and can influence how individuals are perceived by others. Lasers have been extensively used in dermatology for the purpose of rejuvenating skin appearance. This chapter reviews the use of lasers for skin regeneration, healing and summarizes relevant laser physics and laser tissue interaction.

Chapter 11: Aging is defined as a natural, gradual process of biochemical events, leading to gradual damage accumulation and resulting in disease and death. Such changes are hidden as far as the inner organs are concerned and therefore, the skin appears as the first and main teller of these gradual alterations. Skin can be considered the "key hole" to observe the aging process of the whole organism. This chapter reviews key mechanisms involved in skin aging and aging skin as a potential marker of aging in other human tissues.

Chapter 12: During the skin aging process, both the dermis and the epidermis are becoming thinner and the dermal-epidermal junction flattens. In the dermis, the most dramatic changes are the fragmentation and reduction of the extracellular matrix, which leads to the formation of wrinkles. In the epidermis, the proliferation rate of keratinocytes slows down but the most dramatic effect is the change in the protein composition of the cornified envelope. This chapter reviews most recent molecular basis of skin aging with a focus on the cornified envelope.

Taihao Quan

Contents

List of Contributors

Eung Ho Choi

Department of Dermatology, Yonsei University Wonju College of Medicine, 20 Ilsan-dong, Wonju, 220-701, South Korea
E-mail: choieh@yonsei.ac.kr

Alexis Desmoulière

Department of Physiology, Faculty of Pharmacy, University of Limoges, 2 rue du Dr. Marcland, 87025 Limoges cedex, France
E-mail: alexis.desmouliere@unilim.fr

Barbora Dvořánková

Charles University, 1st Faculty of Medicine, Institute of Anatomy, U Nemocnice 3, 128 00 Prague 2, Czech Republic
E-mail: barbora.dvorankova@lf1.cuni.cz

Adam J. Friedman

Department of Dermatology, George Washington School of Medicine and Health Sciences, Washington, DC
E-mail: Ajfriedman@mfa.gwu.edu

Dorothée Girard

University of Limoges, EA (Equiped'Accueil) 6309 "Myelin maintenance and peripheral neuropathies", Faculties of Medicine and Pharmacy, Limoges, France

CHU (Centre Hospitalier Universitaire) Dupuytren de Limoges, Limoges, France
E-mail: dorothee.girard@unilim.fr

Aleksandar Godic

Consultant Dermatologist, Dermatology, University Hospital Lewisham, High Street, London, SE13 6LH, UK
E-mail: aleksandar.godic@gmail.com

Nicolette Nadene Houreld

Laser Research Centre, Faculty of Health Sciences, University of Johannesburg, PO Box 17011, Doornfontein, Johannesburg, 2028, South Africa
E-mail: nhoureld@uj.ac.za

Ondřej Kodet

Charles University, 1st Faculty of Medicine, Institute of Anatomy and Department of Dermatovenerology, U Nemocnice 2 and 3, 128 00 Prague 2, Czech Republic
E-mail: ondrej.kodet@lf1.cuni.cz

Michal Kolář

Institute of Molecular Genetics, Academy of Sciences vvi., Vídeňská 1083,142 20 Prague, Czech Republic
E-mail: kolarmi@img.cas.cz

Eliška Krejčí

Charles University, 1st Faculty of Medicine, Institute of Anatomy, U Nemocnice 3, 128 00 Prague 2, Czech Republic
E-mail: eliska.krejci@lf1.cuni.cz

Lukáš Lacina

Charles University, 1st Faculty of Medicine, Institute of Anatomy and Department of Dermatovenerology, U Nemocnice 2 and 3, 128 00 Prague 2, Czech Republic
E-mail: lukas.lacina@lf1.cuni.cz

Angelo Landriscina

Department of Medicine (Division of Dermatology), Albert Einstein College of Medicine, Bronx, New York

Betty Laverdet

University of Limoges, EA (Equiped' Accueil) 6309 "Myelin maintenance and peripheral neuropathies", Faculties of Medicine and Pharmacy, Limoges, France

CHU (Centre Hospitalier Universitaire) Dupuytren de Limoges, Limoges, France
E-mail: betty.laverdet@etu.unilim.fr

Evgenia Makrantonaki

Departments of Dermatology, Venereology, Allergology and Immunology, Dessau Medical Center, 06847 Dessau, Germany

Geriatry Research Group, Charité Universitaetsmedizin Berlin, 13347 Berlin, Germany

Department of Dermatology and Allergology, University Medical Center Ulm, 89081 Ulm, Germany
E-mail: evgenia.makrantonaki@uni-ulm.de

Hitoshi Masaki

Tokyo University of Technology, School of Bioscience and Biotechnology Advanced Cosmetic Course, Photoaging Research Laboratory 1404-1, Katakura-cho, Hachioji, Tokyo 192-0982, Japan
E-mail: masaki@stf.teu.ac.jp

Ondřej Naňka

Charles University, 1st Faculty of Medicine, Institute of Anatomy, U Nemocnice 3, 128 00 Prague 2, Czech Republic
E-mail: ondrej.nanka@lf1.cuni.cz

Georgios Nikolakis

Departments of Dermatology, Venereology, Allergology and Immunology, Dessau Medical Center, 06847 Dessau, Germany
E-mail: georgios.nikolakis@klinikum-dessau.de

Chunji Quan

Department of Pathology, Affiliated Hospital of Yanbian University, Yanji 133000, Jilin Province, China
E-mail: chunjiquan@163.com

Taihao Quan

Department of Dermatology, University of Michigan Medical School, Ann Arbor, Michigan, USA
E-mail: thquan@umich.edu

Klaus Richter

Department of Cell Biology, Division of Genetics, University of Salzburg, Salzburg 5020, Austria
E-mail: klaus.richter@sbg.ac.at

Mark Rinnerthaler

Department of Cell Biology, Division of Genetics, University of Salzburg, Salzburg 5020, Austria
E-mail: mark.rinnerthaler@sbg.ac.at

Jamie Rosen

Department of Medicine (Division of Dermatology), Albert Einstein College of Medicine, Bronx, New York

Karel Smetana, jr.

Charles University, 1st Faculty of Medicine, Institute of Anatomy, U Nemocnice 3, 128 00 Prague 2, Czech Republic
E-mail: karel.smetana@lf1.cuni.cz

Maria Karolin Streubel

Department of Cell Biology, Division of Genetics, University of Salzburg, Salzburg 5020, Austria
E-mail: mariakarolin.streubel@stud.sbg.ac.at

Hynek Strnad

Institute of Molecular Genetics, Academy of Sciences vvi., Vídeňská 1083,142 20 Prague, Czech Republic
E-mail: strnad@img.cas.cz

Pavol Szabo

Charles University, 1st Faculty of Medicine, Institute of Anatomy, U Nemocnice 3, 128 00 Prague 2, Czech Republic
E-mail: pavol.szabo@lf1.cuni.cz

Christos C. Zouboulis

Departments of Dermatology, Venereology, Allergology and Immunology, Dessau Medical Center, 06847 Dessau, Germany
E-mail: christos.zouboulis@klinikum-dessau.de

1

Molecular Mechanisms of Human Skin Connective Tissue Aging

Taihao Quan

❑ Introduction

Human skin, the outmost organ of the body, is the largest and the heaviest organ of the human body. Human skin serves as a protective barrier from harmful environmental factors, such as heat, solar ultraviolet (UV) irradiation, micro-organisms, wounding and water loss (Chuong et al. 2002; Farage et al. 2010; Kolarzyk and Pach 2000). The human skin is composed of three distinct layers: the outermost epidermis, the thick dermis below the epidermis and the deepest hypodermis below the dermis (Bolognia et al. 2008; Farage et al. 2010). The epidermis is primarily composed of keratinocytes, which produce keratins that are a major component of the protective skin barrier. The dermis is composed of a dense collage-rich connective tissue and stromal cells such as dermal fibroblasts. The subcutaneous hypodermis consists of fat cells dispersed throughout the connective tissue framework. The dermal connective tissue is intimately interacts with the epidermis and subcutaneous hypodermis to support the structural and mechanical integrity of the skin. The dermis is less cellular than the epidermis. The bulk of human skin is composed of dense collagen-rich extracellular matrix (ECM) proteins, such as collagen, elastin, fibronectin and proteoglycans. As human skin is the heaviest organ of the body, dermal collagen represents by far the most abundant protein that constitutes the bulk (90% dry weight) of skin (Bernstein et al. 1996; Uitto 1986). Dermal connective tissue collagen is essentially responsible for the skin's structural and mechanical properties. In human skin, collagen-rich ECM is synthesized, organized

Department of Dermatology, University of Michigan Medical School, Ann Arbor, Michigan, USA.
E-mail: thquan@umich.edu

and maintained by dermal fibroblasts (Farage et al. 2010; Fisher et al. 2008). Dermal fibroblasts secrete the precursors of all the components of the ECM proteins in skin. Therefore, the main function of dermal fibroblasts is to maintain the structural and mechanical integrity of the skin by maintaining collagen homeostasis, such as controlling the turnover of collagen and other ECM proteins. By creating dermal ECM connective tissue, dermal fibroblasts control skin's homeostasis including maintenance of epidermal barrier/ protective functions and regulation of body temperature, sensory reception, vascularization and water balance. Therefore, collagen is the principal structural protein in skin and alteration of dermal fibroblast function has significant impact on homeostasis of collagen.

Collagen is not only the major structural protein of the skin, but also is the most abundant protein, making up about 25% to 35% of the whole-body protein content (Di Lullo et al. 2002). In human, collagen is mostly found in fibrous connective tissue such as bone, tendon, ligament and skin and is also abundant in cornea, cartilage, blood vessels, the gut and intervertebral disc. Type I collagen is by far the main structural protein of the dermal ECM connective tissue and therefore the main component of human skin. Type I collagen forms collagen fibrils in association with other types of collagen (i.e. type III, type V, Type XIV) and other ECM proteins. Collagen fibrils serve two major functions, mechanical support and scaffold for cellular attachment.

Like all proteins, type I collagen undergoes natural breakdown and fragmentation by enzymatic degradation. However, collagen degradation in human skin is very slow, with calculated half-life of 17 years (Verzijl et al. 2000). Humans express several enzymes that are capable of breakdown and fragmentation of type I collagen. These enzymes are members of a family of matrix protein-degrading enzymes, referred to as matrix metalloproteinases (MMPs), as discussed in detail below (Hegedus et al. 2008; Lapiere Ch 2005). MMPs comprise a large family of proteinases that are capable of degrading every type of dermal ECM protein (Page-McCaw et al. 2007). In human skin, dermal fibroblasts are the major source of MMPs production (Brennan et al. 2003; Fisher et al. 2009; Qin et al. 2014).

Human skin, like all other organs, undergoes natural aging process with the passage of time. The prominent molecular feature of aging skin is altered dermal microenvironment characterized by fragmentation of collagen fibrils and declined collagen synthesis (Fisher et al. 2002; Fisher et al. 2009; Fisher et al. 2008; Qin et al. 2014; Varani et al. 2006). Age-related alteration of dermal microenvironment is the driving force for the most prominent clinical features of aged skin. Age-related alteration of dermal microenvironment impairs skin dermis structural and mechanical properties and creates a tissue microenvironment that promotes age-related skin diseases, such as thinning, increased fragility, impaired vasculature support, poor wound healing and a tissue microenvironment that promotes cancer. Therefore, mechanisms that alter the dermal microenvironment are critically important to both the primary clinical features and the pathophysiology of skin aging.

This chapter describes the role of dermal fibroblasts in skin connective tissue aging and in age-related skin diseases.

❑ Human Skin Connective Tissue Aging and Dermal Fibroblasts

Human skin, like all other organs, undergoes natural aging process as a consequence of the passage of time. Meantime, human skin, unlike other organs, continuously experience harmful stress and damage from environmental sources such as solar ultraviolet (UV) radiation and micro-organisms. (Fisher et al. 2008; Yaar and Gilchrest 1998). Ultraviolet irradiation from the sun is a well-recognized, potent environmental insult capable of damaging skin tissue. UV-induced skin damage includes sunburn, immune suppression, cancer and premature skin aging (photoaging) (Biesalski et al. 2003; de Pablo et al. 2000; Fisher et al. 2002; Taylor and Sober 1996; Yaar and Gilchrest 2007). Based on its causes, cutaneous aging can be classified into two types: natural aging, also known as intrinsic aging and photoaging, also known as extrinsic aging. Natural aging refers to those changes observed in all individuals resulting from the passage of time, whereas photoaging refers to those changes attributable to habitual sun exposure. Both processes are cumulative and therefore photoaging is superimposed on intrinsic aging. Therefore, the alterations seen in aged skin are a combination of intrinsic and extrinsic aging. The most clinically noticeable age-related changes occur on face, neck, forearm and lower leg skin (Wlaschek et al. 2001). These areas undergo a combination of natural aging and photoaging and age-related skin diseases occur most often in these areas. Aging skin is recognizable by fine and course wrinkles, skin laxity, coarseness, uneven pigmentation and brown spots. Histological and ultrastructural studies have revealed that the major alterations in photoaged skin are localized in the connective tissue dermis (Fisher et al. 1996a; Fisher et al. 1997a). Biochemical evidence of connective tissue damage in aged human skin includes alterations of collagen and elastin. Since collagen fibrils and elastin are responsible for the strength and resiliency of skin, their degeneration with aging causes skin to become fragile and easily bruised. Histologically, connective tissue damage induced by ultraviolet irradiation manifests as a disorganization of collagen fibrils, massive accumulation of abnormal, amorphous and elastin-containing material. The accumulation of elastotic material is accompanied by degeneration of the surrounding collagen matrix. Naturally-aged skin differs from photoaged skin. The severity of changes in the dermal matrix of naturally-aged skin relative to photoaged skin is less. Only a modest increase in the number and thickness of elastic fibers is observed. However, reflecting the general atrophic state of naturally-aged skin, there are reduced collagen production and increased collagen damage, compared to younger skin (Fisher et al. 2009; Quan and Fisher 2015).

Young Collagen   **Aged Collagen**

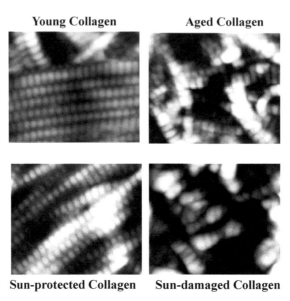

Sun-protected Collagen   Sun-damaged Collagen

FIG. 1   *Alteration of dermal connective tissue collagen is a characteristic feature of naturally aged and photoaged human skin. Nanoscale human skin dermal collagen fibrils are analyzed by atomic force microscopy (AFM). Representative AFM images of dermal collagen fibrils in 21 years old vs 83 years old individuals (top panel) and 54 years old sun-protected underarm vs sun-damaged forearm human skin (lower panel).*

In human skin, collagen-rich ECM is synthesized, organized and maintained by dermal fibroblasts (Farage et al. 2010; Fisher et al. 2008). Figure 1 shows nanoscale topographical images of dermal collagen fibrils assessed by atomic force microscopy (AFM). In young (20-30 years) or sun-protected underarm (50-60 years) human skin, intact and well-organized collagen fibrils are abundant and tightly packed (left panels). In contrast, in aged (80 +years) or sun-exposed forearm (50-60 years) human dermis (right panels), collagen fibrils are fragmented, disorganized and scarce. Therefore, in general, naturally-aged and photoaged skin share common molecular features, characterized by aberrant collagen homeostasis that includes reduced production of collagen and increased collagen degradation (Fisher et al. 2000; Fisher et al. 2002; Fisher et al. 2009; Fisher et al. 2008; Quan and Fisher 2015; Quan et al. 2010b). This aberrant collagen homeostasis results in net collagen deficiency which is characteristic features of skin connective tissue aging. Age-related aberrant collagen homeostasis creates impaired tissue microenvironment by reducing structural/mechanical integrity of the skin and causes age-related skin diseases. Therefore, aberrant collagen homeostasis is central event in human skin connective tissue aging, which is virtually caused by impaired dermal fibroblasts function, as described below.

❑ Impaired Transforming Growth Factor-β (TGF-β) Pathway in Dermal Fibroblasts Contributes to Thin Skin Dermisin Human Skin Connective Tissue Aging

Two interrelated mechanisms are involved in human skin connective tissue aging; reduced collagen biosynthesis and increased collagen fibril fragmentation. These mechanisms result in a net collagen deficiency, which manifests as thin, fragile skin. TGF-β signaling plays a central role in ECM biosynthesis and thus is critical for maintaining of dermal connective tissue structural and mechanical integrity (Ignotz and Massague 1986; Patil et al. 2011; Quan et al. 2010b; Varga et al. 1987). In human dermal fibroblasts, TGF-β not only functions as primary regulator for collagen and other ECM synthesis, but also prevents collagen fragmentation by inhibiting MMP-1 expression (Hall et al. 2003; Quan et al. 2002a). Therefore, impaired TGF-β signaling has significant impact on collagen homeostasis in human skin. In mammals, three isoforms of TGF-β, TGF-β1, TGF-β2, TGF-β3, have been identified (Massague 1990). TGF-β initiates its cellular action by interaction with its cell surface receptor complex, composed of TGF-β type I receptor (TβRI) and TGF-β type II receptor (TβRII) (Massague 2000). Binding of TGF-β allows TβRII to activate TβRI, which in turn phosphorylates intracellular transcription factors, Smad2 and Smad3. Activated Smad2 or Smad3 forms heteromeric complexes with the common partner, Smad4. Activated Smad complexes translocate into nucleus, where they interact with Smad Binding Element (SBE) in the promoter regions of TGF-β target genes, such as collagen, connective tissue growth factor (CCN2/CTGF), fibronectin and MMP-1.

A wealth of evidence indicates that TGF-β plays a central role in stimulation of collagen and other ECM in numerous fibrotic disorders and wound healing, where it is believed to stimulate deposition of collagenous ECM (Mauviel 2005; Varga and Whitfield 2009). While TGF-β-stimulatory action on collagen and other ECM deposition is relatively well studied, there are limited studies about collagen-loss in aged human skin as a consequence of impaired-TGF-β signaling pathway. Studies from Quan et al. demonstrate that impaired TGF-β signaling in aged human skin dermal fibroblasts is a one of the mechanisms of the collagen-loss in aged human skin (Quan et al. 2002a, b, 2004a; Quan et al. 2001; Quan et al. 2010b). Laser capture microdissection (LCM) coupled quantitative real-time RT-PCR indicates that TβRII mRNA level is reduced 59% in aged (80+years) skin dermis, compared to young (20-30 years) skin dermis *in vivo* (Quan et al. 2006; Quan et al. 2010b). Similarly, TβRII mRNA level is reduced 38% in photoaged forearm skin, compared with subject-matched, sun-protected hip skin (Quan et al. 2006). In contrast to TβRII, no change in TβRI mRNA level is observed in young and aged or photoaged and sun-protected human skin *in vivo*. Interestingly, TβRII mRNA expression is substantially reduced in human skin *in vivo* by UV irradiation (Quan et al. 2004), as seen in naturally-aged and photoaged human skin *in vivo*. In contrast, TβRI mRNA expression is not altered by UV irradiation, as observed in naturally-aged and photoaged human skin *in vivo*, suggesting TβRII specific down-regulation by UV irradiation. UV irradiation of cultured adult human dermal fibroblasts indicates that both TβRII mRNA and protein levels are significantly decreased, while UV irradiation had no effect on expression of either TβRI mRNA or protein (Quan et al. 2004). As described above, TGF-β initiates its cellular action by binding to cell surface receptors, TβRI and TβRII. Reduced expression of TβRII causes reduced binding of TGF-β1 to the surface of dermal fibroblasts (Quan et al. 2001). This loss of TGF-β binding results in decreased cellular responsiveness to TGF-β (Quan et al. 2001). In the absence of functional receptor-binding, TGF-β is no longer able to stimulate phosphorylation of its intracellular transcription factors Smad2 and Smad3. Therefore, Smad2 and Smad3 do not translocate into the nucleus or alter transcription of target genes. Electrophoretic Mobility Shift Assays (EMSA), using the Smad 3 Binding Element (SBE) as probe, shows that exposure of human skin to UV irradiation substantially reduces formation of the TGF-β-induced DNA/Smad complex (Quan et al. 2002b). Preventing loss of TβRII by over-expression of TβRII expression vector restores TGF-β activation of Smad3 and therefore protects against UV inhibition of type I procollagen gene expression (Quan et al. 2004).

The mechanism by which UV irradiation specifically reduces TβRII levels in human skin fibroblasts has been studied by investigating the possibility that UV irradiation could affect the stability of TβRII mRNA and protein (Quan et al. 2004). Reduced TβRII expression could result from increased degradation and/or reduced synthesis. Non-irradiated or UV-irradiated skin fibroblasts are treated with actinomycin D or cycloheximide to prevent *de novo* mRNA or protein synthesis, respectively and the half-lives of TβRII mRNA and protein are determined. The half-life of TβRII mRNA and protein is similar, in both non-irradiated and UV-irradiated cells. These data demonstrate that UV irradiation does not alter degradation of either TβRII mRNA or TβRII protein. Given that UV irradiation does not accelerate breakdown of either TβRII mRNA or protein, the observed UV reduction of TβRII mRNA and protein could result from reduced TβRII protein synthesis. The ability of UV irradiation to inhibit TβRII protein synthesis was confirmed by comparison of *de novo* TβRII protein synthesis in sham and UV-irradiated human skin fibroblasts. The protein synthesis of TβRII is significantly lower in UV-irradiated human skin fibroblasts, compared to non-irradiated fibroblasts. Furthermore, UV irradiation reduces TβRII promoter luciferase reporter, confirming the ability of UV irradiation to inhibit TβRII gene transcription. A series of 5′-deletion of TβRII promoter (covering 2 kb of the TβRII proximal promoter) revels that a 137-bp region upstream of the transcriptional start site is responsible for UV-inhibition of TβRII promoter (He et al. 2014a). Mutation of potential transcription factor binding sites within this promoter region reveals that an inverted CCAAT box (-81 bp from transcription start site) is required for promoter activity. Mutation of the CCAAT box completely abolishes UV irradiation regulation of the TβRII promoter. Super shift experiments indicate that nuclear factor Y (NFY) is able to binding to this sequence, however NFY binding is not altered in response to UV irradiation, indicating additional protein(s) are capable of binding this sequence in response to UV irradiation. These data demonstrate that down regulation of TβRII is resulted from inhibition of transcription and protein synthesis, rather than alteration of TβRII mRNA or protein stabilities. These data provide strong support for the new concept that down-regulation of TβRII is a critical event in reduced procollagen synthesis in naturally-aged and photoaged human skin.

Smad proteins function as core intracellular signaling transducer in mediating TGF-β signaling. Smad proteins play pivotal role in TGF-β-dependent regulation of collagen and other ECM production. However, little is known about the role of specific Smad protein in loss of collagen production, which is major contributing factor to age-related thinning of the skin. Two TGF-β receptor-activated Smad transcription factors, Smad2 and Smad3, has been shown to play an important role in mediating TGF-β signaling pathway (Massague 2000). However, less is known whether or which Smad proteins are involved in age-related collagen loss in human skin. The relative contribution of Smad2 and Smad3 to TGF-β-dependent regulation of type I procollagen in human skin dermal fibroblasts has been investigated by siRNA-mediated knockdown approaches. Strikingly, knockdown of endogenous Smad3, but not Smad2, reduces basal and TGF-β1-stimulated type I procollagen and CTGF/CCN2 (connective tissue growth factor), which is primarily regulated by TGF-β and functions as downstream mediator of TGF-β-induced type I procollagen (Quan et al. 2010b; Thompson et al. 2010). Conversely, over-expression Smad3, but not Smad2, increases type I procollagen and CTGF/CCN2 mRNA and protein, suggesting that Smad3, but not Smad2 mediates type I procollagen and CTGF/CCN2 expression in human skin fibroblasts.

Blocking TGF-β type I receptor activation by a selective inhibitor of TβRI kinase (SB431542) (Laping et al. 2002) completely abolishes basal and TGF-β-induced Smad3 phosphorylation and TGF-β/Smad3-dependent reporter activity. Consistently, inhibition of Smad3 activation significantly reduces both basal and TGF-β-induced type I procollagen and CTGF/CCN2 mRNA and protein. Importantly, overexpression of Smad3, but not Smad2, overcomes the reduced type I collagen and CTGF/CCN2 by TβRI kinase inhibitor. These data further demonstrate that Smad3, but not Smad2, is required for type I procollagen and CTGF/CCN2 gene expression in human skin fibroblasts.

Interestingly, the protein level of Smad3, but not Smad2, is markedly reduced in *in vitro* aging model of senescent cells. Consistently, Smad3 reporter activity is significantly reduced in senescent cells. Importantly, this reduced Smad3 activity is coincident with reduced type I procollagen and CTGF/CCN2 in senescent cells, suggesting that Smad3-specific down-regulation mediates the reduced expression of type I procollagen and CTGF/CCN2 in *in vitro* aging model of senescent cells (He et al. 2014b). Restoration of reduce Smad3 by overexpression results in significant increases of Smad3 phosphorylation, type I procollagen and CTGF/CCN2 in senescent dermal fibroblast. These data provide evidence that down-regulation of type I procollagen and CTGF/CCN2 in senescent dermal fibroblast is mediated by reduction of Smad3. The mechanism by which Smad3 protein specific reduction in senescent dermal fibroblasts remains to be determined. One possibility is that elevated ROS and protein oxidation in senescent dermal fibroblasts (He et al. 2014b) may enhance Smad3 protein susceptibility to proteolytic degradation (Davies 1987; Davies and Delsignore 1987; Davies et al. 1987a; Davies and Goldberg 1987a, b; Davies et al. 1987b). TGF-β receptors and Smads proteins have been reported to be degraded via ubiquitin-proteosome and sumoylation pathways turnover (Bonni et al. 2001; Fukuchi et al. 2001; Izzi and Attisano 2004; Kavsak et al. 2000; Lin et al. 2000; Lin et al. 2003a; Lin et al. 2003b; Long et al. 2004; Moustakas et al. 2001). Both protein degradation systems are regulated by ROS (Bossis and Melchior 2006; Manza et al. 2004; Saitoh and Hinchey 2000; Zhou et al. 2004). However, oxidative exposure does not alter the half-life of Smad3 protein, arguing against accelerated protein degradation (He et al. 2014b). It appears more likely that reduced protein synthesis, which has been observed to occur in response to elevated ROS, may account for the observed reduction of Smad3 protein levels.

More importantly, the levels of Smad3, but not Smad2, mRNA and protein is significantly reduced in aged human skin, compared to young human skin *in vivo*. Consistently, this reduced Smad3 is coincident with reduced type I procollagen and CTGF/CCN2 in aged human skin *in vivo*. These data demonstrate that Smad3 is a key molecule in mediating TGF-β stimulation of type I procollagen in human skin fibroblasts and reduced expression of Smad3 likely contributes to loss of type I procollagen in aged human skin fibroblasts *in vivo*.

In general, Smad3 is an essential mediator of TGF-β immediate-early target genes, such as transcription factors, for example JunB, c-fos c-Myc. Inhibition of Smad3 but Smad2 allows keratinocytes to escape from TGF-β induced cell cycle arrest. In contrast, some gene such as matrix metalloproteinase, MMP-2 expression is Smad2 dependent but not Smad3. On the other hand, some genes such as plasminogen activator inhibitor-1 (PIA-1) require both Smad2 and Smad3. One of the significant physical differences between Smad2 and Sma3 is DNA binding ability. Smad3 is able to bind directly to the TGF-β target gene promoter but not Smad2 (Massague et al. 2005). The data from Smad2 and Smad3 knockout mice further suggested that individual Smad plays different roles during embryonic development (Brown et al. 2007). Deletion of Smad2 is embryonic lethal due to failure to establish an anterior-posterior axis, gastrulation and mesoderm formation, whereas Smad3 knockout mice are viable and survival several months, suggesting that Smad3 is dispensable for embryonic development. In supporting our data, targeted disruption of Smad3 significantly attenuates pulmonary, renal and skin fibrosis in a mouse models, suggesting that Smad3 plays an important role in collagen homeostasis (Bonniaud et al. 2004; Flanders et al. 2002; Inazaki et al. 2004; Lakos et al. 2004; Roberts et al. 2001). Apart from Smad-dependent signaling pathway, non-Smad signaling pathways have been implicated in TGF-β stimulation of type I procollagen in variety of cell types. For example, TGF-β-induced collagen is mediated by direct activation of mitogen-activate protein kinase (MAPK) pathway, including extracellular signal-regulated protein kinase (ERK), c-Jun N-terminal kinase (JNK) and p38 (Mulder 2000). In addition to MAPK, TGF-β can activate PI3 kinase and that also mediates TGF-β-dependent collagen synthesis (Asano et al. 2004). TGF-β also activates PKC δ, which in turn mediates TGF-β stimulation of type I collagen (Runyan et al. 2003). However, TGF-β minimally activates these non-Smad pathways including MAPK PI3 kinase and PKC pathways in primary adult human skin fibroblasts. Furthermore, blocking of these pathways by well-known selective inhibitors, such as PD98059 for ERK, SB203580 for p38, JNK inhibitor I for JNK, LY294002 for PI3K/AKT and Calphostin C for PKC does not alter TGF-β stimulation of type I collagen in human skin fibroblasts. In contrast, "switching off" of Smad3 pathway near completely abolished TGF-β-stimulation of type I procollagen, suggesting type I procollagen is primarily mediated by Smad3-dependent mechanism in adult primary human skin fibroblasts.

Thinning of the skin connective tissue dermis takes place commonly in chronologically-aged individuals and one of the most prominent features in aged skin. Loss of type I collagen, the major structural component in human skin, is responsible for thinning of the skin and alteration of skin dermal structural architecture. Smad3 functions a key molecule in mediating TGF-β stimulation of type I procollagen and reduced expression of Smad3 likely contributes to loss of type I procollagen in aged human skin fibroblasts *in vivo*. The mechanism(s) involved in Smad3-sepecific down-regulation in aging skin fibroblasts is unknown. Additional investigation is clearly warranted to explore the mechanisms of reduced expression of Smad3 in aged human skin. One potential clue behind reduced expression of Smad3 in aged human skin is that Smad3 is significantly down-regulated in oxidative stress-induced senescent dermal fibroblasts. As reactive oxygen spaces (ROS) considers as a major driving force in aging process (Balaban et al. 2005; Finkel and Holbrook 2000), oxidative damage is significantly elevated in aged skin dermis and inhibits type I procollagen gene expression (Fisher et al. 2009). These observations suggest that elevated oxidative stress in aging skin likely down-regulates Smad3, which in turn contributes to loss of type I collagen in aging skin. Further studies are needed to understand the mechanisms about how ROS/oxidative stress specifically down-regulates Smad3 in human dermal fibroblasts.

In addition to Smad2 and Smad3, Smad7 functions to interfere with TGF-β-induced activation of Smad2 and Smad3 and thereby acts to block TGF-β signaling. Expression of Smad7 is induced by TGF-β itself, indicating a negative feedback mechanism that regulates TGF-β/Smad signaling (Afrakhte et al. 1998; Hayashi et al. 1997; Itoh et al. 1998; Nakao et al. 1997). Aberrant regulation of Smad7 could impair the delicate balance inherent in TGF-β/Smad signaling and thereby contribute to pathophysiology of certain human diseases (Fiocchi 2001; He et al. 2002; Nakao et al. 2002; Varga 2002). For example, in the fibrotic disease scleroderma, the level of Smad7 expression has been reported to be reduced (Dong et al. 2002). This reduction could allow unbalanced activation of the TGF-β/Smad pathway, resulting in excess production and deposition of ECM, the hallmark of fibrosis. Conversely, Smad7 has been reported to be over-expressed in inflammatory bowel disease (Monteleone et al. 2001). This over-expression could dismiss TGF-β-mediated immunosuppression, resulting in hyper-secretion of proinflammatory cytokines. Smad2, Smad3 and Smad4 are constitutively expressed in human skin and cultured human dermal fibroblasts and that UV irradiation has no significant effect on the protein level of any of these three Smad proteins (Quan et al. 2005). In contrast, exposure of the human skin *in vivo* or *in vitro* cultured dermal fibroblasts to acute solar UV irradiation rapidly induces the expression of Smad7 mRNA and protein (Quan et al. 2005). Importantly, this induction of Smad7 by UV irradiation results inhibition of TGF-β-induced type I procollagen gene expression. UV irradiation potently induces Smad7 promoter reporter activity, indicating that Smad7 induction is, at least in part, regulated at transcription level. The 5'-flanking region of the Smad7 promoter contains binding sequences for transcription factors Smad3 and AP-1 (Brodin et al. 2000). These regulatory elements and flanking sequences of the Smad7 gene promoter are near completely conserved in human, rat and murine genes (Stopa et al. 2000). Transcription factors Smad3 and AP-1 are necessary for optimal induction of Smad7 transcription (Brodin et al. 2000; Nagarajan et al. 1999; von Gersdorff et al. 2000). Disruption of Smad3 element abolishes TGF-β-mediated induction of Smad7, but does not greatly impair basal expression (Quan et al. 2005). Disruption of AP-1 binding site substantially reduces both basal and TGF-β-stimulated Smad7 expression. UV irradiation reduces protein binding to the Smad3 site and increases binding to the AP-1 site. Analysis of proteins bound to the AP-1 site reveals increased binding of AP-1 family members, c-Jun and c-Fos. Deletion of AP-1 binding site in the Smad7 promoter completely abolishes UV stimulation of Smad7 transcription. Furthermore, over-expression of dominant negative c-Jun substantially reduces UV induction of Smad7 transcription (Quan et al. 2005). These data demonstrate that UV irradiation induces Smad7 via activation of transcription factor AP-1 in human dermal fibroblasts. UV irradiation activates multiple cell surface growth factor and cytokine receptors, which initiates intracellular signal transduction cascades (Fisher et al. 1996a; Fisher et al. 2002; Fisher et al. 1997a; Rittie and Fisher 2002). These activated signaling cascades activate target transcription factors, including AP-1. These data strongly suggest that UV-activated AP-1 stimulates Smad7 expression, which impairs TGF-β responsiveness, the primary regulator of type I collagen. Furthermore, Type I (α2) procollagen promoter activity is reduced by UV and further reduced by overexpression of Smad7 (Quan et al. 2001), suggesting that UV inhibition of procollagen gene expression is mediated, at least in part, by induction of Smad7.

As relates to UV inhibition of procollagen biosynthesis, a single exposure to UV irradiation (2MED) causes a near-complete loss of procollagen synthesis which persists for 24 hours, followed by recovery 48-72 hours post UV in human skin *in vivo* (Fisher et al. 1998). In non-irradiated human skin, TGF-β2 is more abundant than TGF-β1 or TGF-β3 (Quan et al. 2002b). Following UV irradiation, there is a rapid and sharp decrease in TGF-β2 that coincides with a UV-induced loss of procollagen synthesis within 24 hours post UV (Quan et al. 2002b). TGF-β1 and TGF-β3 show a gradual increase, starting at 24 hours post UV that coincides with recovery of procollagen synthesis, observed at 48-72 hours post UV. For these reasons, it is postulated that UV-induced reductions in collagen synthesis in human skin *in vivo* could be caused, at least in part, by impairment of TGF-β/Smad signaling pathway. In naturally-aged human skin dermis, TGF-β1 mRNA and protein expression are markedly reduced, compared to young skin dermis (Quan et al. 2010b). Laser capture microdissection confirmed that TGF-β1 mRNA in captured fibroblasts is significantly reduced in aged dermal fibroblasts, compared to young dermal fibroblasts in human skin *in vivo*. Above data provide strong evidence that impairment of TGF-β/Smad signaling in dermal fibroblasts largely contributes to thin dermis of the aged human skin by inhibition of collagen synthesis.

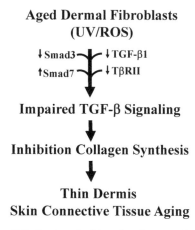

Aged Dermal Fibroblasts
(UV/ROS)

↓Smad3 — ↓TGF-β1
↑Smad7 — ↓TβRII

Impaired TGF-β Signaling
↓
Inhibition Collagen Synthesis
↓
Thin Dermis
Skin Connective Tissue Aging

FIG. 2 *Impaired transforming growth factor-β (TGF-β) pathway in dermal fibroblast contributes to thin skin dermisin human skin connective tissue aging (see text for details).*

In conclusion, as TGF-β signaling plays a key role in ECM biosynthesis, impairment of TGF-β signaling is largely responsible for collagen loss in aged human skin. Figure 2 depicts a model in which impaired TGF-β signaling in aged dermal fibroblasts contributes to human skin connective tissue aging. Unlike other organs, human skin is exposed to reactive oxygen species (ROS) generated from both environmental sources, such as solar ultraviolet irradiation and endogenous oxidative metabolism. Chronic exposure to ROS results in impairment of TGF-β signaling by alterations of multiple TGF-β pathway components: reduced TGF-β1, TGF-β type II receptor and Smad3, as well as up-regulation of Smad7. Impaired TGF-β signaling causes inhibition of collagen synthesis, which eventually results in thin skin dermis, the prominent feature of human skin connective tissue aging.

❏ Elevated Matrix-degrading Metalloproteinases (MMPs) in Dermal Fibroblasts Contributes to Damaged Skin Dermis in Human Skin Connective Tissue Aging

As described above, human skin connective tissue aging is caused by two primary pathways, either by inhibiting procollagen biosynthesis or by stimulating collagen breakdown, resulting in reduced collagen content or disorganized collagen fibrils in skin dermis (Fisher et al. 1998; Fisher et al. 1997a; Quan et al. 2010b). Matrix-degrading metalloproteinases (MMPs), which degrade collagen and other ECM proteins, are elevated in naturally-aged and photoaged and UV-irradiated human skin *in vivo* (Fisher et al. 2009; Fisher et al. 1997a; Quan et al. 2009). Elevated MMPs over years or decades can promote accumulation of dermal ECM fragmentation, the characteristic feature of aged human skin. Therefore, MMPs-mediated ECM fragmentation is considered to be the major contributor to the skin connective tissue damage seen in naturally-aged and photoaged human skin. Although the critical role of MMPs in skin photoaging process is undeniable, some important questions remain: such as what is the underlying molecular mechanism of elevated MMPs in aged dermal fibroblasts and what is the relative contribution of each of MMPs to the overall connective tissue destruction seen in aged skin?

MMPs comprise a family of zinc-containing proteinases with distinct structural and substrate specificities and specifically degrade ECM proteins (Stamenkovic 2003; Sternlicht and Werb 2001). MMPs are classified as collagenases, gelatinases, stromelysins and membrane-type MMPs according to their substrate specificities and whether they are secreted soluble proteins or bound to cell surface membrane (Fu et al. 2008). MMPs are involved in a wide range of proteolytic events in physiological and pathological circumstances including embryogenesis, wound healing, inflammation, angiogenesis and cancer (Egeblad and Werb 2002; Kerkela and Saarialho-Kere 2003; Reibel et al. 1978; Sternlicht and Werb 2001).

To date, the MMP gene family consists of 25 members, 24 of which are expressed in mammals (Egeblad and Werb 2002; Hegedus et al. 2008). In human skin, MMP-8, -10, -12, -20 and -26 are not detectable (Quan et al. 2009).

MMP-14, -2, -3, -28, -7 and -15 are the most highly expressed, while remaining MMPs are expressed at lower levels. In human skin, MMP-1 appears to be primary enzyme involved in normal turnover of dermal collagen (Brennan et al. 2003; Fisher et al. 1996a; Fisher et al. 1997a). In healthy young skin, MMP-1 expression is exceedingly low, near the limit of detection by the RT-PCR (Fisher et al. 2009; Quan et al. 2009). However, MMP-1 is potently induced by wide range of stimulus such as UV irradiation and reactive oxygen species (Fisher et al. 2009; Quan et al. 2009). After primary cleavage of collagen at a single site by MMP-1, collagen denatures and then undergoes further degradation by other members of the MMP family (Brennan et al. 2003; Fisher et al. 1996b; Fisher et al. 1997b). In addition, skin expresses natural MMP inhibitors, including tissue inhibitors of matrix metalloproteinases (TIMPs) and the proteoglycan decorin. These inhibitors further act to retard collagen breakdown (Gomez et al. 1997). Although dermal collagen in human skin is stable, dermal collagen undergoes progressive gradual alterations and accumulations of damage through over years or decades, which eventually cause skin connective tissue aging seen in aged skin.

Studies over the past several years have revealed that solar UV radiation elevates at least three different MMPs in human skin *in vivo*, i.e., interstitial collagenase (MMP-1), stromelysin-1 (MMP-3) and 92kDa gelatinase (MMP- 9) (Brenneisen et al. 2002; Quan et al. 2009). MMP-1 and MMP-3 mRNA levels are rapidly and potently induced by several thousand-fold, whereas MMP-9 is modestly induced in human skin *in vivo*. MMP-1 initiates cleavage of collagen fibrils, typically type I and III in skin, at a single site within its central triple helix. Once cleaved by MMP-1, collagen fibrils can be further degraded by MMP-3 and MMP-9 (Brennan et al. 2003; Fisher et al. 1996a). The combined actions of MMP-1, 3 and 9 have the capacity to degrade most of the proteins that comprise the skin dermal collagenous ECM. Exposure of sun-protected human skin to purified human MMP-1 in organ culture causes collagen fragmentation and alterations in the structure and organization of collagen fibrils in the dermis that resemble those observed in naturally-aged and photoaged skin (Fisher et al. 2009; Fligiel et al. 2003; Varani et al. 2001). These studies suggest that MMP-1, MMP-3 and MMP-9 are primary UV-inducible collagenolytic enzymes and MMP-1 is the major protease capable of initiating degradation of native fibrillar collagens in human skin *in vivo*. Laser capture microdissection (LCM) coupled with real-time RT-PCR indicates that all three UV irradiation inducible MMPs, are primarily produced by the epidermis, rather than dermis in human skin *in vivo* (Quan et al. 2009). Epidermal keratinocytes are the major cellular source of MMPs that are produced in response to exposure of human skin to solar UV irradiation. Although collagen-degrading MMP-1, 3 and 9 are primarily induced in the epidermis, the secreted MMPs are able to diffuse into the dermis and degrade collagenous ECM. In addition, it is conceivable that dermal cells may also play a role in epidermal production of MMPs, through indirect paracrine mechanisms, by secretion of growth factors or cytokines, which in turn modulate MMP stimulation by epidermal keratinocytes. It is also noteworthy that solar UV radiation readily reaches the reticular dermis, rendering dermal fibroblasts accessible targets (Farage et al. 2008; Wlaschek et al. 2001). As dermal fibroblasts are the major cell type of the dermal compartment, UV-inducible MMPs are also induced by dermal stromal cell including fibroblasts (Kolarzyk et al. 2000).

Compared to acute UV irradiation, a larger variety of MMPs, including UV-inducible MMPs, are constantly elevated in chronic photodamaged skin (Quan et al. 2009). Among the 18 MMPs expressed in human skin, seven were significantly elevated in photodamaged forearm, compared to sun-protected underarm skin (MMP-9, 5.3-fold; MMP-27, 5.1-fold; MMP-3, 3.0-fold; MMP-11, 2.7-fold; MMP-17, 2.2-fold; MMP-1, 1.9-fold; MMP-2, 1.6-fold). To quantify the relative contributions to elevated MMPs, epidermis and dermis were separated by laser capture microdissection (LCM). Interestingly, compared to acute UV irradiation, in which the epidermis is the major source of transiently induced MMPs (Quan et al. 2009), the dermis is the major source of elevated MMPs in chronic photodamaged skin (Quan et al. 2013a). MMPs and TIMPs are often coordinately regulated as a means to control excess MMP activity. Compared to acute UV irradiation, in which TIMP-1 is significantly upregulated (Fisher et al. 1997a), elevated multiple MMPs in photoaged skin are not accompanied by alterations of TIMPs expression. The observed preferential induction of MMPs relative to TIMPs is demonstrated by degraded collagen fibrils assessed by *in situ* zymography. Therefore, photodamaged dermis constitutively expresses elevated levels of multiple MMPs, which likely lead to chronic, progressive degradation of the dermal collagenous ECM in photodamaged human skin.

Similarly, multiple MMPs (MMP-1, MMP-2, MMp-3, MMp-9, MMp-23, MMP-24 and MMP-27) are elevated in naturally-aged human skin dermis other than epidermis (Quan, unpublished data), suggesting the combined actions of the wide variety of MMPs that are constitutively elevated in naturally-aged and photodamaged dermis are involved in progressive degradation of dermal ECM.

MMPs are strongly regulated by transcription factor AP-1, which is rapidly induced and activated by UV irradiation in human skin *in vivo* (Birkedal-Hansen et al. 1993; Farage et al. 2007; Fisher et al. 1996a; Mauviel 1993). UV irradiation rapidly up-regulates c-Jun expression by activating the mitogen activated protein (MAP) kinase pathway. Elevated levels of c-Jun, in association with constitutively expressed c-Fos, increase levels of transcription factor activator-1 (AP-1), which is required for transcription of matrix metalloproteinases. Interestingly, the ERK MAP kinase pathway is reduced whereas the stress-activated MAP kinase pathway is increased in aged, compared to young human skin *in vivo* (Chung et al. 2000). The transcription factor c-Jun is elevated two-fold in aged skin compared to young skin, suggesting c-Jun/AP1 may drive up-regulation of MMPs in aging skin (Chung et al. 2000). In addition, the c-Jun transcription factor negatively regulates type

I procollagen (Fisher et al. 1998). Type I (α2) procollagen promoter activity is reduced by UV and is further reduced by overexpression of wild type c-Jun. Overexpression of dominant negative mutant c-Jun completely abrogates UV inhibition of type I (α2) procollagen promoter activity (Fisher et al. 1998). It follows that UV inhibition of type I procollagen synthesis is mediated, at least in part, by UV-induced c-Jun. The coordinated regulation of collagen breakdown and collagen synthesis involves the transcription factor c-Jun. These data provide evidence that elevated c-Jun/AP1 activity in aged skin contributes to reduced collagen synthesis and increased collagen degradation in human skin connective tissue aging.

To explore MMP-1 function in skin aging, a transgenic mice with catalytically-active human MMP-1 has been generated (Xia et al. 2015). The skin of adult MMP-1 transgenic mouse shows normal gross appearance, but histology demonstrates significant fragmentation and disorganization of collagen fibrils, confirmed by Masson's Trichrome staining and atomic force microscopy. Collagen fibrils in control mice are intact, abundant and well-organized, similar to young skin; however, collagen fibrils in MMP-1 transgenic mice are fragmented, sparse and disorganized, as observed in aged skin. Transmission electron microscope further indicates that collagen fibrils are densely packed and well-organized in control mice, but are loosely packed, fragmented and disorganized in MMP-1 transgenic mice. This work provides evidence that elevated MMP-1 drives collagen fragmentation and disorganization.

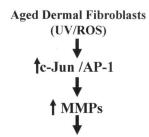

Aged Dermal Fibroblasts
(UV/ROS)

↑c-Jun /AP-1

↑ MMPs

Damaged Collagenous ECM
Skin Connective Tissue Aging

FIG. 3   *Elevated matrix-degrading metalloproteinases (MMPs) in dermal fibroblasts contributes to damaged skin dermis in human skin connective tissue aging (see text for details).*

In conclusion, elevated MMPs in dermal fibroblasts are responsible for skin connective tissue damage in aged human skin. Figure 3 depicts a model in which elevated MMPs in aged dermal fibroblasts contributes to human skin connective tissue aging. Human skin is exposed to reactive oxygen species (ROS) generated from both environmental sources (UV irradiation) and endogenous oxidative metabolism. Chronic exposure to ROS upregulates multiple MMPs by activation of c-Jun/AP-1, the primary regulator of MMPs expression. Elevated multiple MMPs damage dermal collagenous ECM, which eventually results in fragmented and disorganized collagen fibrils, the prominent feature of human skin connective tissue aging. Therefore, targeting MMPs inhibition could benefit skin health in the elderly.

❑ MMPs and Lysyl Oxidase (LOX) in Diabetic Human Skin

Interestingly, aged-appearing skin is more common in diabetes. Aged-appearing skin has a profound effect on the development of skin disorders in diabetic patients. Diabetes affects every organ system of the body including the skin, the largest organ in the body (Duff et al. 2015). It is estimated that more than two-thirds (79.2%) of diabetic patients experience a skin problem at some stage throughout the course of their disease (Demirseren et al. 2014). Many of these skin conditions can occur in anyone, but are acquired more easily in diabetics (Demirseren et al. 2014; Duff et al. 2015; Levy and Zeichner 2012). For example, in comparison to the general population, diabetic patients more commonly experience aged-appearing skin as well as more skin infections such as those secondary to foot ulcers. In fact, such skin problems are sometimes the first warning indicator for internal complications of diabetes and may allow an astute physician to initiate diagnostic testing. Among all known human MMPs, diabetic skin shows elevated levels of MMP-1 and MMP-2 (gelatinase A), the major protease that digests denatured collagen. These data support the concept that the combined actions of MMP-1 and MMP-2, which are constitutively elevated in diabetic skin, likely lead to chronic, progressive alterations of dermal collagenous ECM and thus contribute to old-looking skin in diabetes. Laser capture microdissection (LCM) coupled real-time PCR further indicates that elevated MMPs in diabetic skin are primarily expressed in the dermis.

Elevated MMPs is evidenced by significant alterations of dermal collagen structure, characterized by nanoscale fragmentation and disorganization of collagen fibrils in diabetic skin. Furthermore, diabetic skin shows increased lysyl oxidase (LOX) expression and higher cross-linked collagens. These alterations of collagen integrity could result in changes in mechanical properties. Atomic force microscopy (AFM) further indicates that fragmented and disorganized collagen fibrils in diabetic skin are stiffer and harder than intact and well-organized collagen fibrils in non-diabetic skin. The persistent elevation of MMPs and LOX over the years is thought to result in the accumulation of fragmented and cross-linked collagen and thus impairs dermal collagen structural integrity and mechanical properties in diabetes. These data provide the molecular basis of aged-appearing skin in diabetes and partially explain why old-looking skin is more common in diabetic patients.

Some skin problems are more common in diabetes, such as diabetic foot ulcers, which are a frequent and disabling complication resulting in significant morbidity (Apelqvist et al. 1993; Boyko et al. 1996). Chronic and progressive alterations of the dermal collagenous microenvironment due to constitutive elevation of MMPs and LOX may have a profound effect on non-healing in diabetic foot ulceration. The aberrant collagen microenvironment due to elevated MMPs, LOX and alteration of dermal mechanical properties could serve as risk factors for diabetic foot ulceration. Understanding the quality of diabetic skin may help us to predict those who are predisposed to the development of diabetic foot ulceration and other skin problems in diabetes.

Figure 4 depicts a model in which alterations of the structural and mechanical properties of dermal collagen contribute to the aged appearance of skin in diabetes. Diabetic dermis constitutively expresses elevated levels of MMP-1/MMP-2 and LOX, which results in increased collagen fragmentation, crosslinking and consequently alterations of mechanical properties of the dermis. Constitutive elevation of MMPs and LOX over the years is thought to result in accumulation of fragmented and cross-linked collagen fragments and thus contributes to aged-appearing skin in diabetes. This model provides the molecular foundations for diabetes-related aged appearance of skin and the molecular basis for the impaired the structural integrity and aberrant collagen microenvironment, which may have a profound effect on the development of skin disorders in diabetic patients.

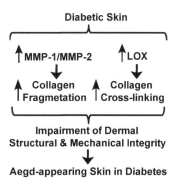

FIG. 4 *Alterations of the structural and mechanical properties of dermal collagen contribute to the aged appearance of skin in diabetes (see text for details).*

❑ Age-associated Reduction of Cellular Spreading/Mechanical Force Up-regulates Matrix Metalloproteinase-1 Expression in Human Dermal Fibroblasts

As collagen fragmentation and disorganization are an inevitable process in human skin connective tissue aging, fragmentation of collagen fibrils impairs fibroblast attachment and thereby reduces fibroblast spreading and shape/size. (Fisher et al. 2009; Fisher et al. 2008; Qin et al. 2014; Varani et al. 2004). Collagen fragmentation is largely initiated by MMP-1, which becomes elevated during the aging process in human skin (Fisher et al. 2009; Fisher et al. 2008).

Reduced fibroblast spreading/mechanical tension up-regulates MMP-1 expression as observed in aged human skin dermal fibroblasts *in vivo* (Fisher et al. 2009; Fisher et al. 2008; Quan et al. 2013a). Multiphoton fluorescence microscopy demonstrates the contracted morphology and reduced cell size of dermal fibroblasts in aged human skin, compared to the stretched appearance of fibroblasts in young skin (Qin et al. 2014). While cell shape and mechanical forces are known to regulate many cellular functions, the molecular basis of their impact on dermal fibroblast function and skin connective tissue aging are not well understood.

Investigation of the relationship between fibroblast shape/mechanical force indicates that MMP-1 expression is largely regulated by cell shape/size and mechanical force (Qin et al. 2014). Atomic force microscopy indicates that the key cellular mechanical properties of traction force and tensile strength are markedly reduced by loss of fibroblast shape/size. Interestingly, reduced cell spreading/mechanical force substantially upregulates MMP-1 expression, which led to collagen fibril fragmentation and disorganization in three dimensional collagen lattices. To further investigate the molecular events underlying this process, Qin et al. used glass substrates whose surface is coated with patterned arrays of discrete spots of type I collagen (Qin et al. 2014). These spots serve as attachment sites for fibroblasts, which otherwise could not attach to the glass surface. The spots are spaced to create four different geometric shapes of specific size, which is approximately one-third the size of fully spread fibroblasts. Thus, attachment to the type I collagen spots determines fibroblast size and shape. Reducing fibroblast size, without impairing actin cytoskeleton assembly, results in significant up-regulation of MMP-1 expression. This induction is observed regardless of fibroblast shape, which included circle, diamond, triangle and square. The molecular mechanism underlying these findings indicates that reduced spreading/ mechanical force upregulated transcription factor c-Jun and its binding to a canonical AP-1 binding site in the MMP-1 proximal promoter. c-Jun, which are typically comprise the AP-1 transcription factor complex, has been shown to principal regulator of MMP-1 transcription, under a variety of conditions (Birkedal-Hansen et al. 1993; Gutman and Wasylyk 1990; Mauviel 1993). A Blocking c-Jun function with dominant negative mutant c-Jun (Li et al. 2000; Quan et al. 2010a) markedly reduce selevation of MMP-1 expression in response to reduced spreading/mechanical force. Furthermore, restoration of fibroblast spreading/mechanical force led to decline of c-Jun and MMP-1 levels and eliminated collagen fibril fragmentation and disorganization. These data reveal a novel mechanism by which alterations of fibroblast shape/mechanical force upregulates MMP-1 via activation of c-Jun/AP-1 and consequent collagen fibril fragmentation. These data further suggest that elevated MMP-1 expression in aged human skin arises, at least in part, from reduced spreading/mechanical force of dermal fibroblasts. This mechanism provides a foundation for understanding the cellular and molecular basis of age-related collagen fragmentation in human skin connective tissue aging.

Cell shape/mechanical force impacts multiple cellular processes including signal transduction, gene expression and metabolism (Alenghat et al. 2004; Ingber 2006; Silver et al. 2003; Wang et al. 1993). Currently, mechanisms by which reduced cell spreading/mechanical force induces c-Jun/AP-1 remains elusive. AP-1 activity is regulated by a wide range of stimuli including reactive oxygen species (ROS) (Shaulian and Karin 2002). Fibroblasts that have reduced spreading/mechanical force due to fragmentation of surrounding collagen fibrils display increase levels of ROS (Fisher et al. 2009). ROS is considered to be a major driving force for the aging process (Golden et al. 2002; Stadtman 1992). Indeed, it has been reported that protein oxidation, a marker of oxidative stress, is increased in aged human dermis *in vivo* (Fisher et al. 2009). These data suggest that elevated ROS generation may be mediate induction of c-Jun and AP-1 activity in response to reduced fibroblast spreading/mechanical force. Further studies are needed to elucidate the mechanisms that couple fibroblast spreading/mechanical force to oxidative stress and the role of these mechanisms in skin connective tissue aging.

In human skin, dermal fibroblasts are embedded in a collagen-rich ECM microenvironment and interact with collagen fibrils to maintain their cell shape/size and mechanical force. Accumulating evidence indicates that cell shape/size and mechanical force regulate essential cell functions (Hynes 2009). Cell shape and mechanical force are largely regulated by interactions with surrounding ECM proteins. The ECM proteins not only provide structural support for the tissues integrity but also provide binding sites for cells and mechanical resistance to cellular traction forces (Geiger et al. 2009; Ingber 2006). During aging, accumulation of fragmented collagen fibrils has functional consequences including altered cell shape that affect dermal fibroblast functions in collagen homeostasis (Fisher et al. 2009; Quan et al. 2013a; Quan et al. 2012). In healthy human dermis, intact collagen interacts with intracellular cytoskeleton through collagen-binding integrins and helps cells maintain their spread cell shape. However, in aged human skin dermis, fragmented collagen fibrils fail to interact with intracellular cytoskeleton; cells become rounded and unspread (Fisher et al. 2009; Fisher et al. 2008). Loss of dermal fibroblast cell shape in aged human skin is caused by MMP-1-mediated fragmented collagen. This is evidenced by recent mouse model of skin connective tissue aging, MMP-1 transgenic mouse model (Xia et al. 2015). In this mouse model, MMP-1-medaited fragmentation of collagen fibrils cannot support and maintain normal fibroblast spreading and morphology. Compared to control mice, fibroblasts from MMP-1 transgenic mice display loss of cell spreading/shape/size. Interestingly, expression of human MMP-1 in mouse skin epidermis causes dermal collagen fibril fragmentation and disorganization. While UV irradiation induces several 1,000-fold MMP-1 in epidermis, the major collagenase activity is actually seen in the human dermis *in vivo* (Quan et al. 2009). These data provide evident that elevated MMP-1 in epidermis is secreted and diffuses into the dermis to degrade collagen.

Elevated MMP-1 in aged skin breaks down collagenous ECM fibrils, thereby weakening the structural integrity and impairing attachment of fibroblasts to the dermal ECM. These conditions cause reduced fibroblast spreading and mechanical force. This reduced cell spreading/mechanical tension further stimulates MMP-1 through activation of c-Jun/AP-1 (Figure 5). The positive feedback (or vicious cycle) relationship between elevated MMP-1 and reduced cell spreading/mechanical tension is consistent with the biology of aging, which is epitomized by continual reduction of homeostatic control. Targeting AP-1 may improve the structure and function of aged human skin thereby mitigating age-related skin diseases.

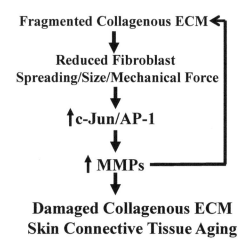

FIG. 5 *A model in which age-associated reduction of cellular spreading/mechanical force up-regulates matrix metalloproteinase-1 expression in human dermal fibroblasts (see text for details).*

❑ Age-associated Reduction of Cellular Spreading/ Mechanical Force Down-regulates Type I Collagen Expression in Human Dermal Fibroblasts

The primary dermal fibroblasts from aged (>80 years) or young (>30 years) individuals, which are cultured in monolayer, in *in vitro* tissue culture plastic dishes, are indistinguishable from each other with respect to cell shape/ size and mechanical force, as well as the gene expression levels of MMP-1, type I collagen and key regulatory pathways including c-Jun/AP-1, ROS and

TGF-β signaling (Fisher et al. 2009). In contrast, human dermal fibroblasts, obtained from individuals of any age (21-86 years of age), cultured in three dimensional collagen lattices that have been partially-fragmented by treatment with exogenous MMP-1, have a reduced spreading/size and contracted appearance, consistent with reduced mechanical tension. These "collapsed" fibroblasts have elevated levels of MMP-1 and reduced collagen production, compared to "stretched" fibroblasts cultured in intact collagen lattices. These observations suggest that the dermal collagenous ECM microenvironment is largely responsible for age-related loss of fibroblast spreading/shape/size and impaired function in aged human skin *in vivo*.

As the structural and mechanical integrity of human skin is largely dependent on the dermal extracellular matrix (ECM), fragmented collagen fibrils are unable to support cell-ECM interaction and mechanical force and thus impairs cell spreading/shape/size. Primary adult human dermal fibroblasts are cultured in either mechanically constrained or unconstrained three dimensional collagen matrices. Mechanical constraint is achieved by incorporating a nylon mesh disk within the matrices (Kessler et al. 2001). The rigidity of the disk counter acted the traction force of the fibroblasts and thereby prevented contraction of the matrices. Fibroblasts in restrained matrices displayed elongated, spread morphology and prominent actin filaments. In contrast, fibroblasts in unconstrained matrixes displayed a rounded, contracted appearance, lacking distinct actin filaments. Quantitative morphometric analysis revealed that fibroblast surface area was reduced 76% in unconstrained matrices, compared to fibroblasts in constrained matrices. Reduced size of fibroblasts in mechanically unrestrained three-dimensional collagen lattices coincides with reduced mechanical force, measured by atomic force microscopy. Atomic force microscopy (AFM) indicates that the key cellular mechanical properties; traction force and tensile strength were reduced 56% and 55%, respectively, while deformation is increased 2-fold, in unconstrained compared to constrained matrices. Interestingly, dermal fibroblast size/mechanical force down-regulates key ECM components such as type I collagen, fibronectin and connective tissue growth factor (CTGF/CCN2) (Kessler et al. 2001; Quan et al. 2010b).

Importantly, TGF-β signaling, the major regulator of ECM production (Quan et al. 2010b; Verrecchia and Mauviel 2002), is significantly impaired when the cells lose their size and mechanical force. Both basal and TGF-β-induced TGF-β/Smad3-dependent luciferase reporter (SBEX4) (Quan et al. 2001) are markedly reduced in fibroblasts with reduced size/mechanical force. Consistent with these results, both basal and TGF-β-induced binding of Smad3 to its DNA response element are substantially inhibited by reduced fibroblast size/mechanical force. Furthermore, TGF-β-dependent Smad3 phosphorylation, which is required for transcriptional activity, is significantly inhibited by reduced size/mechanical force. Importantly, reduced size/mechanical force specifically down-regulates TGF-β type II receptor (TβRII) and thus impairs TGF-β/Smad signaling pathway (Figure 6).

Reduced size/mechanical force does not alter TβRI mRNA or protein levels, as observed in aged human skin *in vivo*. Other TGF-β pathway components such as TGF-β ligands and Smads also remain unchanged. In contrast, TβRII mRNA and protein levels are significantly decreased by 57% and 72%, respectively. TβRII is necessary for TGF-β ligand binding to TGF-β receptor complex, the initial step of TGF-β signaling. TGF-β1-binding to fibroblasts is reduced approximately 90% by reduced size/mechanical force. Disruption of the actin cytoskeleton resulted in reduced fibroblast size and specifically down-regulates TβRII gene expression, but not TβRI. These data suggest that reduced fibroblast size/mechanical force results in specific down-regulation of TβRII.

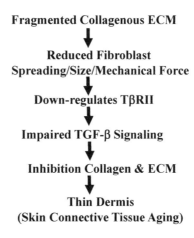

Fragmented Collagenous ECM

↓

**Reduced Fibroblast
Spreading/Size/Mechanical Force**

↓

Down-regulates TβRII

↓

Impaired TGF-β Signaling

↓

Inhibition Collagen & ECM

↓

**Thin Dermis
(Skin Connective Tissue Aging)**

FIG. 6   *A model in which age-associated reduction of cellular spreading/mechanical force down-regulates type I collagen expression through impairment of TGF-β signaling in human dermal fibroblasts (see text for details).*

Furthermore, down-regulation of TβRII is associated with significantly decreased phosphorylation, DNA-binding and transcriptional activity of its key down-stream effector Smad3 and reduced expression of Smad3-regulated essential ECM components type I collagen, fibronectin and connective tissue growth factor (CTGF/CCN2). Restoration of TβRII expression does not change the fibroblasts morphology. However, compared to fibroblasts transfected with control vector, expression of TβRII increases basal and TGF-β1-induced Smad3 phosphorylation. Restoration of TβRII also elevates basal and TGF-β1-induced protein levels of type I procollagen, fibronectin and CTGF/CCN2. These data demonstrate that down-regulation of TβRII is key event that mediates impaired TGF-β signaling and consequently decreased ECM production in response to reduced fibroblast size/mechanical force. Furthermore, reduced expression of TβRII and ECM components in response to reduced fibroblast size/mechanical force is fully reversed by restoring cell size/mechanical force.

More importantly, dermal fibroblasts obtained from young (21-30 years old) and aged (>80 years old) human buttocks skin by laser capture microdissection laser capture microdissection demonstrates that dermal fibroblast size is associated with reduced expression of TβRII, type I collagen, fibronectin, in aged human skin. TβRII gene expression was reduced nearly 60% in aged, compared to young skin. This reduction is also associated with decreased activation of TβRII downstream effector Smad3, measured by electrophoretic mobility shift assay, using nuclear extracts from young and aged dermis.

Currently, the mechanism by which loss of cell spreading/shape/size and mechanical force specifically down-regulates TβRII remains elusive. Clearly, further studies are needed to elucidate how fibroblast spreading/mechanical force regulates TβRII and the role of these mechanisms in skin connective tissue aging. Reduced size/mechanical force significantly reduces TβRII promoter activity, suggesting reduced TβRII mRNA and protein results, at least in part, from decreased gene transcription. In addition to transcriptional regulation, TβRII is regulated by post-transcriptional mechanisms. Recently, it has been reported that microRNA-21 (miR-21) reduces TβRII expression through direct interaction with 3' non-translated sequences in the TβRII transcript (Kim et al. 2009; Yu et al. 2012). Interestingly, miR21 was significantly induced by reduced size/mechanical force. Furthermore, addition of miR-21 mimic results in down-regulation of TβRII, but not TβRI expression. These data indicate that the level of miR-21 is responsive to size/mechanical force and may participate in the mechanism of down-regulation of TβRII expression.

❑ Age-associated Dermal ECM Microenvironment and Age-related Skin Diseases

As the population in the United States ages, prevention of age-related diseases and improvement of quality of life for the elderly are becoming increasingly prominent public health issues. Age-associated morbidity and diseases impose significant financial burdens on our nation's healthcare system (Gehrs et al. 2006; Hartman et al. 2008; Johnson 1989). Indeed, healthcare cost per capita for the elderly population is over three times higher than that of a working-aged person. Aging affects all individuals and is the highest risk factor for many common chronic diseases. There is strong association of aging with increased risk of age-related common diseases, such as cancer, diabetes, atherosclerosis, cataracts, metabolic syndrome, sarcopenia osteoporosis and decline in immune system function (Bourla and Young 2006; Campisi 2008; Kaufman 2009; Kudravi and Reed 2000). Skin aging is also associated with numerous deleterious alterations, such as impaired wound healing, increased frailty, greater risk of cancer development and increased susceptibility to contact dermatitis (Fisher et al. 1997a; Holt et al. 1992; Kudravi and Reed 2000; Zhao et al. 2010). The recent survey identified that skin cancer is the most common type of cancer in the United States, with more 3.5 million skin cancers in over two million people are diagnosed annually (Kahlos et al. 2000; Paalman et al. 2000). Although mortality from skin cancer is low, skin cancer often entails significant medical costs, loss of function and disfigurement. The annual cost of treatment in the U.S. is estimated to be $1 billion (Calderon et al. 2000). These findings are directly relevant to public health care in the largest sense, yet knowledge regarding the mechanisms by which solar UV radiation damages skin is far from complete. As cancer is an age-related disease, one fundamental but critical question is that why the cancers more frequently occur in elderly but not in young population. This connection between aging and disease is especially true for epithelial (i.e. non-melanoma) skin cancer, which is the most common form of cancer in the USA. For example, one in five Americans will develop skin cancer in the course of a lifetime and 40-50% of Americans who lives to age 65 will have skin cancer at least once (Gloster and Brodland 1996; Kahlos et al. 2000; National Cancer Institute (U.S.), 2005). Ultraviolet (UV) irradiation from the sun is a key initiating factor for development of most keratinocyte skin cancer. UV irradiation causes DNA damage that can lead to mutations, which can accumulate as a result of repeated sun exposures. Although accumulation of mutations by UV irradiation with age has been implicated as a significant contributor to keratinocyte skin cancer, it does not fully explain why keratinocyte skin cancer is so common in the elderly. Beyond accumulation of mutations, other age-associated mechanisms that promote keratinocyte skin cancer are far from clear. One possibility of development of skin cancer associated with chronic solar exposure is that alteration in the dermal ECM microenvironment by UV irradiation may contribute to age-related skin carcinogenesis. UV irradiation not only causes DNA mutations, but also significantly damages collagen-rich dermal connective tissues. Collagen degradation products are known to promote migration of such cells as vascular smooth muscle cells, wound healing keratinocytes and the immortal keratinocyte cell line, HaCaT (Carmeliet 2000; Holt et al. 1992). Complex alterations of the composition of the ECM are associated with invasive melanoma (Aikawa et al. 2006; Grether-Beck and Krutmann 2000; Krutmann 2000). It is, thus, possible that UV alterations in the dermal collagen matrix in photodamaged skin may provide the microenvironment for the development of various invasive skin cancers. Indeed, it has been suggested that alterations in dermal ECM/stroma that occur during skin aging process provide a microenvironment that supports the development of skin cancers (Fisher et al. 2009; Valera et al. 2000). Emerging evidence indicates that young tissue microenvironment (healthy architecture and normal tissue homeostasis) provides tumor-suppressive signals (Bissell and Hines 2011;

Campisi 2008). However, as tissue homeostasis becomes disrupted with aging, such as age-associated dermal microenvironment in elderly, the tissue microenvironment can become a tumor promoter (Bissell and Hines 2011; Hulsmann et al. 2000; Tomita et al. 2000). Indeed, recent publications indicate that alterations in the stromal microenvironment, such as loss of dermal fibroblast Notch (Urtiaga et al. 2000) or TGF-β signaling (Paas and Scannell 2000; Romeo et al. 2000), can induce epithelial tumorigenesis. Furthermore, elevated WNT (Pace and Porro 2000) and HGF (Valera et al. 2000) signaling in stromal fibroblasts can promote cancer drug resistance and control drug sensitivity. In addition to stromal cell associated soluble factors, alterations of stromal ECM mechanical force promote tumorigenesis, suggesting targeting ECM as an important potential implications for anticancer therapies (Arendt and Kuperwasser 2015; Seo et al. 2015). Although the influence of the stromal microenvironment on tumor progression is well recognized, little is known about the role of age-related aberrant dermal ECM microenvironment in skin cancer development.

Age-related dermal ECM microenvironment such as alterations of collagen increases fragility and impairs wound healing. Impaired or delayed wound healing is common in the elderly and presents a significant clinical and economic problem. It has been suggested that impaired dermal fibroblast function is a key factor in the non-healing of chronic wounds in the elderly (Mendez et al. 1998; Wall et al. 2008). Dermal fibroblasts proliferation is reduced in response to various wound in aged animal models (Pace et al. 2000; Reed et al. 2001). Additionally, dermal collagen synthesis, angiogenesis and epidermal reepithelialization all exhibit an age-related delay in response to wound in aged animals (Swift et al. 1999). There is a general decrease in the number and size of dermal fibroblasts with age, the primary cells that are responsible for collagen synthesis and turnover in skin (Cuchacovich et al. 2000). In skin, dermal fibroblasts interact with and attach to collagen fibrils, thereby maintain normal cell shape/mechanical tension for function (Fisher et al. 2008; Qin et al. 2014; Varani et al. 2006). Both in aged human skin *in vivo* and *in vitro* 3D collagen matrix, dermal fibroblasts are unable to maintain normal cell shape/mechanical tension in damaged collagen microenvironment and therefore lost their functions in collagen homeostasis; produce more MMPs and less collagen, that are central event of the skin connective tissue aging (Fisher et al. 2009; Fisher et al. 2008) (Figure 7). It has been shown that dermal fibroblasts cultured from individuals of different age are largely indistinguishable in collagen homeostasis *in vitro* monolayer culture (Fisher et al. 2009). However, in 3D culture, fragmented collagen alters dermal fibroblast function to shift the balance to produce more MMPs and less collagen in aged skin (Fisher et al. 2009). ECM microenvironment of the dermis is largely responsible for the morphological and functional differences that observed between fibroblasts in young versus aged human skin *in vivo* (Fisher et al. 2009; Fisher et al. 2008; Quan et al. 2012).

Therefore, it is conceivable that alteration of dermal collagen network due to loss of dermal collagen structural and mechanical properties in aged skin is unable to support normal mechanical tension within fibroblasts. In contrast, age-related reduced production of collagen is largely reversed by enhancing structural support of the ECM (Quan et al. 2012; Wang et al. 2007). Injection of dermal filler, cross-linked hyaluronic acid, into the aged skin stimulates fibroblasts to activate TGF-β pathway and produce more type I collagen (Quan et al. 2013b; Wang et al. 2007). This stimulation is associated with localized increased of mechanical tension, indicated by fibroblast elongation/spreading and mediated by up-regulation of TβRII and CTGF/CCN2. Interestingly, enhanced mechanical support of the collagen ECM also stimulates fibroblast proliferation, expands vasculature and increases epidermal thickness. Injection of filler into dermal equivalent cultures causes elongation of fibroblasts, coupled with type I collagen synthesis, which is dependent on the TGF-β signaling pathway. Thus, fibroblasts in aged human skin retain their capacity for functional activation, which is restored by enhancing mechanical and structural support of the ECM. As the mechanical properties of the skin is largely dependent on collagen, a wealth of evidence indicates that mechanical properties of tissue microenvironment regulate a variety of cellular functions including signal transduction, gene expression and tissue homeostasis (Fisher et al. 2009; Ingber 1997a; Spencer et al. 2007; Underhill et al. 2012; Varani et al. 2004; Wang et al. 2008). Alterations of the dermal ECM mechanical and structural microenvironment in aged skin have significant consequences on regulation of collagen homeostasis by fibroblasts (Fisher et al. 2009; Qin et al. 2014; Quan et al. 2012). Currently, it is not clear that how the cells sense and transduce signals in response to changes of surrounding microenvironment, such as damaged collagen network in aged skin. Fragmented collagen is unable to support normal cell spreading, shape and mechanical force within fibroblasts and this loss of cell shape and mechanical tension is closely associated with increased c-Jun and transcription factor AP-1 (Fisher et al. 2009). As transcription factor c-Jun/AP-1 functions as a major driving force for multiple MMPs and potent negative regulator of type I procollagen expression (Fisher et al. 1996a; Fisher et al. 1998; Quan et al. 2010a), it is conceivable that elevated AP-1 activity significantly contributes to the multiple elevated MMPs and loss of type I collagen expression in aged skin. Additionally, alterations of dermal collagen network in aged skin may also impair mechanical properties of the adhesion substrate, ECM-integrin mechanical sensing and subsequent integrin signaling events associated with aberrant collagen homeostasis in aged skin.

A wealth of information indicates that the interaction of cells with their surrounding ECM environment is critical for cellular function (Ingber 1997a, b; Lambert et al. 2001; Thomas et al. 2000; Underhill et al. 2012). In human skin, dermal fibroblasts physically interact with and attach to the three-dimensional collagen network through a class of cell membrane receptor, integrins (Boudreau and Bissell 1998; Giancotti and Ruoslahti 1999; Miranti and Brugge 2002). Integrin receptors form structural and functional linkages between the ECM and intracellular cytoskeletal linker proteins. Integrins interact with the actin/myosin-based cytoskeleton to form cellular machinery that is capable of physically contracting the pliable ECM. This contraction operates against the tensile properties of the ECM to generate mechanical forces which define cell morphology. Alterations of collagen network in aged dermis impair mechanical properties of the adhesion substrate, ECM-integrin mechanical sensing and subsequent integrin signaling events. Damaged collagen network in aged skin is unable to support normal mechanical tension within fibroblasts and this loss of mechanical tension is closely associated with altered dermal fibroblast function in collagen homeostasis. In human skin dermis, fibroblasts are surrounded by collagen-rich ECM environment and physically interact with the collagenous ECM through collagen-binding integrins. Currently, four collagen-binding integrins, $\alpha 1$, $\alpha 2$, $\alpha 10$ and $\alpha 11$, are identified and all belong to the integrin $\beta 1$ subfamily (Popova et al. 2007; Zhu et al. 2007)). However, little is known about the expression and functions of these collagen-binding integrins in human skin. Nevertheless, future studies must be carried out to understand the role of these collagen-binding integrins in human skin connective tissue aging.

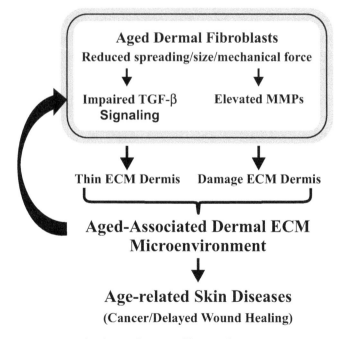

FIG. 7 *Molecular mechanisms of human skin connective tissue aging (see Conclusion for details).*

❏ Conclusion

Aberrant homeostasis of dermal connective tissue collagen, which is caused by impaired dermal fibroblast function, is primary responsible for the human skin connective tissue aging. Figure 7 depicts a model for how aged dermal fibroblasts contribute to human skin connective tissue aging and age-related skin diseases. Dermal fibroblast functions in aged skin are significantly impaired in collagen homeostasis as evidence of impaired TGF-β signaling, the major regulator of collagen production and elevated multiple MMPs. This age-dependent loss of fibroblast function causes dermal collagen loss and accumulation of damaged collagen, which is characteristic feature of skin connective tissue aging. Loss of dermal collagen in aged skin alters dermal ECM microenvironment by reducing structural integrity and mechanical properties. Reduced structural integrity and mechanical properties create an age-associated dermal ECM microenvironment that causes age-related skin diseases, such as increased fragility and poor wound healing and promotes skin cancer. These structural and mechanical alterations of dermis likely also impact epidermal function, contributing to epidermal thinning, which is another prominent feature of aged skin.

On the other hand, age-related aberrant ECM microenvironment (altered dermal collagen structural and mechanical property) has a significant impact on dermal fibroblasts function by reducing attachment to collagen fibers, reduced spreading/size and reduced mechanical tension. Therefore, this working model reveals an inherent self-perpetuating positive feedback nature between impaired dermal fibroblast function and alteration of dermal collagen structural and mechanical environment. Aged dermal fibroblast weakens the structural integrity and mechanical properties of the dermal ECM. The weakened dermal ECM microenvironment (age-associated dermal ECM microenvironment) provides less resistance to the mechanical forces exerted on it by dermal fibroblasts, thereby reducing the mechanical tension and cell spreading/size in the fibroblasts. This reduced mechanical tension and spreading/size in the fibroblasts results in further impairing dermal fibroblast function in collagen homeostasis and weakening the structural integrity and mechanical properties of the dermal ECM. The essential positive feedback between impaired dermal fibroblast function and loss of the integrity of dermal ECM network is consistent with the biology of aging, which is represented by gradual and progressive loss of homeostatic control within tissues.

❏ Acknowledgments

This study is supported by the National Institutes of Health (Bethesda, MD) Grants: ES014697 and ES014697 30S1 to Taihao Quan, AG019364 to Gary J. Fisher and Taihao Quan, AG031452 and AG025186 to Gary J. Fisher. The author would like to thank Drs Gary J. Fisher and John J. Voorhees for their help and support. The author also thanks Drs Zhaoping Qin, Tianyuan He, Yuan Shao, Patrick Robichaud and Trupta Purohit for technical assistance.

❏ References

Afrakhte, M., A. Moren, S. Jossan, S. Itoh, K. Sampath, B. Westermark, et al. 1998. Induction of inhibitory Smad6 and Smad7 mRNA by TGF-beta family members. Biochem Biophys Res Commun 249: 505-511.

Aikawa, T., J. Gunn, S.M. Spong, S.J. Klaus and M. Korc. 2006. Connective tissue growth factor-specific antibody attenuates tumor growth, metastasis and angiogenesis in an orthotopic mouse model of pancreatic cancer. Mol Cancer Ther 5: 1108-1116.

Alenghat, F.J., S.M. Nauli, R. Kolb, J. Zhou and D.E. Ingber. 2004. Global cytoskeletal control of mechanotransduction in kidney epithelial cells. Exp Cell Res 301: 23-30.

Apelqvist, J., J. Larsson and C.D. Agardh. 1993. Long-term prognosis for diabetic patients with foot ulcers. J Intern Med 233: 485-491.

Arendt, L.M. and C. Kuperwasser. 2015. Working stiff: How obesity boosts cancer risk. Sci Transl Med 7: 301fs334.

Asano, Y., H. Ihn, K. Yamane, M. Jinnin, Y. Mimura and K. Tamaki. 2004. Phosphatidylinositol 3-kinase is involved in alpha2(I) collagen gene expression in normal and scleroderma fibroblasts. J Immunol 172: 7123-7135.

Balaban, R.S., S. Nemoto and T. Finkel. 2005. Mitochondria, oxidants and aging. Cell 120: 483-495.

Bernstein, E.F., Y.Q. Chen, J.B. Kopp, L. Fisher, D.B. Brown, P.J. Hahn, et al. 1996. Long-term sun exposure alters the collagen of the papillary dermis. Comparison of sun-protected and photoaged skin by northern analysis, immunohistochemical staining and confocal laser scanning microscopy. J Am Acad Dermatol 34: 209-218.

Biesalski, H.K., M. Berneburg, T. Grune, M. Kerscher, J. Krutmann, W. Raab, et al. 2003. Hohenheimer Consensus Talk. Oxidative and premature skin ageing. Exp Dermatol 12 Suppl 3: 3-15.

Birkedal-Hansen, H., W.G. Moore, M.K. Bodden, L.J. Windsor, B. Birkedal-Hansen, A. DeCarlo, et al. 1993. Matrix metalloproteinases: a review. Crit Rev Oral Biol Med 4: 197-250.

Bissell, M.J. and W.C. Hines. 2011. Why don't we get more cancer? A proposed role of the microenvironment in restraining cancer progression. Nat Med 17: 320-329.

Bolognia, J., J.L. Jorizzo and R.P. Rapini. 2008. Dermatology. pp. Mosby/Elsevier, [St. Louis, Mo.].

Bonni, S., H.R. Wang, C.G. Causing, P. Kavsak, S.L. Stroschein, K. Luo, et al. 2001. TGF-beta induces assembly of a Smad2-Smurf2 ubiquitin ligase complex that targets SnoN for degradation. Nat Cell Biol 3: 587-595.

Bonniaud, P., M. Kolb, T. Galt, J. Robertson, C. Robbins, M. Stampfli, et al. 2004. Smad3 null mice develop airspace enlargement and are resistant to TGF-beta-mediated pulmonary fibrosis. J Immunol 173: 2099-2108.

Bossis, G. and F. Melchior. 2006. Regulation of SUMOylation by reversible oxidation of SUMO conjugating enzymes. Mol Cell 21: 349-357.

Boudreau, N. and M. Bissell. 1998. Extracellular matrix signaling: integration of form and function in normal and malignant cells. Curr Opin Cell Biol 10: 640-646.

Bourla, D.H. and T.A. Young. 2006. Age-related macular degeneration: a practical approach to a challenging disease. J Am Geriatr Soc 54: 1130-1135.

Boyko, E.J., J.H. Ahroni, D.G. Smith and D. Davignon. 1996. Increased mortality associated with diabetic foot ulcer. Diabet Med: a journal of the British Diabetic Association 13: 967-972.

Brennan, M., H. Bhatti, K.C. Nerusu, N. Bhagavathula, S. Kang, G.J. Fisher, et al. 2003. Matrix metalloproteinase-1 is the major collagenolytic enzyme responsible for collagen damage in UV-irradiated human skin. Photochem Photobiol 78: 43-48.

Brenneisen, P., H. Sies and K. Scharffetter-Kochanek. 2002. Ultraviolet-B irradiation and matrix metalloproteinases: from induction via signaling to initial events. Ann N Y Acad Sci 973: 31-43.

Brodin, G., A. Ahgren, P. ten Dijke, C.H. Heldin and R. Heuchel. 2000. Efficient TGF-beta induction of the Smad7 gene requires cooperation between AP-1, Sp1 and Smad proteins on the mouse Smad7 promoter. J Biol Chem 275: 29023-29030.

Brown, K.A., J.A. Pietenpol and H.L. Moses. 2007. A tale of two proteins: differential roles and regulation of Smad2 and Smad3 in TGF-beta signaling. J Cell Biochem 101: 9-33.

Calderon, N.L., L.H. Paasch and T.I. Fortoul. 2000. Ultrastructural glomerular changes in experimental infection with the classical swine fever virus. Vet Res 31: 447-453.

Campisi, J. 2008. Aging and cancer cell biology. Aging Cell 7: 281-284.

Carmeliet, P. 2000. Mechanisms of angiogenesis and arteriogenesis. Nat Med 6: 389-395.

Chung, J.H., S. Kang, J. Varani, J. Lin, G.J. Fisher and J.J. Voorhees. 2000. Decreased extracellular-signal-regulated kinase and increased stress-activated MAP kinase activities in aged human skin *in vivo*. J Invest Dermatol 115: 177-182.

Chuong, C.M., B.J. Nickoloff, P.M. Elias, L.A. Goldsmith, E. Macher, P.A. Maderson, et al. 2002. What is the 'true' function of skin? Exp Dermatol 11: 159-187.

Cuchacovich, T.M., P. Pacheco, G. Merino, P. Gallardo, H. Gatica, H. Valenzuela, et al. 2000. [Clinical features and response to systemic treatment of primary and secondary episcleritis and scleritis resistant to local treatment]. Rev Med Chil 128: 1205-1214.

Davies, K.J. 1987. Protein damage and degradation by oxygen radicals. I. general aspects. J Biol Chem 262: 9895-9901.

Davies, K.J. and M.E. Delsignore. 1987. Protein damage and degradation by oxygen radicals. III. Modification of secondary and tertiary structure. J Biol Chem 262: 9908-9913.

Davies, K.J., M.E. Delsignore and S.W. Lin. 1987. Protein damage and degradation by oxygen radicals. II. Modification of amino acids. J Biol Chem 262: 9902-9907.

Davies, K.J. and A.L. Goldberg. 1987a. Oxygen radicals stimulate intracellular proteolysis and lipid peroxidation by independent mechanisms in erythrocytes. J Biol Chem 262: 8220-8226.

Davies, K.J. and A.L. Goldberg. 1987b. Proteins damaged by oxygen radicals are rapidly degraded in extracts of red blood cells. J Biol Chem 262: 8227-8234.

Davies, K.J., S.W. Lin and R.E. Pacifici. 1987. Protein damage and degradation by oxygen radicals. IV. Degradation of denatured protein. J Biol Chem 262: 9914-9920.

de Pablo, M.A., M.A. Puertollano, A. Galvez, E. Ortega, J.J. Gaforio and G. Alvarez de Cienfuegos. 2000. Determination of natural resistance of mice fed dietary lipids to experimental infection induced by Listeria monocytogenes. FEMS Immunol Med Microbiol 27: 127-133.

Demirseren, D.D., S. Emre, G. Akoglu, D. Arpaci, A. Arman, A. Metin, et al. 2014. Relationship between skin diseases and extracutaneous complications of diabetes mellitus: clinical analysis of 750 patients. Am J Clin Dermatol 15: 65-70.

Di Lullo, G.A., S.M. Sweeney, J. Korkko, L. Ala-Kokko and J.D. San Antonio. 2002. Mapping the ligand-binding sites and disease-associated mutations on the most abundant protein in the human, type I collagen. J Biol Chem 277: 4223-4231.

Dong, C., S. Zhu, T. Wang, W. Yoon, Z. Li, R.J. Alvarez. et al. 2002. Deficient Smad7 expression: a putative molecular defect in scleroderma. Proc Natl Acad Sci USA 99: 3908-3913.

Duff, M., O. Demidova, S. Blackburn and J. Shubrook. 2015. Cutaneous manifestations of diabetes mellitus. Clin Diabetes 33: 40-48.

Egeblad, M. and Z. Werb. 2002. New functions for the matrix metalloproteinases in cancer progression. Nat Rev Cancer 2: 161-174.

Farage, M., P. Elsner and H. Maibach. 2007. Influence of usage practices, ethnicity and climate on the skin compatibility of sanitary pads. Archives of gynecology and obstetrics 275: 415-427.

Farage, M.A., K.W. Miller, P. Elsner and H.I. Maibach. 2008. Functional and physiological characteristics of the aging skin. Aging Clin Exp Res 20: 195-200.

Farage, M.A., K.W. Miller, H.I. Maibach and SpringerLink (Online service). 2010. Textbook of Aging Skin, pp. Springer-Verlag, Berlin Heidelberg, Berlin, Heidelberg.

Finkel, T. and N.J. Holbrook. 2000. Oxidants, oxidative stress and the biology of ageing. Nature 408: 239-247.

Fiocchi, C. 2001. TGF-beta/Smad signaling defects in inflammatory bowel disease: mechanisms and possible novel therapies for chronic inflammation. J Clin Invest 108: 523-526.

Fisher, G.J., S.C. Datta, H.S. Talwar, Z.Q. Wang, J. Varani, S. Kang, et al. 1996a. Molecular basis of sun-induced premature skin ageing and retinoid antagonism. Nature 379: 335-339.

Fisher, G.J., S.C. Datta, H.S. Talwar, Z.Q. Wang, J. Varani, S. Kang, et al. 1996b. Molecular basis of sun-induced premature skin ageing and retinoid antagonism. Nature 379: 335-339.

Fisher, G.J., Z.Q. Wang, S.C. Datta, J. Varani, S. Kang and J.J. Voorhees. 1997a. Pathophysiology of premature skin aging induced by ultraviolet light. N Engl J Med 337: 1419-1428.

Fisher, G.J., Z.Q. Wang, S.C. Datta, J. Varani, S. Kang and J.J. Voorhees. 1997b. Pathophysiology of premature skin aging induced by ultraviolet light. New Eng J Med 337: 1419-1428.

Fisher, G.J., H.S. Talwar, J. Lin, P. Lin, F. McPhillips, Z. Wang. et al. 1998. Retinoic acid inhibits induction of c-Jun protein by ultraviolet radiation that occurs subsequent to activation of mitogen-activated protein kinase pathways in human skin *in vivo*. J Clin Invest 101: 1432-1440.

Fisher, G.J., S. Datta, Z. Wang, X.Y. Li, T. Quan, J.H. Chung, et al. 2000. c-Jun-dependent inhibition of cutaneous procollagen transcription following ultraviolet irradiation is reversed by all-trans retinoic acid. J Clin invest 106: 663-670.

Fisher, G.J., S. Kang, J. Varani, Z. Bata-Csorgo, Y. Wan, S. Datta, et al. 2002. Mechanisms of photoaging and chronological skin aging. Arch Dermatol 138: 1462-1470.

Fisher, G.J., J. Varani and J.J. Voorhees. 2008. Looking older: fibroblast collapse and therapeutic implications. Arch Dermatol 144: 666-672.

Fisher, G.J., T. Quan, T. Purohit, Y. Shao, M.K. Cho, T. He, et al. 2009. Collagen fragmentation promotes oxidative stress and elevates matrix metalloproteinase-1 in fibroblasts in aged human skin. Am J Pathol 174: 101-114.

Flanders, K.C., C.D. Sullivan, M. Fujii, A. Sowers, M.A. Anzano, A. Arabshahi, et al. 2002. Mice lacking Smad3 are protected against cutaneous injury induced by ionizing radiation. Am J Pathol 160: 1057-1068.

Fligiel, S.E., J. Varani, S.C. Datta, S. Kang, G.J. Fisher and J.J. Voorhees. 2003. Collagen degradation in aged/photodamaged skin *in vivo* and after exposure to matrix metalloproteinase-1 *in vitro*. J Invest Dermatol 120: 842-848.

Fu, X., W.C. Parks and J.W. Heinecke. 2008. Activation and silencing of matrix metalloproteinases. Semin Cell Dev Biol 19: 2-13.

Fukuchi, M., T. Imamura, T. Chiba, T. Ebisawa, M. Kawabata, K. Tanaka, et al. 2001. Ligand-dependent degradation of Smad3 by a ubiquitin ligase complex of ROC1 and associated proteins. Mol Biol Cell 12: 1431-1443.

Gehrs, K.M., D.H. Anderson, L.V. Johnson and G.S. Hageman. 2006. Age-related macular degeneration–emerging pathogenetic and therapeutic concepts. Ann Med 38: 450-471.

Geiger, B., J.P. Spatz and A.D. Bershadsky. 2009. Environmental sensing through focal adhesions. Nat Rev Mol Cell Biol 10: 21-33.

Giancotti, F. and E. Ruoslahti. 1999. Integrin Signaling. Science 285: 1028-1032.

Gloster, H.M., Jr. and D.G. Brodland. 1996. The epidemiology of skin cancer. Dermatol Surg 22: 217-226.

Golden, T.R., D.A. Hinerfeld and S. Melov. 2002. Oxidative stress and aging: beyond correlation. Aging Cell 1: 117-123.

Gomez, D., H. Alonso, H. Yoshiji and U. Thorgeirsson. 1997. Tissue inhibitors of metalloproteinases: structure, regulation and biological functions. Eur J Cell Biol 74: 111-112.

Grether-Beck, S. and J. Krutmann. 2000. Gene regulation by ultraviolet A radiation and singlet oxygen. Methods Enzymol 319: 280-290.

Gutman, A. and B. Wasylyk. 1990. The collagenase gene promoter contains a TPA and oncogene-responsive unit encompassing the PEA3 and AP-1 binding sites. EMBO J 9: 2241-2246.

Hall, M.C., D.A. Young, J.G. Waters, A.D. Rowan, A. Chantry, D.R. Edwards, et al. 2003. The comparative role of activator protein 1 and Smad factors in the regulation of Timp-1 and MMP-1 gene expression by transforming growth factor-beta 1. J Biol Chem 278: 10304-10313.

Hartman, M., A. Catlin, D. Lassman, J. Cylus and S. Heffler. 2008. U.S. Health spending by age, selected years through 2004. Health Aff (Project Hope) 27: w1-w12.

Hayashi, H., S. Abdollah, Y. Qiu, J. Cai, Y.Y. Xu, B.W. Grinnell, et al. 1997. The MAD-related protein Smad7 associates with the TGFbeta receptor and functions as an antagonist of TGFbeta signaling. Cell 89: 1165-1173.

He, T., T. Quan and G.J. Fisher. 2014. Ultraviolet irradiation represses TGF-beta type II receptor transcription through a 38-bp sequence in the proximal promoter in human skin fibroblasts. Exp Dermatol 23 Suppl 1: 2-6.

He, T., T. Quan, Y. Shao, J.J. Voorhees and G.J. Fisher. 2014. Oxidative exposure impairs TGF-beta pathway via reduction of type II receptor and SMAD3 in human skin fibroblasts. Age (Dordr) 36: 9623.

He, W., A.G. Li, D. Wang, S. Han, B. Zheng, M.J. Goumans, et al. 2002. Overexpression of Smad7 results in severe pathological alterations in multiple epithelial tissues. EMBO J 21: 2580-2590.

Hegedus, L., H. Cho, X. Xie and G.L. Eliceiri. 2008. Additional MDA-MB-231 breast cancer cell matrix metalloproteinases promote invasiveness. J Cell Physiol 216: 480-485.

Holt, D.R., S.J. Kirk, M.C. Regan, M. Hurson, W.J. Lindblad and A. Barbul. 1992. Effect of age on wound healing in healthy human beings. Surgery 112: 293-297; discussion 297-298.

Hulsmann, M., T. Stefenelli, R. Berger, B. Sturm, A. Parkner, A. Zuckermann, et al. 2000. Response of right ventricular function to prostaglandin E1 infusion predicts outcome for severe chronic heart failure patients awaiting urgent transplantation. J Heart Lung Transplant 19: 939-945.

Hynes, R.O. 2009. The extracellular matrix: not just pretty fibrils. Science 326: 1216-1219.

Ignotz, R.A. and J. Massague. 1986. Transforming growth factor β stimulates the expression of fibronectin and collagen and their incorporation into the extracellular matrix. J Biol Chem 261: 4337-4345.

Inazaki, K., Y. Kanamaru, Y. Kojima, N. Sueyoshi, K. Okumura, K. Kaneko, et al. 2004. Smad3 deficiency attenuates renal fibrosis, inflammation and apoptosis after unilateral ureteral obstruction. Kidney Int 66: 597-604.

Ingber, D.E. 1997a. Integrins, tensegrity and mechanotransduction. Gravit Space Biol Bull 10: 49-55.

Ingber, D.E. 1997b. Tensegrity: the architectural basis of cellular mechanotransduction. Annu Rev Physiol 59: 575-599.

Ingber, D.E. 2006. Cellular mechanotransduction: putting all the pieces together again. FASEB J 20: 811-827.

Itoh, S., M. Landstrom, A. Hermansson, F. Itoh, C.H. Heldin, N.E. Heldin, et al. 1998. Transforming growth factor beta1 induces nuclear export of inhibitory Smad7. J Biol Chem 273: 29195-29201.

Izzi, L. and L. Attisano. 2004. Regulation of the TGFbeta signalling pathway by ubiquitin-mediated degradation. Oncogene 23: 2071-2078.

Johnson, M.L. 1989. Aging of the United States population. The dermatologic implications. Clin Geriatr Med 5: 41-51.

Kahlos, K., Y. Soini, P. Paakko, M. Saily, K. Linnainmaa and V.L. Kinnula. 2000. Proliferation, apoptosis and manganese superoxide dismutase in malignant mesothelioma. Int J Cancer 88: 37-43.

Kaufman, S.R. 2009. Developments in age-related macular degeneration: Diagnosis and treatment. Geriatrics 64: 16-19.

Kavsak, P., R.K. Rasmussen, C.G. Causing, S. Bonni, H. Zhu, G.H. Thomsen, et al. 2000. Smad7 binds to Smurf2 to form an E3 ubiquitin ligase that targets the TGF beta receptor for degradation. Mol Cell 6: 1365-1375.

Kerkela, E. and U. Saarialho-Kere. 2003. Matrix metalloproteinases in tumor progression: focus on basal and squamous cell skin cancer. Exp Dermatol 12: 109-125.

Kessler, D., S. Dethlefsen, I. Haase, M. Plomann, F. Hirche, T. Krieg, et al. 2001. Fibroblasts in mechanically stressed collagen lattices assume a "synthetic" phenotype. J Biol Chem 276: 36575-36585.

Kim, Y.J., S.J. Hwang, Y.C. Bae and J.S. Jung. 2009. MiR-21 regulates adipogenic differentiation through the modulation of TGF-beta signaling in mesenchymal stem cells derived from human adipose tissue. Stem Cells 27: 3093-3102.

Kolarzyk, E. and J. Pach. 2000. [Comparison of ventilatory efficiency in alcohol and opiate abusers]. Pneumonol Alergol Pol 68: 303-311.

Kolarzyk, E., D. Targosz, D. Pach and L. Misiolek. 2000. Nervous regulation of breathing in opiate dependent patient. Part I. Respiratory system efficiency and breathing regulation in the first stage of controlled abstinence. Przegl Lek 57: 531-535.

Krutmann, J. 2000. Ultraviolet A radiation-induced biological effects in human skin: relevance for photoaging and photodermatosis. J Dermatol Sci 23: Suppl 1: S22-26.

Kudravi, S.A. and M.J. Reed. 2000. Aging, cancer and wound healing. *In vivo* 14: 83-92.

Lakos, G., S. Takagawa, S.J. Chen, A.M. Ferreira, G. Han, K. Masuda, et al. 2004. Targeted disruption of TGF-beta/Smad3 signaling modulates skin fibrosis in a mouse model of scleroderma. Am J Pathol 165: 203-217.

Lambert, C.A., A.C. Colige, C. Munaut, C.M. Lapiere and B.V. Nusgens. 2001. Distinct pathways in the over-expression of matrix metalloproteinases in human fibroblasts by relaxation of mechanical tension. Matrix Biol 20: 397-408.

Lapiere Ch, M. 2005. Tadpole collagenase, the single parent of such a large family. Biochimie 87: 243-247.

Laping, N.J., E. Grygielko, A. Mathur, S. Butter, J. Bomberger, C. Tweed, et al. 2002. Inhibition of transforming growth factor (TGF)-beta1-induced extracellular matrix with a novel inhibitor of the TGF-beta type I receptor kinase activity: SB-431542. Mol Pharmacol 62: 58-64.

Levy, L. and J.A. Zeichner. 2012. Dermatologic manifestation of diabetes. J Diabetes 4: 68-76.

Li, J.J., Y. Cao, M.R. Young and N.H. Colburn. 2000. Induced expression of dominant-negative c-jun downregulates NFkappaB and AP-1 target genes and suppresses tumor phenotype in human keratinocytes. Mol Carcinog 29: 159-169.

Lin, X., M. Liang and X.H. Feng. 2000. Smurf2 is a ubiquitin E3 ligase mediating proteasome-dependent degradation of Smad2 in transforming growth factor-beta signaling. J Biol Chem 275: 36818-36822.

Lin, X., M. Liang, Y.Y. Liang, F.C. Brunicardi and X.H. Feng. 2003. SUMO-1/Ubc9 promotes nuclear accumulation and metabolic stability of tumor suppressor Smad4. J Biol Chem 278: 31043-31048.

Lin, X., M. Liang, Y.Y. Liang, F.C. Brunicardi, F. Melchior and X.H. Feng. 2003. Activation of transforming growth factor-beta signaling by SUMO-1 modification of tumor suppressor Smad4/DPC4. J Biol Chem 278: 18714-18719.

Long, H., T. Shi, P.J. Borm, J. Maatta, K. Husgafvel-Pursiainen, K. Savolainen, et al. 2004. ROS-mediated TNF-alpha and MIP-2 gene expression in alveolar macrophages exposed to pine dust. Part Fibre Toxicol 1: 3.

Manza, L.L., S.G. Codreanu, S.L. Stamer, D.L. Smith, K.S. Wells, R.L. Roberts, et al. 2004. Global shifts in protein sumoylation in response to electrophile and oxidative stress. Chem Res Toxicol 17: 1706-1715.

Massague, J. 1990. The transforming growth factor-beta family. Annu Rev Cell Biol 6: 597-641.

Massague, J. 2000. How cells read TGF-beta signals. Nat Rev Mol Cell Biol 1: 169-178.

Massague, J., J. Seoane and D. Wotton. 2005. Smad transcription factors. Genes & Dev 19: 2783-2810.

Mauviel, A. 1993. Cytokine regulation of metalloproteinase gene expression. J Cell Biochem 53: 288-295.

Mauviel, A. 2005. Transforming growth factor-beta: a key mediator of fibrosis. Methods Mol Med 117: 69-80.

Mendez, M.V., A. Stanley, H.Y. Park, K. Shon, T. Phillips and J.O. Menzoian. 1998. Fibroblasts cultured from venous ulcers display cellular characteristics of senescence. J Vasc Surg 28: 876-883.

Miranti, C. and J. Brugge. 2002. Sensing the environment: a historical perspective on integrin signal transduction. Nature Cell Biol 4: 83-90.

Monteleone, G., A. Kumberova, N.M. Croft, C. McKenzie, H.W. Steer and T.T. MacDonald. 2001. Blocking Smad7 restores TGF-beta1 signaling in chronic inflammatory bowel disease. J Clin Invest 108: 601-609.

Moustakas, A., S. Souchelnytskyi and C.H. Heldin. 2001. Smad regulation in TGF-beta signal transduction. J Cell Sci 114: 4359-4369.

Mulder, K.M. 2000. Role of Ras and Mapks in TGFbeta signaling. Cytokine Growth Factor Rev 11: 23-35.

Nagarajan, R.P., J. Zhang, W. Li and Y. Chen. 1999. Regulation of Smad7 promoter by direct association with Smad3 and Smad4. J Biol Chem 274: 33412-33418.

Nakao, A., M. Afrakhte, A. Moren, T. Nakayama, J.L. Christian, R. Heuchel, et al. 1997. Identification of Smad7, a TGFbeta-inducible antagonist of TGF-beta signalling. Nature 389: 631-635.

Nakao, A., K. Okumura and H. Ogawa. 2002. Smad7: a new key player in TGF-beta-associated disease. Trends Mol Med 8: 361-363.

National Cancer Institute (U.S.). 2005. Cancer trends progress report, pp. National Cancer Institute, NIH, DHHS, Bethesda, MD.

Paalman, M.H., R.G. Cotton and H.H. Kazazian, Jr. 2000. VARIATION, DATABASES and DISEASE: new directions for human mutation. Hum Mutat 16: 97-98.

Paas, T. and N.J. Scannell. 2000. Financing Estonia's unemployment insurance system: problems and prospects. J Cult Divers 7: 84-88.

Pace, F. and G.B. Porro. 2000. Gastroesophageal reflux and Helicobacter pylori: a review. World J Gastroenterol 6: 311-314.

Pace, F., V. Annese, P. Ceccatelli and L. Fei. 2000. Ambulatory oesophageal pH-metry. Position paper of the Working Team on Oesophageal pH-metry by the GISMAD (Gruppo Italiano di Studio sulla Motilita dell'Apparato Digerente). Dig Liver Dis 32: 357-364.

Page-McCaw, A., A.J. Ewald and Z. Werb. 2007. Matrix metalloproteinases and the regulation of tissue remodelling. Nat Rev Mol Cell Biol 8: 221-233.

Patil, A.S., R.B. Sable and R.M. Kothari. 2011. An update on transforming growth factor-beta (TGF-beta): sources, types, functions and clinical applicability for cartilage/bone healing. J Cell Physiol 226: 3094-3103.

Popova, S.N., M. Barczyk, C.F. Tiger, W. Beertsen, P. Zigrino, A. Aszodi, et al. 2007. Alpha11 beta1 integrin-dependent regulation of periodontal ligament function in the erupting mouse incisor. Mol Cell Biol 27: 4306-4316.

Qin, Z., J.J. Voorhees, G.J. Fisher and T. Quan. 2014. Age-associated reduction of cellular spreading/mechanical force up-regulates matrix metalloproteinase-1 expression and collagen fibril fragmentation via c-Jun/AP-1 in human dermal fibroblasts. Aging Cell 13: 1028-1037.

Quan, T. and G.J. Fisher. 2015. Role of Age-Associated Alterations of the Dermal Extracellular Matrix Microenvironment in Human Skin Aging: A Mini-Review. Gerontology 61: 427-34.

Quan, T., T. He, J.J. Voorhees and G.J. Fisher. 2001. Ultraviolet irradiation blocks cellular responses to transforming growth factor-beta by down-regulating its type-II receptor and inducing Smad7. J Biol Chem 276: 26349-26356.

Quan, T., T. He, S. Kang, J.J. Voorhees and G.J. Fisher. 2002a. Connective tissue growth factor: expression in human skin *in vivo* and inhibition by ultraviolet irradiation. J Invest Dermatol 118: 402-408.

Quan, T., T. He, S. Kang, J.J. Voorhees and G.J. Fisher. 2002b. Ultraviolet irradiation alters transforming growth factor beta/smad pathway in human skin *in vivo*. J Invest Dermatol 119: 499-506.

Quan, T., T. He, S. Kang, J.J. Voorhees and G.J. Fisher. 2004. Solar ultraviolet irradiation reduces collagen in photoaged human skin by blocking transforming growth factor-beta type II receptor/Smad signaling. Am J Pathol 165: 741-751.

Quan, T., T. He, J.J. Voorhees and G.J. Fisher. 2005. Ultraviolet irradiation induces Smad7 via induction of transcription factor AP-1 in human skin fibroblasts. J Biol Chem 280: 8079-8085.

Quan, T., T. He, Y. Shao, L. Lin, S. Kang, J.J. Voorhees, et al. 2006. Elevated cysteine-rich 61 mediates aberrant collagen homeostasis in chronologically aged and photoaged human skin. Am J Pathol 169: 482-490.

Quan, T., Z. Qin, W. Xia, Y. Shao, J.J. Voorhees and G.J. Fisher. 2009. Matrix-degrading metalloproteinases in photoaging. J Investig Dermatol Symp Proc 14: 20-24.

Quan, T., Z. Qin, Y. Xu, T. He, S. Kang, J.J. Voorhees, et al. 2010. Ultraviolet irradiation induces CYR61/CCN1, a mediator of collagen homeostasis, through activation of transcription factor AP-1 in human skin fibroblasts. J Invest Dermatol 130: 1697-1706.

Quan, T., Y. Shao, T. He, J.J. Voorhees and G.J. Fisher. 2010. Reduced expression of connective tissue growth factor (CTGF/CCN2) mediates collagen loss in chronologically aged human skin. J Invest Dermatol 130: 415-424.

Quan, T., F. Wang, Y. Shao, L. Rittie, W. Xia, J.S. Orringer, et al. 2013. Enhancing Structural Support of the Dermal Microenvironment Activates Fibroblasts, Endothelial Cells and Keratinocytes in Aged Human Skin *in vivo*. J Invest Dermatol 133: 658-667.

Quan, T., E. Little, H. Quan, Z. Qin, J.J. Voorhees and G.J. Fisher. 2013a. Elevated matrix metalloproteinases and collagen fragmentation in photodamaged human skin: impact of altered extracellular matrix microenvironment on dermal fibroblast function. J Invest Dermatology 133: 1362-1366.

Quan, T., F. Wang, Y. Shao, L. Rittié, W. Xia, J.S. Orringer, et al. 2013b. Enhancing structural support of the dermal microenvironment activates fibroblasts, endothelial cells and keratinocytes in aged human skin *in vivo*. Journal of Investigative Dermatology 133: 658-667.

Reed, M.J., N.S. Ferara and R.B. Vernon. 2001. Impaired migration, integrin function and actin cytoskeletal organization in dermal fibroblasts from a subset of aged human donors. Mech Ageing Dev 122: 1203-1220.

Reibel, J., E. Dabelsteen, H. Birkedal-Hansen, B. Ellegaard and I. Mackenzie. 1978. Demonstration of actin in oral epithelial cells. Scand J Dent Res 86: 470-477.

Rittie, L. and G.J. Fisher. 2002. UV-light-induced signal cascades and skin aging. Ageing Res Rev 1: 705-720.

Roberts, A.B., E. Piek, E.P. Bottinger, G. Ashcroft, J.B. Mitchell and K.C. Flanders. 2001. Is Smad3 a major player in signal transduction pathways leading to fibrogenesis? Chest 120: 43S-47S.

Romeo, E., E. Pompili, F. di Michele, M. Pace, R. Rupprecht, G. Bernardi, et al. 2000. Effects of fluoxetine, indomethacine and placebo on 3 alpha, 5 alpha tetrahydroprogesterone (THP) plasma levels in uncomplicated alcohol withdrawal. World J Biol Psychiatry 1: 101-104.

Runyan, C.E., H.W. Schnaper and A.C. Poncelet. 2003. Smad3 and PKCdelta mediate TGF-beta1-induced collagen I expression in human mesangial cells. Am J Physiol Renal Physiol 285: F413-422.

Saitoh, H. and J. Hinchey. 2000. Functional heterogeneity of small ubiquitin-related protein modifiers SUMO-1 versus SUMO-2/3. J Biol Chem 275: 6252-6258.

Seo, B.R., P. Bhardwaj, S. Choi, J. Gonzalez, R.C. Andresen Eguiluz, K. Wang, et al. 2015. Obesity-dependent changes in interstitial ECM mechanics promote breast tumorigenesis. Sci Transl Med 7: 301ra130.

Shaulian, E. and M. Karin. 2002. AP-1 as a regulator of cell life and death. Nat Cell Biol 4: E131-136.

Silver, F.H., L.M. Siperko and G.P. Seehra. 2003. Mechanobiology of force transduction in dermal tissue. Skin Res Technol 9: 3-23.

Spencer, V.A., R. Xu and M.J. Bissell. 2007. Extracellular matrix, nuclear and chromatin structure and gene expression in normal tissues and malignant tumors: a work in progress. Adv Cancer Res 97: 275-294.

Stadtman, E.R. 1992. Protein oxidation and aging. Science 257: 1220-1224.

Stamenkovic, I. 2003. Extracellular matrix remodelling: the role of matrix metalloproteinases. J Pathol 200: 448-464.

Sternlicht, M.D. and Z. Werb. 2001. How matrix metalloproteinases regulate cell behavior. Annu Rev Cell Dev Biol 17: 463-516.

Stopa, M., D. Anhuf, L. Terstegen, P. Gatsios, A.M. Gressner and S. Dooley. 2000. Participation of Smad2, Smad3 and Smad4 in transforming growth factor beta (TGF-beta)-induced activation of Smad7. THE TGF-beta response element of the promoter requires functional Smad binding element and E-box sequences for transcriptional regulation. J Biol Chem 275: 29308-29317.

Swift, M.E., H.K. Kleinman and L.A. DiPietro. 1999. Impaired wound repair and delayed angiogenesis in aged mice. Lab Invest 79: 1479-1487.

Taylor, C.R. and A.J. Sober. 1996. Sun exposure and skin disease. Annu Rev Med 47: 181-191.

Thomas, G., F. de Pablo, J. Schlessinger and J. Moscat. 2000. The ins and outs of protein phosphorylation. Workshop report: control of signaling by protein phosphorylation. EMBO Rep 1: 11-15.

Thompson, K., D.W. Hamilton and A. Leask. 2010. ALK5 inhibition blocks TGFss-induced CCN2 expression in gingival fibroblasts. J Dent Res 89: 1450-1454.

Tomita, G.M., Y. Wang, M.J. Paape, B. Poultrel and P. Rainard. 2000. Influence of bispecific antibodies on the *in vitro* bactericidal activity of bovine neutrophils against Staphylococcus aureus. J Dairy Sci 83: 2269-2275.

Uitto, J. 1986. Connective tissue biochemistry of the aging dermis. Age-related alterations in collagen and elastin. Dermatol Clin 4: 433-446.

Underhill, G.H., G. Peter, C.S. Chen and S.N. Bhatia. 2012. Bioengineering methods for analysis of cells *in vitro*. Annu Rev Cell Dev Biol 28: 385-410.

Urtiaga, M., N. de Pablo and S. Martinez. 2000. [Surveillance report on Diseases of Compulsory Notification in Navarra. 1999]. An Sist Sanit Navar 23: 293-299.

Valera, E.T., R. Cipolotti, J.E. Bernardes, R.C. Pacagnella, D.M. Lima, L.G. Tone, et al. 2000. [Transient pancytopenia induced by parvovirus B19 in a child with hereditary spherocytosis]. J Pediatr (Rio J) 76: 323-326.

Varani, J., D. Spearman, P. Perone, S.E. Fligiel, S.C. Datta, Z.Q. Wang, et al. 2001. Inhibition of type I procollagen synthesis by damaged collagen in photoaged skin and by collagenase-degraded collagen *in vitro*. Am J Pathol 158: 931-942.

Varani, J., L. Schuger, M.K. Dame, C. Leonard, S.E. Fligiel, S. Kang, et al. 2004. Reduced fibroblast interaction with intact collagen as a mechanism for depressed collagen synthesis in photodamaged skin. J Invest Dermatol 122: 1471-1479.

Varani, J., M.K. Dame, L. Rittie, S.E. Fligiel, S. Kang, G.J. Fisher, et al. 2006. Decreased collagen production in chronologically aged skin: roles of age-dependent alteration in fibroblast function and defective mechanical stimulation. Am J Pathol 168: 1861-1868.

Varga, J. 2002. Scleroderma and Smads: dysfunctional Smad family dynamics culminating in fibrosis. Arthritis Rheum 46: 1703-1713.

Varga, J. and M.L. Whitfield. 2009. Transforming growth factor-beta in systemic sclerosis (scleroderma). Front Biosci (Schol Ed) 1: 226-235.

Varga, J., J. Rosenbloom and S.A. Jimenez. 1987. Transforming growth factor beta (TGF beta) causes a persistent increase in steady-state amounts of type I and type III collagen and fibronectin mRNAs in normal human dermal fibroblasts. Biochem J 247: 597-604.

Verrecchia, F. and A. Mauviel. 2002. Transforming growth factor-beta signaling through the Smad pathway: role in extracellular matrix gene expression and regulation. J Invest Dermatol 118: 211-215.

Verzijl, N., J. DeGroot, S.R. Thorpe, R.A. Bank, J.N. Shaw, T.J. Lyons, et al. 2000. Effect of collagen turnover on the accumulation of advanced glycation end products. J Biol Chem 275: 39027-39031.

von Gersdorff, G., K. Susztak, F. Rezvani, M. Bitzer, D. Liang and E.P. Bottinger. 2000. Smad3 and Smad4 mediate transcriptional activation of the human Smad7 promoter by transforming growth factor beta. J Biol Chem 275: 11320-11326.

Wall, I.B., R. Moseley, D.M. Baird, D. Kipling, P. Giles, I. Laffafian, et al. 2008. Fibroblast dysfunction is a key factor in the non-healing of chronic venous leg ulcers. J Invest Dermatol 128: 2526-2540.

Wang, F., L.A. Garza, S. Kang, J. Varani, J.S. Orringer, G.J. Fisher, et al. 2007. *In vivo* stimulation of de novo collagen production caused by cross-linked hyaluronic acid dermal filler injections in photodamaged human skin. Arch Dermatol 143: 155-163.

Wang, F., L.A. Garza, S. Cho, R. Kafi, C. Hammerberg, T. Quan, et al. 2008. Effect of increased pigmentation on the antifibrotic response of human skin to UV-A1 phototherapy. Arch Dermatol 144: 851-858.

Wang, N., J.P. Butler and D.E. Ingber. 1993. Mechanotransduction across the cell surface and through the cytoskeleton. Science 260: 1124-1127.

Wlaschek, M., I. Tantcheva-Poor, L. Naderi, W. Ma, L.A. Schneider, Z. Razi-Wolf, et al. 2001. Solar UV irradiation and dermal photoaging. J Photochem Photobiol B 63: 41-51.

Xia, W., T. Quan, C. Hammerberg, J.J. Voorhees and G.J. Fisher. 2015. A mouse model of skin aging: fragmentation of dermal collagen fibrils and reduced fibroblast spreading due to expression of human matrix metalloproteinase-1. J Dermatol Sci 78: 79-82.

Yaar, M. and B.A. Gilchrest. 1998. Aging versus photoaging: postulated mechanisms and effectors. J Investig Dermatol Symp Proc 3: 47-51.

Yaar, M. and B.A. Gilchrest. 2007. Photoageing: mechanism, prevention and therapy. Br J Dermatol 157: 874-887.

Yu, Y., S.S. Kanwar, B.B. Patel, P.S. Oh, J. Nautiyal, F.H. Sarkar, et al. 2012. MicroRNA-21 induces stemness by downregulating transforming growth factor beta receptor 2 (TGFbetaR2) in colon cancer cells. Carcinogenesis 33: 68-76.

Zhao, B., L. Li and K.L. Guan. 2010. Hippo signaling at a glance. J Cell Sci 123: 4001-4006.

Zhou, W., J.J. Ryan and H. Zhou. 2004. Global analyses of sumoylated proteins in Saccharomyces cerevisiae. Induction of protein sumoylation by cellular stresses. J Biol Chem 279: 32262-32268.

Zhu, C.Q., S.N. Popova, E.R. Brown, D. Barsyte-Lovejoy, R. Navab, W. Shih, et al. 2007. Integrin alpha 11 regulates IGF2 expression in fibroblasts to enhance tumorigenicity of human non-small-cell lung cancer cells. Proc Natl Acad Sci USA 104: 11754-11759.

2

(Myo)fibroblasts/Extracellular Matrix in Skin Wound and Aging

Dorothée Girard,[1,2,a] *Betty Laverdet*[1,2,b] and *Alexis Desmoulière*[1,2,#,*]

❑ Introduction

The skin is the primary protection of the body against external injuries and is essential in the maintenance of general homeostasis. The dermis, located beneath the epidermis, represents the thickest compartment of the skin and is mainly composed of a dense collagen network supporting specific dermal apparatus such as hair follicles, sebaceous and sweat glands. Dermal (myo)fibroblasts play a major role in the synthesis and maintenance of the extracellular matrix (ECM) as well as in the wound healing process. During aging, the dermal ECM and associated resident cells undergo senescence affecting both the structure of the dermis and its role in skin repair. In addition, extrinsic factors such as ultraviolet (UV) irradiation and intrinsic factors such as diabetes or medicines can further accelerate this phenomenon. Thus, aging has direct consequences on the dermis via both the alteration of ECM components and the impairment of (myo)fibroblast function.

[1] University of Limoges, EA (Equiped'Accueil) 6309 "Myelin maintenance and peripheral neuropathies", Faculties of Medicine and Pharmacy, Limoges, France.
[2] CHU (Centre Hospitalier Universitaire) Dupuytren de Limoges, Limoges, France.
[a] E-mail: dorothee.girard@unilim.fr
[b] E-mail: betty.laverdet@etu.unilim.fr
[#] Address for Correspondence: Department of Physiology, Faculty of Pharmacy, University of Limoges, 2 rue du Dr. Marcland, 87025 Limoges cedex, France.
[*] Corresponding author: alexis.desmouliere@unilim.fr

❑ Skin Extracellular Matrix and Myofibroblastic Differentiation

Skin Extracellular Matrix

Dermal fibroblasts are responsible for the synthesis and maintenance of the ECM. The ECM is a complex network composed of macromolecules such as collagens, elastin and glycoproteins that strongly interact with each other and with resident cells to maintain the structural integrity and function of the skin (Table 1). The ECM of the dermal layer is composed mostly of fibrillar collagens with type I collagen being the most abundant followed by type III collagen. Type IV collagen which forms network of beaded filaments is also found (Kielty and Shuttleworth 1997) as well as fibril-associated collagens with interrupted triple helices (FACIT) collagens such as collagens XII and XIV (Gelse et al. 2003; Agarwal et al. 2012) and type V collagen to a lesser extent (Chanut-Delalande et al. 2004). Collagen fibers make up 70% of the dermis, giving it structural strength, tensile mechanical property and toughness. Another important component of the dermal ECM is elastin which maintains normal elasticity, stretching and flexibility. Proteoglycans and glycosaminoglycans represent another essential part of the ECM and provide viscosity and hydration to the skin (Mikesh et al. 2013). The dermis consists of two regions, the papillary dermis (or upper dermis) closer to the epidermis and the reticular dermis (or deep dermis), thicker than the papillary dermis, overlying the hypodermis. The papillary dermis is composed of thin elastin and collagen fibers mainly oriented perpendicularly to the skin surface, while the reticular dermis is composed of thicker and multidirectional fibers (Watt and Fujiwara 2011).

TABLE 1 Structure and roles of dermal extracellular matrix components. Molecules composing the extracellular matrix provide specific structural properties to the dermis such as elasticity, tensile strength and compressibility and are also involved in cell communication and signaling regulation via for example transforming growth factor-β and integrin signaling pathways (Schultz et al. 2005; Egbert et al. 2014).

Family	Name	Structure	Roles
Collagens	Types I, II, III, VI, V	Fibrillar/microfibrillar	Tensile strength
	Types XII, XIV, XVI	Fibril-associated collagen with interrupted triple helix	
Elastin		Elastic fiber	Stretching and resilience

Table 1 Contd.

Family	Name	Structure	Roles
Glycoproteins	Fibrillin	Glycoprotein	Maintenance of elastic fiber integrity
	Fibronectin	High molecular weight glycoprotein	Promotion of cell adhesion and communication
Glycosaminoglycans	Hyaluronic acid	Repetition of disaccharide units	Hydration and resistance to compression
Proteoglycans	Decorin, versican, heparan sulfate, dermatan sulfate, small leucine-rich proteoglycans	Glycosaminoglycan conjugated protein	Hydration and cell signaling regulation
Periostin		Matricellular protein	Regulation of collagen fibrillogenesis

Myofibroblastic Differentiation

Fibroblasts are spindle-shaped cells with long cytoplasmic prolongations and derive from multipotent mesenchymal cells. Fibroblasts form a heterogeneous cell population which plays a major role, as mentioned above, in the deposition of ECM components. Indeed, in the skin, fibroblasts are able to organize a complex ECM network responsible for dermal architecture and remarkable cutaneous biomechanical properties. Following internal or external injury signals, skin fibroblasts can acquire a myofibroblastic phenotype, presenting critical properties for wound healing, repair and "firmness" of aged and damaged skin.

Myofibroblastic differentiation of fibroblastic cells begins with the appearance of the proto-myofibroblast, whose stress fibers contain only β- and γ-cytoplasmic actin. Proto-myofibroblasts evolve, but not always necessarily, into the differentiated myofibroblast, the most common variant of this cell, with stress fibers containing α-smooth muscle (SM) actin (Hinz et al. 2012). Myofibroblasts can, according to the experimental or clinical situation, express other SM cell contractile proteins, such as SM-myosin heavy chains or desmin; however, the presence of α-SM actin represents the most reliable marker of the myofibroblastic phenotype (Desmoulière et al. 2005).

During the healing process, after the inflammatory and vascular phase, the granulation tissue develops with the appearance of myofibroblasts which synthesize and deposit ECM components which will replace the provisional matrix (Darby et al. 2014). These cells exhibit contractile properties, due to the expression of α-SM actin and play a major role in the contraction and the maturation of the granulation tissue (Hinz et al. 2001). During the resolution phase of healing, the cell number is dramatically reduced by apoptosis of vascular cells and myofibroblasts (Desmoulière et al. 1995) (Fig. 1).

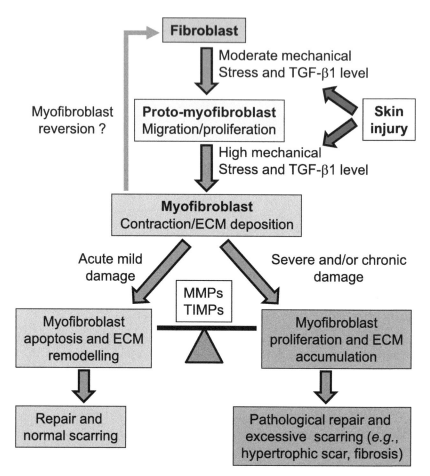

FIG. 1   Fibroblast-myofibroblast modulation during normal or pathological repair. *Proto-myofibroblasts express stress fibers containing cytoplasmic actins and develop focal adhesions. Myofibroblasts express stress fibers containing α-smooth muscle actin and develop supermature focal adhesions. Mechanical stress is a major inducer of myofibroblast differentiation via the extracellular matrix (ECM) and modifications of ECM are involved in transforming growth factor (TGF)-β1 activation leading to a vicious circle in pathological situations. In addition, the balance between matrix metalloproteinases (MMPs) and their inhibitors (TIMPs for tissue inhibitor of metalloproteinases) plays an essential role in ECM deposition/remodeling. During granulation tissue resolution, the reversion of the myofibroblast phenotype to the fibroblast phenotype remains to be demonstrated. (adapted from Desmoulière et al. 2003).*

In few cases, a pathological wound healing course of events can be encountered (Desmoulière et al. 2003). These abnormal repair processes are the result of an impaired remodeling of the granulation tissue leading for example to abnormal cutaneous repair in hypertrophic or keloid scars and to fibrosis in internal organs (Fig. 1). In cutaneous excessive scarring, the normal healing process is not achieved and the granulation tissue continues to grow, due to an abnormal and excessive secretion of growth factors and/or to the lack of molecules inducing apoptosis or ECM remodeling. In internal organs, when the noxious stimulus responsible for a lesion persists, an excessive ECM deposition is observed leading to the development of organ fibrosis. As in pathological cutaneous wounding, the installation and persistence of fibrosis are the consequences of an imbalanced ECM synthesis and degradation by the myofibroblasts. In this situation, the balance between matrix metalloproteinases (MMPs) and their inhibitors (TIMPs for tissue inhibitor of metalloproteinases) plays an essential role.

❑ (Myo)fibroblasts and Extracellular Matrix During Normal Wound Repair

Main Pathways Controlling Extracellular Matrix Deposition and Myofibroblast Differentiation

Myofibroblasts are interconnected by gap junctions and are also connected to the ECM by a specialized structure called fibronexus, a transmembrane complex involving intracellular microfilaments in continuity with extracellular fibronectin fibers (Eyden 2008). More recently, the fibronexus has been assimilated to the mature or supermature focal contact, *i.e.* three-dimensional transcellular structure containing the fibronectin isoform ED-A and α-SM actin; these are organized by intracellularly and extracellularly originated forces and play a role in the establishment and modulation of the myofibroblastic phenotype (Dugina et al. 2001). It has also been shown that α-SM actin is crucial for focal adhesion maturation in myofibroblasts (Hinz et al. 2003).

Various cytokines and growth factors are involved in skin homeostasis and wound healing (Barrientos et al. 2008). Among all these soluble factors, some directly act on fibroblast activity and granulation tissue formation, especially the transforming growth factor (TGF)-β1, a potent inducer of myofibroblastic differentiation (Desmoulière et al. 1993). Beyond a specific effect on the induction of α-SM actin expression, TGF-β1 also promotes the deposition of large amounts of ECM; in fact, TGF-β1 not only induces synthesis of ECM but it also reduces MMP activity by promoting TIMP expression. It is interesting to underline that TGF-β1 action on myofibroblastic differentiation is only possible in the presence of ED-A fibronectin which underlines the fact that close relationships exist between ECM components, growth factor activation and cell function regulation.

Interestingly and less studied, it is now clear that innervation and neuropeptides play an important role for skin homeostasis and during wound healing. For example, substance P, which is released from nerve endings after injury, induces inflammation and mediates angiogenesis, keratinocyte proliferation and fibrogenesis. It is suggested that poorly healing wounds such as diabetic wounds have insufficient substance P levels to promote a neuroinflammatory response necessary for normal wound repair, while, conversely, increased nerve numbers and neuropeptide levels could induce exuberant inflammation and excessive scarring (Scott et al. 2007). In aged patients, cutaneous repair processes are less efficient (Sgonc and Gruber 2013) and it could be partly due to a deterioration of the peripheral nervous system at the skin level (for review, see Laverdet et al. 2015). We have analyzed the effects of location and aging on intra-epidermal nerve fiber density (IENFD) (unpublished observations). Our results showed that hip (proximal) and ankle (distal) young skins are innervated with equivalent densities. Surprisingly, there was no difference between young and aged proximal skin biopsies in terms of IENFD. However, a significant location effect on IENFD was observed in aged patients. Actually, in aged patients, IENFD was significantly decreased in distal biopsies compared with proximal biopsies. This decrease of the IENFD, mainly involving type C and Aδ nerve fibers in skin biopsies performed in aged patients and far from the cell bodies of the sensory neurons (distal biopsies), can provide new insights into the skin breakdown appearing with aging and/or photo-aging, particularly in lower extremities where wounds are often difficult to repair.

Mechanical Forces

Fibroblasts and myofibroblasts, because of their contractile properties and privileged relationships with the ECM, can modify their activity depending on the mechanical environment. Myofibroblastic differentiation features, such as stress fibers, ED-A fibronectin or α-SM actin expression, appear earlier in granulation tissue subjected to an increase in mechanical tension by splinting a full-thickness wound with a plastic frame as compared to normally healing wounds (Hinz et al. 2001). Fibroblasts cultured on substrates of variable stiffness present different phenotypes (Achterberg et al. 2014). Cultured fibroblasts do not express stress fibers on soft surfaces; when the stiffness of the substrate increases, a sudden change in cell morphology occurs and stress fibers appear (Yeung et al. 2005). Shear forces exerted by fluid flow are able to induce TGF-β1 production and differentiation of fibroblasts cultured in collagen gels in the absence of other exterior stimuli such as cytokine treatment (Ng et al. 2005) and ECM pre-strain regulates the bioavailability of TGF-β1 (Klingberg et al. 2014). The role of mechanical stress in stimulating myofibroblast activity has also been shown in experiments where dermal wounds in mice are mechanically stressed by stretching or splinting the wound; this mechanical load increased myofibroblast activity resulting in increased scar formation and mimicking to some extent human hypertrophic scarring (Aarabi et al. 2007). In aged skin, it is suggested that old fibroblasts have an age-dependent reduction in the capacity for collagen synthesis and simultaneously experience a loss of mechanical stimulation resulting from the decrease of intact collagen fibers (Fisher et al. 2008; Vedrenne et al. 2012).

❑ (Myo)fibroblasts and Extracellular Matrix Dysregulation in Aging

Intrinsic skin aging factors are typically non modifiable and include ethnicity, anatomical site differences and chronological changes such as the hormonal alterations following menopause; on the other side, extrinsic skin aging factors are largely modifiable with lifestyle choices (*e.g.*, smoking and alcohol consumption) but mainly UV light exposure accounting for up to 80% of visible skin aging (Farage et al. 2008; Vedrenne et al. 2012). Thus, aged human skin is characterized by a flattening of the dermal-epidermal junction, reduced mechanical tension and loss of elasticity mainly due to marked reduction of dermal collagen and elastin contents.

Senescence, Aging Fibroblasts and Extracellular Matrix

Like other organs in the body, skin undergoes alterations due to the passage of time commonly called senescence. The main phenomenon is based on the observation that diploid cells, such as fibroblasts, have a finite life-span and limited rounds of cell division also called replicative senescence. Although senescent cells remain viable, cellular senescence is associated with altered gene expression, genome instability and mitochondrial dysfunction. The progressive and inevitable decline of dermal fibroblast cellular integrity leads to functional impairment as well as degenerative changes in the dermis with a direct impact on ECM composition (Fisher et al. 2008; Tigges et al. 2014).

Senescent dermal fibroblasts are characterized by a decreased collagen-synthetic capacity leading to disorganized collagen fibers (Varani et al. 2006). In addition, aged fibroblasts switch from a matrix-producing to a matrix-degrading phenotype. It is translated by increased expression of MMPs (mainly MMP-1) associated with decreased expression of TIMPs (Hornebeck 2003; Fisher et al. 2009; Qin et al. 2014). This phenomenon further disrupts the organization of collagen fibrils as well as elastin network and has a deleterious impact on fibroblasts themselves. The loss of ECM structural integrity leads to decreased mechanical tension, reduced cellular interaction and impaired stimulation of fibroblasts.

Glycation and Oxidative Stress

Nonenzymatic protein glycation (or Maillard reaction) is a cascade of reactions yielding a heterogeneous class of compounds, collectively termed advanced glycation end-products (AGEs). The generation of AGEs is a complex process that initially involves a condensation reaction between proteins and glucose, followed by Amadori rearrangement, cyclization, polymerization, cleavage and oxidation processes. AGEs have been implicated in the pathogenesis of diabetes where hyperglycemia is a main contributing factor, renal failure and aging (Brownlee 1995). Protein glycation contributes to skin aging as it deteriorates collagen and elastin network within the dermis by crosslinking and has consequently a deleterious impact on fibroblast function. Oxidative processes are part of the protein glycation mechanism and oxidative stress itself is another mechanism that contributes to skin aging. Skin is damaged due to free radicals (reactive oxygen species or ROS) that accumulate during the lifespan of an individual, especially when the skin is exposed to UV irradiation. This phenomenon is called the Free Radical theory and leads to irreversible cellular functional impairment. ROS can target proteins, as well as lipids and nucleic acids, leading to an accumulation of cellular oxidative damage and the formation of carbonyl groups which are well identified as biomarkers of oxidative stress. Thus, fibroblasts can be directly targeted as well as ECM components leading to further destruction and fragmentation of both collagen and elastin networks (Fisher et al. 2009).

Hormones/Menopause

It is now well admitted that many of the adverse effects associated with cutaneous aging are also inducible by glucocorticoids (GC) (Tiganescu et al. 2011). Systemically or after therapeutic administration, cortisol binds to the ubiquitously expressed GC receptor to modulate gene transcription. Within target tissues, cortisol concentrations are regulated at a pre-receptor level by isozymes of the 11β-hydroxysteroid dehydrogenase (11β-HSD) and the 11β-HSD type 1 activates cortisol from inactive cortisone (Tomlinson et al. 2004). 11β-HSD type 1 increases with age in human skins and in human dermal fibroblasts from both photo-protected and photo-exposed sites and 11β-HSD type 1 also increased with donor age (Tiganescu et al. 2011). Then, the age-associated increase in dermal 11β-HSD type 1 which induces an increased local GC activation, may contribute to the adverse changes in skin morphology and functions associated with chronological aging and photo-aging.

Interestingly, the 11β-HSD type 1 expression is increased in post-menopausal skin. The resulting increased level of GC induces the thinning of the dermis and epidermis, reduced proliferative capacities of keratinocytes and dermal fibroblasts and modifications of the ECM; these changes compromise barrier function, tensile strength and structural integrity resulting in a skin that is thinner, dryer and more prone to shearing. In addition, blockade of the age-related increase in 11β-HSD type 1 activity may promote improved structural and functional properties in aging skin (Tiganescu et al. 2013). It could be suggested that selective 11β-HSD type 1 inhibitors could be used to reverse or prevent menopause related skin fragility. In addition, estrogen deficiency following menopause results in atrophic skin changes and acceleration of skin aging (Thornton 2013).

Aggravating Factors

Different factors are known to be implicated in the acceleration of skin aging. Among these are environmental factors such as tobacco smoking or sun exposure and medical factors related to specific diseases or their associated treatments.

Tobacco Smoking

Tobacco smoking is one of the most known environmental aggravating factors. Indeed, tobacco causes premature skin aging via different mechanisms. Tobacco acts directly on the dermis by inducing abnormal accumulation of elastic fibers and a decrease of collagen synthesis caused by an up regulation of MMP-1 and MMP-3 (Yin et al. 2000). Moreover, tobacco smoking has an effect on TGF-β1 expression which has a role in epidermal homeostasis and induces the synthesis of ECM proteins in the dermis. Tobacco smoking induces a non-functional latent form of TGF-β1 and down regulates TGF-β1 receptors (Yin et al. 2000). Thus, tobacco smokers display the so-called characteristic "smoker's face" that includes facial wrinkles, skin atrophy and grey appearance.

Ultra Violet/Environment

UV irradiation is also well known to induce premature skin aging. Abnormal skin exposure to UV has deleterious effects on fibroblasts and keratinocytes. The primary mechanism by which UV radiation induces molecular response is via the generation of ROS. Different studies have been realized to study the impact of UVB on fibroblast senescence *in vitro*. For example, a study has shown that exposure of dermal fibroblasts to sub-lethal doses of UVB induces premature senescence (Chainiaux et al. 2002). These cells expressed specific biomarkers of senescence such as decreased proliferation, senescence-associated β galactosidase (SA-βgal) activity and altered gene expression. These premature senescent fibroblasts also display increased TGF-β1, MMP-1 and MMP-2 mRNA expression (Debacq-Chainiaux et al. 2005). Concerning the effect of UVA on fibroblasts, it has been shown that this treatment induces growth arrest, increased expression of SA-βgal and alteration of cell morphology (Herrmann et al. 1998). UV irradiation acts also on collagen. Exposure to UV irradiation induces an increase of MMP levels (Fisher et al. 1996) which consequently promotes collagen degradation and a decrease of collagen production.

Diabetes

Diabetes is a chronic disease which is characterized by an inability to use insulin in response to hyperglycemia (type II diabetes). Diabetic patients can have different complications such as vasculopathy (microangiopathy and macroangiopathy) or neuropathy. This neuropathy induces a loss of sensitivity and generally begins on foot. When diabetic patients injure their foot, the wound is not painful and it can progress to an ulcer which may lead to amputation. As described above, diabetes complications can be attributed to reaction of glycation which can modify the mechanical properties of human skin. The AGEs induce a loss of skin plasticity and skin is thinner in diabetic patients compared to healthy patients (Hashmi et al. 2006). AGEs also stimulate fibroblast apoptosis (Alikhani et al. 2005) and promote senescence phenomenon (Ravelojaona et al. 2009). ECM is also modulated by AGEs: mRNA expression of TGF-β1 is increased and the MMP-1/TIMP-1 ratio is higher in diabetic skin tissues. ECM protein expression is also modified in diabetic skin tissues with an increased expression of MMP-9 and TGF-β1 (Ren et al. 2013).

❑ Effect of Age on Wound Repair

Definitively, age-related impairment in wound healing is a well-accepted fact. However, the mechanisms underlying this deficiency are not completely understood (Gould et al. 2015). Numerous alterations in aging skin can have an impact on wound repair, including in particular fibroblast senescence, the altered quality of the ECM and the decreased capacities of the fibroblasts to manage ECM deposition and remodeling leading to lower mechanical properties of the skin (see above and Quan and Fisher 2015). In this section, alterations in the repair process of aged skin and general factors associated with elderly that might impair cutaneous healing will be discussed.

Alterations in one of the steps which follow one another during the repair process can lead to a defect in healing. Aging alters the inflammatory and endothelial cell adhesion molecule profiles during human cutaneous wound healing (Ashcroft et al. 1998), the macrophage phagocytic function (Swift et al. 2001) and more generally decreases the inflammasome proteins (Stojadinovic et al. 2013). These alterations lead to delayed wound closure with diminished granulation tissue formation, decreased angiogenesis, decreased collagen and growth factor synthesis and reduced numbers of myofibroblasts (Mirza et al. 2009) (Fig. 2). In 2013, Sgonc and Gruber underlined that in young individuals, temporary hypoxia stimulates wound healing by inducing cytokine and growth factor production and by increasing granulation tissue formation while in elderlies, the response to hypoxia seems to be impaired. A reduced response to hypoxia linked to a defect in hypoxia inducible factor-1α signaling could affect angiogenesis through reduced vascular endothelial cell growth factor levels. In addition, aged fibroblasts present impaired migratory capacities with complete loss of responsiveness to hypoxia and deficits in the migratory and signal transduction responsiveness to TGF-β1 that may partly explain diminished healing capabilities often observed in aged patients (Mogford et al. 2002). An up-regulation of MMP-2 and MMP-9 in cutaneous wounds of healthy elderlies and a down-regulation of TIMP-1 and TIMP-2 are observed; in addition, the levels of TGF-β1 which favors collagen deposition are decreased (Ashcroft et al. 2002). Finally, this situation impairs ECM deposition resulting in impaired healing and certainly represents an essential factor leading to age-related delayed wound repair. However, it has been shown that the rate of scar maturation vary with age, with older subjects (>55 years) displaying accelerated maturation, whereas a prolonged high turnover state and a retarded rate of maturation are observed in younger subjects (<30 years) (Bond et al. 2008). Interestingly, it is observed that young patients easily develop hypertrophic scar after burns while it is rare in adult and elderly persons. We can suggest with others that in aging, even if early phases of wound healing are affected, the remodeling and maturation phases are better controlled leading to an improved scarring process. Obviously, it is true in healthy persons. If adverse situations are present, *i.e.* malnutrition, vascular or immune problems, kidney or liver pathologies, diabetes, non-healing wounds can develop usually secondary to chronic inflammation (Eming et al. 2007).

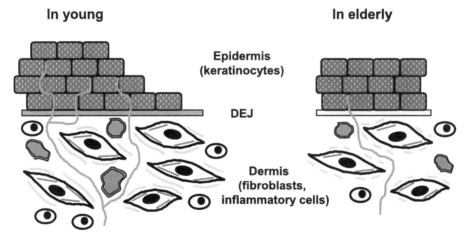

FIG. 2 **Effects of aging on wound healing.** *In elderly compared with young persons, an inflammation defect is present, reepithelialization (keratinocyte proliferation and migration), neoangiogenesis, reinnervation (brown lines), TGF-β1 levels and myofibroblastic differentiation (expression of α-smooth muscle actin; red bares in the fibroblast cytoplasm) are decreased and extracellular matrix (green lines) deposition is less effective with decreased secretion, increased matrix metalloproteinase levels and decreased tissue inhibitor of metalloproteinase levels. The quality of the dermal-epidermal junction (DEJ) is also affected.*

It is also important to underline that alterations in aging skin can have an impact on wound healing, but also modify the skin susceptibility to injury. As underlined above, for example, the skin fragility and the altered innervation increase the risk of skin lesion after mechanical stress or burn. In addition, the contribution of estrogen versus aging in age-associated delayed human wound healing seems essential (Hardman and Ashcroft 2008) and knowing that estrogens have a role in all phases of wound healing by modifying the inflammatory response, accelerating re-epithelialisation, stimulating granulation tissue formation and regulating proteolysis (Emmerson and Hardman 2012), impaired wound healing associated with aging is coupled with estrogen deficiency (Thornton 2013). Moreover, elevated 11β-HSD type 1 activity in aging skin leading to increased local GC generation (see above), may account for adverse changes occurring in the elderly (Tiganescu et al. 2013).

❑ Models of Aged Skin

Investigating on how aging affects the skin as well as wound healing requires experimental models. Although studies on human biopsies and/or clinical trials remain the gold standard, several *in vivo* and *in vitro* models represent a precious alternative shedding lights on age-related mechanisms affecting (myo)fibroblast function and the ECM.

Animal Models

Research studies have been undertaken *in vivo* using animal models. Small mammals such as rat, mouse and rabbit models are the most currently used. They can be easily housed, are well-characterized and have the advantage to age relatively fast. However, the skin morphology and physiology of these models are quite different from the human skin and the extrapolation of conclusions from these studies to human condition has its limits. Large mammal models of aging and wound healing such as porcine models would be a more suitable alternative as their skin morphology is closer to human (Sullivan et al. 2001). Yet, limitations in the feasibility of using larger animals can be too detrimental to be overcome. Thus, many studies have used rat and mouse models and in a recent review article, Kim et al. (2015) have highlighted that these studies had assessed the deleterious effect of aging on wound healing and more particularly on dermal healing by investigating the granulation tissue remodeling process, ECM proteins content and/or tensile strength.

In vitro Reconstructed Skin

Studies performed *in vivo* have limitations and they can raise cultural and ethical issues. Therefore, *in vitro* models represent another valuable experimental asset. Human reconstructed skin or tissue-engineered skin, using either immortalized cell lines or primary cell culture, is now a well-established model that can recapitulate many morphological and molecular characteristics of normal human skin (Ali et al. 2015). Fibroblasts are cultured within a collagen matrix that can be supplemented with chitin to mimic the dermal layer. Different experimental strategies can be considered; cells can be isolated from patient skin biopsies and be exposed to stimuli promoting aging and senescence such as UV irradiation, AGEs and oxidative stress (Marionnet et al. 2010; Pageon et al. 2014; Cadau et al. 2015).

❑ Therapeutic Options

Cosmetics

A wide range of cosmetics are available to try to limit visible effects of skin aging. Effects of several of these molecules are controversial but the efficiency of a few molecules on skin aging is confirmed by both *in vitro* and *in vivo* studies. Among these molecules, two types of products are mainly used in anti-aging cosmetics: retinoids and antioxidants. Sun blockers are also important to limit consequences of photo-aging. Actions on the dermal ECM of these different molecules are detailed in Table 2.

TABLE 2 **Overview of the principal molecules used in anti-aging cosmetics.**

Molecules	Effects on Dermal Cells and Extracellular Matrix	References
Retinoids	↗Production of collagen, elastin and glycosaminoglycans ↘ Expression of matrix metalloproteinase-1 No ultraviolet-protection	Ramos-e-Silva et al. 2001 Kligman 1996 Varani et al. 2000 Chapman 2012
Alpha hydroxy acids	Promote growth and cell differentiation ↗ Production of dermal glycosaminoglycan	Ramos-e-Silva et al. 2001 Smith 1996 Ramos-e-Silva et al. 2004
Alpha lipoic acid	Exfoliant No ultraviolet protection	Beitner 2003
L-ascorbic acid	↗ Synthesis of collagens types I and III Ultraviolet-protection	Farris 2005 Nusgens et al. 2001
Vitamin E	Ultraviolet-protection	Maalouf et al. 2002
Ubiquinone	↗Production of collagen, dermal extracellular matrix protection	Burke 2005
Vitamine B3	↗ Skin elasticity, skin color improvement	Bissett et al. 2005
Hormone replacement therapy	↗Production of collagen, dermal thickness improvement ↗ Skin elasticity	Brincat 2004 Sator et al. 2007
Hyaluronic acid injection	↗Skin hydration and fibroblast activation ↗Synthesis of collagen type I, matrix metalloproteinase-1 and tissue inhibitor of metalloproteinase-1	Yoneda et al. 1988 Jäger et al. 2012

Wound Healing

Different therapeutic options exist in order to improve wound healing. The action of these treatments is mediated among others by an effect on (myo)fibroblasts. Thus, for chronic wounds such as ulcers, an option is to stimulate the activity of (myo)fibroblasts to induce wound contraction and promote wound healing. Today, only one treatment is available and can be used only on diabetic foot ulcers. Regranex ® (becaplermin) is a gel containing recombinant human platelet-derived growth factor-BB. This product increases ECM synthesis and improves wound healing (Pierce et al. 1992; Wu et al. 1997). Different trials have been performed on patients. For example, Wieman et al. (1998) have shown that wound healing of diabetic foot ulcers treated with Regranex ® is better than with placebo. Hindsight, Regranex ® commercialization was stopped in certain countries because there were a limited number of prescriptions and other alternatives were available.

Concerning hypertrophic scars, the opposite strategy is used: it is necessary to inhibit myofibroblast activities to stop ongoing fibrosis. Different factors are known to be suppressors of myofibroblast activities such as NF-κB (Mann et al. 2010), specific miRNAs such as miR-29 (Maurer et al. 2010) and miR-200a (Wang et al. 2011), interferon-γ (Pittet et al. 1994) and CXCL-10 (Jiang et al. 2010) for example. Likewise, pharmacological products can be used to reduce cellular division such as bleomycin or 5-fluorouracil (Aggarwal et al. 2008; Sadeghinia and Sadeghinia 2012). It is also possible to use corticosteroid injections into the scar to induce inhibition of fibroblast growth (Cruz and Korchin 1994) and to enhance collagen and fibroblast degeneration (Boyadjiev et al. 1995).

❏ Conclusion

An important aspect which remains to be clearly elucidated is the origin of myofibroblasts. It is well admitted that the major contribution for myofibroblast production originates from local recruitment of connective tissue fibroblasts. However, mesenchymal stem cells, circulating fibrocytes and bone marrow-derived cells, local pericytes, as well as resident epithelial cells through epithelial-to-mesenchymal transition may represent alternative sources of myofibroblasts when local fibroblasts are not able to comply with the request. Depending on the situation and the cellular microenvironment, these diverse cell types probably contribute to the appearance of (myo)fibroblast subpopulations whose phenotype can be modulated by their interactions with neighboring cells and the ECM. Moreover, research on skin progenitor cells which can differentiate in many different cell types and which are always present within the skin of elderly patients could represent an interesting source of cells able to promote, when correctly stimulated, the repair process of difficult-to-heal wounds. Finally, deleterious effects of exogenous factors such as UV exposure and AGEs on skin health during aging, affecting particularly dermal fibroblasts and the ECM, must be underlined to prevent the appearance of skin problems which can become dramatic with age.

❑ Acknowledgements

This work was supported in part by the French Armaments Procurement Agency (DGA, No 2013 94 0903). Betty Laverdet and Dorothée Girard were supported by fellowships (doctoral and postdoctoral respectively) from the French Armaments Procurement Agency.

❑ References

Aarabi, S., K.A. Bhatt, Y. Shi, J. Paterno, E.I. Chang, S.A. Loh, et al. 2007. Mechanical load initiates hypertrophic scar formation through decreased cellular apoptosis. FASEB J 21: 3250-3261.

Achterberg, V.F., L. Buscemi, H. Diekmann, J. Smith-Clerc, H. Schwengler, J.J. Meister, et al. 2014. The nano-scale mechanical properties of the extracellular matrix regulate dermal fibroblast function. J Invest Dermatol 134: 1862-1872.

Agarwal, P., D. Zwolanek, D.R. Keene, J.N. Schulz, K. Blumbach, D. Heinegård, et al. 2012. Collagen XII and XIV, new partners of cartilage oligomeric matrix protein in the skin extracellular matrix suprastructure. J Biol Chem 287: 22549-22559.

Aggarwal, H., A. Saxena, P.S. Lubana, R.K. Mathur and D.K. Jain. 2008. Treatment of keloids and hypertrophic scars using bleom. J Cosmet Dermatol 7: 43-49.

Ali, N., M. Hosseini, S. Vainio, A. Taieb, M. Cario-André and H.R. Rezvani. 2015. Skin equivalents: skin from reconstructions as models to study skin development & diseases. Br J Dermatol 173: 391-403.

Alikhani, Z., M. Alikhani, C.M. Boyd, K. Nagao, P.C. Trackman and D.T. Graves. 2005. Advanced glycation end products enhance expression of pro-apoptotic genes and stimulate fibroblast apoptosis through cytoplasmic and mitochondrial pathways. J Biol Chem 280: 12087-12095.

Ashcroft, G.S., M.A. Horan and M.W. Ferguson. 1998. Aging alters the inflammatory and endothelial cell adhesion molecule profiles during human cutaneous wound healing. Lab Invest 78: 47-58.

Ashcroft, G.S., S.J. Mills and J.J. Ashworth. 2002. Ageing and wound healing. Biogerontology 3: 337-345.

Barrientos, S., O. Stojadinovic, M.S. Golinko, H. Brem and M. Tomic-Canic. 2008. Growth factors and cytokines in wound healing. Wound Repair Regen 16: 585-601.

Beitner, H. 2003. Randomized, placebo-controlled, double blind study on the clinical efficacy of a cream containing 5% alpha-lipoic acid related to photoageing of facial skin. Br J Dermatol 149: 841-849.

Bissett, D.L., J.E. Oblong and C.A. Berge. 2005. Niacinamide: A B vitamin that improves aging facial skin appearance. Dermatol Surg 31: 860-865.

Bond, J.S., J.A. Duncan, A. Sattar, A. Boanas, T. Mason, S. O'Kane, et al. 2008. Maturation of the human scar: an observational study. Plast Reconstr Surg 121: 1650-1658.

Boyadjiev, C., E. Popchristova and J. Mazgalova. 1995. Histomorphologic changes in keloids treated with Kenacort. J Trauma 38: 299-302.

Brincat, M.P. 2004. Oestrogens and the skin. J Cosmet Dermatol 3: 41-49.

Brownlee, M. 1995. The pathological implications of protein glycation. Clin Invest Med 18: 275-281.

Burke, K.E. 2005. Nutritional antioxidants. pp. 125-132. *In*: Draelos, Z.D. [ed.]. Cosmeceuticals. Elsevier Health Sciences, Philadelphia, USA.

Cadau, S., S. Leoty-Okombi, S. Pain, N. Bechetoille, V. André-Frei and F. Berthod. 2015. In vitro glycation of an endothelialized and innervated tissue-engineered skin to screen anti-AGE molecules. Biomaterials 51: 216-225.

Chainiaux, F., J.P Magalhaes, F. Eliaers, J. Remacle and O. Toussaint. 2002. UVB-induced premature senescence of human diploid skin fibroblasts. Int J Biochem Cell Biol 34: 1331-1339.

Chanut-Delalande, H., C. Bonod-Bidaud, S. Cogne, M. Malbouyres, F. Ramirez, A. Fichard, et al. 2004. Development of a functional skin matrix requires deposition of collagen V heterotrimers. Mol Cell Biol 24: 6049-6057.

Chapman, M.S. 2012. Vitamin A: history, current uses and controversies. Semin. Cutan Med Surg 31: 11-16.

Cruz, N.I. and L. Korchin. 1994. Inhibition of human keloid fibroblast growth by Isotretinoin and Triamcinolone acetonide in vitro. Ann Plast Surg 33: 401-405.

Darby, I.A., B. Laverdet, F. Bonté and A. Desmoulière. 2014. Fibroblasts and myofibroblasts in wound healing. Clin Cosmet Investig Dermatol 7: 301-311.

Debacq-Chainiaux, F., C. Borlon, T. Pascal, V. Royer, F. Eliaers, N. Ninane, et al. 2005. Repeated exposure of human skin fibroblasts to UVB at subcytotoxic level triggers premature senescence through the TGF-beta1 signaling pathway. J Cell Sci 118: 743-758.

Desmoulière, A., A. Geinoz, F. Gabbiani and G. Gabbiani. 1993. Transforming growth factor-beta 1 induces alpha-smooth muscle actin expression in granulation tissue myofibroblasts and in quiescent and growing cultured fibroblasts. J Cell Biol 122: 103-111.

Desmoulière, A., M. Redard, I. Darby and G. Gabbiani. 1995. Apoptosis mediates the decrease in cellularity during the transition between granulation tissue and scar. Am J Pathol 146: 56-66.

Desmoulière, A., I.A. Darby and G. Gabbiani. 2003. Normal and pathologic soft tissue remodeling: role of the myofibroblast, with special emphasis on liver and kidney fibrosis. Lab Invest 83: 1689-1707.

Desmoulière, A., C. Chaponnier and G. Gabbiani. 2005. Tissue repair, contraction and the myofibroblast. Wound Repair Regen 13: 7-12.

Dugina, V., L. Fontao, C. Chaponnier, J. Vasiliev and G. Gabbiani. 2001. Focal adhesion features during myofibroblastic differentiation are controlled by intracellular and extracellular factors. J. Cell Sci 114: 3285-3296.

Egbert, M., M. Ruetze, M. Sattler, H. Wenck, S. Gallinat, R. Lucius, et al. 2014. The matricellular protein periostin contributes to proper collagen function and is downregulated during skin aging. J Dermatol Sci 73: 40-48.

Eming, S.A., T. Krieg and J.M. Davidson. 2007. Inflammation in wound repair: molecular and cellular mechanisms. J Invest Dermatol 127: 514-525.

Emmerson, E. and M.J. Hardman. 2012. The role of estrogen deficiency in skin ageing and wound healing. Biogerontology 13: 3-20.

Eyden, B. 2008. The myofibroblast: phenotypic characterization as a prerequisite to understanding its functions in translational medicine. J Cell Mol Med 12: 22-37.

Farage, M.A., K.W. Miller, P. Elsner and H.I. Maibach. 2008. Intrinsic and extrinsic factors in skin ageing: a review. Int J Cosmet Sci 30: 87-95.

Farris, P.K. 2005. Topical vitamin C: a useful agent for treating photoaging and other dermatologic conditions. Dermatol Surg 31: 814-817.

Fisher, G. J., S.C. Datta, H.S. Talwar, Z.Q. Wang, J. Varani, S. Kang, et al. 1996. Molecular basis of sun-induced premature skin ageing and retinoid antagonism. Nature 379: 335-339.

Fisher, G.J., J. Varani and J.J. Voorhees. 2008. Looking older: fibroblast collapse and therapeutic implications. Arch Dermatol 144: 666-672.

Fisher, G.J., T. Quan, T. Purohit, Y. Shao, M.K. Cho, T. He, et al. 2009. Collagen fragmentation promotes oxidative stress and elevates matrix metalloproteinase-1 in fibroblasts in aged human skin. Am J Pathol 174: 101-114.

Gelse, K., E. Pöschl and T. Aigner. 2003. Collagens–structure, function and biosynthesis. Adv Drug Deliv Rev 28: 1531-1546.

Gould, L., P. Abadir, H. Brem, M. Carter, T. Conner-Kerr, J. Davidson, et al. 2015. Chronic wound repair and healing in older adults: current status and future research. Wound Repair Regen 23: 1-13.

Hardman, M.J. and G.S. Ashcroft. 2008. Estrogen, not intrinsic aging, is the major regulator of delayed human wound healing in the elderly. Genome Biol 9: R80.

Hashmi, F., J. Malone-Lee and E. Hounsell. 2006. Plantar skin in type II diabetes: an investigation of protein glycation and biomechanical properties of plantar epidermis. Eur J Dermatol 16: 23-32.

Herrmann, G., P. Brenneisen, M. Wlaschek, J. Wenk, K. Faisst, G. Quel, et al. 1998. Psoralen photoactivation promotes morphological and functional changes in fibroblasts in vitro reminiscent of cellular senescence. J Cell Sci 111: 759-767.

Hinz, B., D. Mastrangelo, C.E. Iselin, C. Chaponnier and G. Gabbiani. 2001. Mechanical tension controls granulation tissue contractile activity and myofibroblast differentiation. Am J Pathol 159: 1009-1020.

Hinz, B., V. Dugina, C. Ballestrem, B. Wehrle-Haller and C. Chaponnier. 2003. Alpha-smooth muscle actin is crucial for focal adhesion maturation in myofibroblasts. Mol Biol Cell 14: 2508-2519.

Hinz, B., S.H. Phan, V.J. Thannickal, M. Prunotto, A. Desmoulière, J. Varga, et al. 2012. Recent developments in myofibroblast biology: paradigms for connective tissue remodeling. Am J Pathol 180: 1340-1355.

Hornebeck, W. 2003. Down-regulation of tissue inhibitor of matrix metalloprotease-1 (TIMP-1) in aged human skin contributes to matrix degradation and impaired cell growth and survival. Pathol Biol 51: 569-573.

Jäger, C., C. Brenner, J. Habicht and R. Wallich. 2012. Bioactive reagents used in mesotherapy for skin rejuvenation in vivo induce diverse physiological processes in human skin fibroblasts in vitro- a pilot study. Exp Dermatol 21: 72-75.

Jiang, D., J. Liang, G.S. Campanella, R. Guo, S. Yu, T. Xie, et al. 2010. Inhibition of pulmonary fibrosis in mice by CXCL10 requires glycosaminoglycan binding and syndecan-4. J Clin Invest 120: 2049-2057.

Kielty, C.M. and C.A. Shuttleworth. 1997. Microfibrillar elements of the dermal matrix. Microsc Res Tech 38: 413-427.

Kim, D.J., T. Mustoe and R.A. Clark. 2015. Cutaneous wound healing in aging small mammals: a systematic review. Wound Repair Regen 23: 318-339.

Kligman, A.M. 1996. Topical retinoic acid (tretinoin) for photoaging: conceptions and misperceptions. Cutis 57: 142-144.

Klingberg, F., M.L. Chow, A. Koehler, S. Boo, L. Buscemi, T.M. Quinn, et al. 2014. Prestress in the extracellular matrix sensitizes latent TGF-β1 for activation. J Cell Biol 207: 283-297.

Laverdet, B., A. Danigo, D. Girard, L. Magy, C. Demiot and A. Desmoulière. 2015. Skin innervation: important roles during normal and pathological cutaneous repair. Histol Histopathol 30: 875-892.

Maalouf, S., M. El-Sabban, N. Darwiche and H. Gali-Muhtasib. 2002. Protective effect of vitamin E on ultraviolet B light-induced damage in keratinocytes. Mol Carcinog 34: 121-130.

Mann, J., D.C.K. Chu, A. Maxwell, F. Oakley, N.L. Zhu, H. Tsukamoto, et al. 2010. MeCP2 controls an epigenetic pathway that promotes myofibroblast transdifferentiation and fibrosis. Gastroenterology 138: 705-714.

Marionnet, C., C. Pierrard, F. Lejeune, J. Sok, M. Thomas and F. Bernerd. 2010. Different oxidative stress response in keratinocytes and fibroblasts of reconstructed skin exposed to non extreme daily-ultraviolet radiation. PLoS ONE 5: e12059.

Maurer, B., J. Stanczyk, A. Jüngel, A. Akhmetshina, M. Trenkmann, M. Brock, et al. 2010. MicroRNA-29, a key regulator of collagen expression in systemic sclerosis. Arthritis Rheum 62: 1733-1743.

Mikesh, L.M., L.R. Aramadhaka, C. Moskaluk, P. Zigrino, C. Mauch and J.W. Fox. 2013. Proteomic anatomy of human skin. J Proteomics 84: 190-200.

Mirza, R., L.A. DiPietro and T.J. Koh. 2009. Selective and specific macrophage ablation is detrimental to wound healing in mice. Am J Pathol 175: 2454-2462.

Mogford, J.E., N. Tawil, A. Chen, D. Gies, Y. Xia and T.A. Mustoe. 2002. Effect of age and hypoxia on TGFbeta1 receptor expression and signal transduction in human dermal fibroblasts: impact on cell migration. J Cell Physiol 190: 259-265.

Ng, C.P., B. Hinz and M.A. Swartz. 2005. Interstitial fluid flow induces myofibroblast differentiation and collagen alignment in vitro. J Cell Sci 118: 4731-4739.

Nusgens, B.V., P. Humbert, A. Rougier, A.C. Colige, M. Haftek, C.A. Lambert, et al. 2001. Topically applied vitamin C enhances the mRNA level of collagens I and III, their processing enzymes and tissue inhibitor of matrix metalloproteinase 1 in the human dermis. J Invest Dermatol 116: 853-859.

Pageon, H., H. Zucchi, F. Rousset, V.M. Monnier and D. Asselineau. 2014. Skin aging by glycation: lessons from the reconstructed skin model. Clin Chem Lab Med 52: 169-174.

Pierce, G.F., J.E. Tarpley, D. Yanagihara, T.A. Mustoe, G.M. Fox and A. Thomason. 1992. Platelet-derived growth factor (BB Homodimer), transforming growth factor-beta 1 and basic fibroblast growth factor in dermal wound healing. Neovessel and matrix formation and cessation of repair. Am J Pathol 140: 1375-1388.

Pittet, B., L. Rubbia-Brandt, A. Desmoulière, A.P. Sappino, P. Roggero, S. Guerret, et al. 1994. Effect of gamma-interferon on the clinical and biologic evolution of hypertrophic ccars and Dupuytren's disease: an open pilot study. Plast Reconstr Surg 93: 1224-1235.

Qin, Z., J.J. Voorhees, G.J. Fisher and T. Quan. 2014. Age-associated reduction of cellular spreading/mechanical force up-regulates matrix metalloproteinase-1 expression and collagen fibril fragmentation via c-Jun/AP-1 in human dermal fibroblasts. Aging Cell 13: 1028-1037.

Quan, T. and G.J. Fisher. 2015. Role of age-associated alterations of the dermal extracellular matrix microenvironment in human skin aging: a mini-review. Gerontology (in press).

Ramos-e-Silva, M., D.M. Hexsel, M.S. Rutowitsch and M. Zechmeister. 2001. Hydroxy acids andretinoids in cosmetics. Clin Dermatol 19: 460-466.

Ramos-e-Silva, M., M.C. Ribeiro de Castro, S.C. da Silva Carneiro and W.C. Lambert. 2004. Alpha-hydroxy acids: unapproved uses or indications. SKINmed 3: 141-148.

Ravelojaona, V., A.M. Robert and L. Robert. 2009. Expression of senescence-associated beta-galactosidase (SA-beta-Gal) by human skin fibroblasts, effect of advanced glycation end-products and fucose or rhamnose-rich polysaccharides. Arch Gerontol Geriatr 48: 151-154.

Ren, M., S. Hao, C. Yang, P. Zhu, L. Chen, D. Lin, et al. 2013. Angiotensin II regulates collagen metabolism through modulating tissue inhibitor of metalloproteinase-1 in diabetic skin tissues. Diab Vasc Dis Res 10: 426-435.

Sadeghinia, A. and S. Sadeghinia. 2012. Comparison of the efficacy of intralesional triamcinolone acetonide and 5-fluorouracil tattooing for the treatment of keloids. Dermatol Surg 38: 104-109.

Sator, P.G., M.O. Sator, J.B. Schmidt, H. Nahavandi, S. Radakovic, J.C. Huber, et al. 2007. A prospective, randomized, double-blind, placebo-controlled study on the influence of a hormone replacement therapy on skin aging in postmenopausal women. Climacteric 10: 320-334.

Schultz, G.S., G. Ladwig and A. Wysocki. 2005. Extracellular matrix: review of its role in acute and chronic wounds. http://www.worldwidewounds.com/2005/august/Schultz/Extrace-Matric-Acute-Chronic-Wounds.html.

Scott J.R., P. Muangman and N.S. Gibran. 2007. Making sense of hypertrophic scar: a role for nerves. Wound Repair Regen. 15 Suppl 1: S27-S31.

Sgonc, R. and J. Gruber. 2013. Age-related aspects of cutaneous wound healing: a mini-review. Gerontology 59: 159-164.

Smith, W.P. 1996. Epidermal and dermal effects of topical lactic acid. J Am Acad Dermatol 35: 388-391.

Stojadinovic, O., J. Minkiewicz, A. Sawaya, J.W. Bourne, P. Torzilli, J.P. de RiveroVaccari, et al. 2013. Deep tissue injury in development of pressure ulcers: a decrease of inflammasome activation and changes in human skin morphology in response to aging and mechanical load. PLoS ONE 8: e69223.

Sullivan, T.P., W.H. Eaglstein, S.C. Davis and P. Mertz. 2001. The pig as a model for human wound healing. Wound Repair Regen 9: 66-76.

Swift, M.E., A.L. Burns, K.L. Gray and L.A. DiPietro. 2001. Age-related alterations in the inflammatory response to dermal injury. J Invest Dermatol 117: 1027-1035.

Thornton, M.J. 2013. Estrogens and aging skin. Dermatoendocrino 5: 264-270.

Tiganescu, A., E.A. Walker, R.S. Hardy, A.E. Mayes and P.M. Stewart. 2011. Localization, age- and site-dependent expression and regulation of 11β-hydroxysteroid dehydrogenase type 1 in skin. J Invest Dermatol 131: 30-36.

Tiganescu, A., A.A. Tahrani, S.A. Morgan, M. Otranto, A. Desmoulière, L. Abrahams, et al. 2013. 11β-Hydroxysteroid dehydrogenase blockade prevents age-induced skin structure and function defects. J Clin Invest 123: 3051-3060.

Tigges, J., J. Krutmann, E. Fritsche, J. Haendeler, H. Schaal, J.W. Fischer, et al. 2014. The hallmarks of fibroblast ageing. Mech Ageing Dev 138: 26-44.

Tomlinson, J.W., E.A. Walker, I.J. Bujalska, N. Draper, G.G. Lavery, M.S. Cooper, et al. 2004.11beta-hydroxysteroid dehydrogenase type 1: a tissue-specific regulator of glucocorticoid response. Endocr Rev 25: 831-866.

Varani, J., R.L. Warner, M. Gharaee-Kermani, S.H. Phan, S. Kang, J.H. Chung, et al. 2000. Vitamin A antagonizes decreased cell growth and elevated collagen-degrading matrix metalloproteinases and stimulates collagen accumulation in naturally aged human skin. J Invest Dermatol 114: 480-486.

Varani, J., M.K. Dame, L. Rittie, S.E.G. Fligiel, S. Kang, G.J. Fisher, et al. 2006. Decreased collagen production in chronologically aged skin. Am J Pathol 168: 1861-1868.

Vedrenne, N., B. Coulomb, A. Danigo, F. Bonté and A. Desmoulière. 2012. The complex dialogue between (myo) fibroblasts and the extracellular matrix during skin repair processes and ageing. Pathol Biol 60: 20-27.

Wang, B., P. Koh, C. Winbanks, M.T. Coughlan, A. McClelland, A. Watson, et al. 2011. miR-200a prevents renal fibrogenesis through repression of TGF-β2 expression. Diabetes 60: 280-287.

Watt, F.M. and H. Fujiwara. 2011. Cell-extracellular matrix interactions in normal and diseased skin. Cold Spring Harb Perspect Biol 3: a005124.

Wieman, T.J., J.M. Smiell and Y. Su. 1998. Efficacy and safety of a topical gel formulation of recombinant human platelet-derived growth factor-BB (becaplermin) in patients with chronic neuropathic diabetic ulcers. A phase III randomized placebo-controlled double-blind study. Diabetes Care 21: 822-827.

Wu, L., M. Brucker, E. Gruskin, S.I. Roth and T.A. Mustoe. 1997. Differential effects of platelet-derived growth factor BB in accelerating wound healing in aged versus young animals: the impact of tissue hypoxia. Plast. Reconstruct Surg 99: 815-822.

Yeung, T., P.C. Georges, L.A. Flanagan, B. Marg, M. Ortiz, M. Funaki, et al. 2005. Effects of substrate stiffness on cell morphology, cytoskeletal structure and adhesion. Cell Motil Cytoskeleton 60: 24-34.

Yin, L., A. Morita and T. Tsuji. 2000. Alterations of extracellular matrix induced by tobacco smoke extract. Arch Dermatol Res 292: 188-194.

Yoneda, M., S. Shimizu, Y. Nishi, M. Yamagata, S. Suzuki and K. Kimata. 1988. Hyaluronic acid-dependent change in the extracellular matrix of mouse dermal fibroblasts that is conducive to cell proliferation. J Cell Sci 90: 275-286.

3
CHAPTER

Changes of Skin Barrier with Aging

Eung Ho Choi, M.D., Ph.D.

❑ Introduction of Skin Barrier

A concept of skin barrier has been developed after an introduction of two compartment organization such as the 'bricks and mortar' model (Elias and Wakefield 2011). Skin barrier mainly resides in the stratum corneum (SC) composed of corneocytes ('bricks') surrounded by intercellular lipid lamellae ('mortar') and attached by corneodesmosome (CD) ('rivet'). It has recently included a tight junction (TJ) attached to lateral walls of keratinocytes in the upper stratum granulosum (SG). The corneocytes contribute to structural stability and elasticity because of their main composition such as keratin fibrils. SC intercellular lipids composed of ceramides, cholesterol and free fatty acids function as inhibitors of transpidermal water loss (TEWL) and a barrier to transcutaneous penetration of external harmful agents (Elias et al. 2003) (Fig. 1).

Keratin filaments occupy 80-90% of corneocytes and form the macrofibrils by cross-linking with the cornified envelope (CE) of the corneocytes. The SC lipid layer is covalently attached to the external surface of the CE proteins of fully differentiated corneocytes. This cornified lipid envelop (CLE) consists of ω-hydroxyceramide covalently attached to CE proteins such as involucrin (Wertz et al. 1989). The ω-hydroxyl group on the ceramides is required for CLE formation (Behne et al. 2000). Thus the CE contributes the effective physical barrier and water impermeable barrier.

Department of Dermatology, Yonsei University Wonju College of Medicine, 20 Ilsan-ro, Wonju, 26426, South Korea.
E-mail: choieh@yonsei.ac.kr

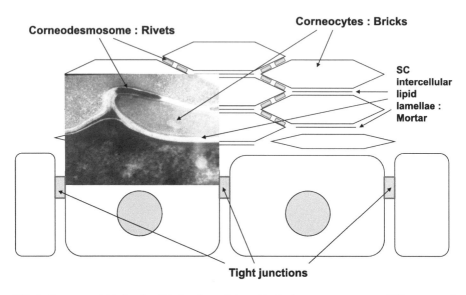

FIG. 1 *Structure of skin barrier. Skin barrier mainly resides in the stratum corneum (SC) composed of corneocytes ('bricks') surrounded by intercellular lipid lamellae ('mortar') and attached by corneodesmosome (CD) ('rivet'). It recently has been shown to include a tight junction (TJ) attaching to lateral walls of keratinocytes in the upper stratum granulosum (SG).*

SC intercellular lipid membrane orginates from lamellar bodies (LB) produced from the Golgi complex in the keratinocytes. Lipid precursors such as phospholipids, sphingomyelin, cholesterol sulfate, glucosylceramide, acylglucocylceramide that are stored in the LB are secreted into the SC-SG inter-space. Thereafter lipid precursors are processed to ceramide (about 50% by weight), cholesterol (25%) and free fatty acids (25%) by hydrolases to form the mature multilamellar structure (Schurer and Elias 1991). They are diploid in molar ratio about 1:1:1 (Mao-Qiang et al. 1993). The SC normally has an acidic pH, referred to as the "acid mantle" (Hachem et al. 2003). This acidic pH contributes to the protective functions of skin, such as permeability barrier homeostasis (Fluhr et al. 2001; Hachem et al. 2003; Mauro et al. 1998), SC integrity/cohesion (Fluhr et al. 2001; Hachem et al. 2003), epidermal antimicrobial defense (Hachem et al. 2003; Korting et al. 1990) and primary cytokine activation (Hachem et al. 2002). Three endogenous pathways as well as exogenous insults contribute to the acidic environment of the SC: (1) the Na^+/H^+ antiporter, NHE1 (Behne et al. 2002), (2) the free fatty acids generated from phospholipids by secretory phospholipase A_2 ($sPLA_2$) (Fluhr et al. 2001; Mao-Qiang et al. 1996), (3) the urocanic acid degraded from histidine by histidase. Deterioration of any of these pathways can elevate SC pH, which is linked to the alteration of permeability barrier homeostasis and SC integrity/cohesion. Maintenance of SC acidity contributes to permeability barrier homeostasis by increasing the activity of the two key ceramide-generating enzymes such as β-glucocerebrosidase (βGlcCer'ase) and acidic sphingomyelinase (aSMase) (Fluhr et al. 2004; Hachem et al. 2005; Holleran et al. 2006) and supports SC integrity and cohesion by decreasing the activity of serine proteases (SPs). SPs not only inactivate lipid-processing enzymes (Hachem et al. 2005), but also degrade the CDs (Hachem et al. 2003) and inhibit LB secretion (Hachem et al. 2006).

Lysis of CD is involved in the desquamation of corneocytes, which is influenced by pH in the SC. In normal epidermis, the upper SC presents with pH 4.5-5.0, but the lower SC presents with pH 6.5-7.0, which normally makes a pH gradient in the SC (Choi et al. 2007). SPs, specific enzymes in the epidermis, such as SCCE (stratum corneum chymotryptic enzyme encoded by *KLK7*) and SCTE (stratum corneum tryptic enzyme encoded by *KLK5*) are activated under an environment of neutral pH and then contribute to the desquamation of corneocytes and the disruption of skin barrier (Briot et al. 2009).

TJ proteins, a major regulator of barrier function in simple epithelia, were identified in human skin (Brandner and Proksch 2006). In the inflammatory diseases of the intestine, many cytokines affect the TJ barrier status. TJs localize in SG (Brandner et al. 2002) and contribute to epidermal barrier formation. Among TJ proteins, claudin (Cldn)-1 and Cldn-4 have a role in the barrier function of the skin (Furuse et al. 2002; Yuki et al. 2011). Cldn-1 null mutant mice showed normal SC structure, however died shortly after birth with an increased TEWL (Furuse et al. 2002). Results of a recent study suggest that Cldn-4 also plays a role in barrier function by observing that the diffusion of 550 Da tracer which is normally stopped at TJ areas was no longer blocked in skin incubated with ochratoxin A that removes Cldn-4 from the TJ structure (Yuki et al. 2011). TJs are highly dynamic structures which transiently open and close in response to numerous stimuli such as pathogens (Ohnemus et al. 2008), UV irradiation (Yuki et al. 2011) and wounding (Malminen et al. 2003). Recently, observation has shown that the alteration of the epidermal Ca^{2+} gradient caused by barrier perturbation affects the TJ structure and function and the faster recovery of TJ as compared to the SC barrier may imply the protective homeostatic mechanism of the skin barrier (Baek et al. 2013). TJs are also involved in antigen presentation of Langerhans cells in the epidermis (Kubo et al. 2009).

The antimicrobial barrier as well as epidermal permeability barrier are the main function of the epidermal barrier. Those are considered as discrete, protective functions of mammalian skin (Elias et al. 2003). Although permeability barrier homeostasis and the outer antimicrobial shield are both localize to the SC, the structural and biochemical basis for each differs (Elias and Choi 2005). The outermost antimicrobial shield is attributed to the low water content, acidic surface pH (Fluhr and Elias 2002), resident microflora and certain proteins of eccrine and sebaceous gland origin (Schroder and Harder 2006). Human SC also contain at least four AMPs such as S100 protein, S100A7 (psoriasin), RNase7, cathelicidin (hCAP18) carboxy-terminal fragment, LL-37 and human β-defensin2 (hBD2) (Elias 2007). HBD2 and LL-37 are inducible by UV-B, chronic inflammation, pathogen challenge and/or during wound healing although expressed at low levels under basal conditions (Aberg et al. 2008). Both hBD2 and LL-37 are packaged within LB in the epidermis (Oren et al. 2003; Braff et al. 2005). Therefore, the epidermal permeability barrier and the antimicrobial barriers are linked (Elias and Choi 2005) and do not have disparate, but rather interdependent processes (Aberg et al. 2008).

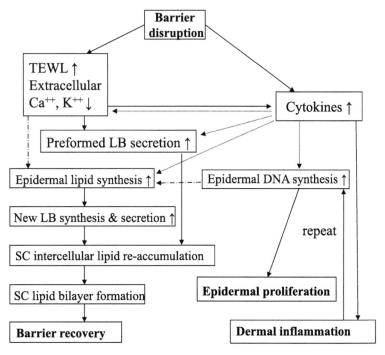

FIG. 2 *Homeostatic response of skin barrier after barrier disruption. After barrier disruption, TEWL occurs immediately. In turn, the loss of epidermal calcium ion follows, which acts as a signal for the homeostasis of skin barrier. Immediately after barrier disruption, pre-formed LBs including lipid precursors are secreted. In turn, new LBs are produced and replenish the disrupted lamellar structures to restore a normalized barrier. On the other hand, epidermal keratinocytes secret pro-inflammatory cytokines which directly stimulate epidermal proliferation and dermal inflammatory cells. Cytokines secreted from dermal inflammatory cells indirectly provoke epidermal proliferation due to an increase of DNA synthesis of keratinocytes.*

Epidermal permeability barrier is regulated by a change in the epidermal calcium ion (Lee et al. 1992). Epidermal calcium gradient in normal and young skin is characterized by low levels of calcium ion in both the basal and spinous layers, with an increase in extracellular and intracellular calcium ion that peaks in the outer SG (Menon et al. 1985). This calcium ion gradient serves many functions in the epidermis, which include the induction of terminal differentiation (Elias et al. 2002), formation of the cornified envelop, epidermal lipid synthesis, exocytosis of LBs and regulation of the last events of terminal differentiation that together form the barrier (Menon et al. 1994; Lee et al. 1998; Choi et al. 2003). After the skin barrier is disrupted by external physico-chemical stress, TEWL occurs and in turn, the loss of epidermal calcium ion follows. The loss of epidermal calcium ion acts as a signal for the homeostasis of skin barrier. Immediately after barrier disruption, pre-formed LBs including lipid precursors for SC intercellular lipid membranes are secreted and, in turn, new LBs are produced and replenish the disrupted lamellar structures to restore a normalized barrier (Menon et al. 1994). Epidermal keratinocytes secret pro-inflammatory cytokines which directly stimulate epidermal proliferation and dermal inflammatory cells. Cytokines secreted from dermal inflammatory cells indirectly provoke epidermal proliferation due to an increase of DNA synthesis of keratinocytes (Wood et al. 1992). Homeostasis of skin barrier function is maintained through above mechanism (Fig. 2).

❑ Structural Changes of Aging Skin Barrier

Skin aging has been commonly divided into intrinsic and extrinsic. Intrinsic aging (chronological aging) presents functional changes rather than macroscopic or morphological changes and extrinsic aging (photoaging) presents structural and physiological changes due to chronic sun exposure. Aged epidermis shows various changes implying skin barrier impairment such as increased transdermal drug delivery, increased sensivity to irritants, aggravation of xerosis and occurrence of pruritus. (Chung et al. 2003; Fisher et al. 2002). The structural changes of aged skin result from combined and cumulative effects of intrinsic aging and extrinsic aging (photo-aging) (Fisher et al. 2002). The epidermis shows remarkable morphologic changes with aging, which include epidermal thinning, flattening of the rete riges and orthokeratosis. Photo-aged epidermis presents more disorganized cellular maturation with some cytologic atypia, a significant decrease in Langerhans cells and an uneven distribution of melanocytes in the basal layer (Reed et al. 1997). The number of SC layers is significantly increased in senile xerosis compared to younger skin. Individual keratohyaline granules are much smaller and distributed more broadly throughout the SG cells with aging (Tezuka 1983). In aged epidermis, SC integrity is impaired and the barrier recovery after acute perturbation with tape stripping is delayed (Ghadially et al. 1995).

The permeability barrier abnormality in aged skin results from the reduced delivery of secreted lipids to the SC. The decrease of lipid secretion, in turn, results in a reduction in the number of SC intercellular lamellar bilayers shown in electron-microscope (EM) findings. Finally,

the extracellular matrix of SC could be more porous in the aged skin (Ghadially et al. 1995). The mechanism responsible for this decreased LB secretion has been suggested as a loss of the epidermal calcium gradient. The distribution of calcium in the epidermis becomes abnormally broad with aging (Forslind et al. 1999). Denda et al. reported that there is an alteration of calcium distribution in the epidermis after the observation of the distribution of calcium ion in the epidermis from young (13, 26, 29, 34 y old), middle aged (48 y old) and elderly (70, **71, 77, 79 y old) subjects. They observed that calcium ion was distributed throughout the epidermis in the epidermis of elderly subjects. Moreover, the epidermal calcium gradient in the middle-aged subjects appeared intermediate between that of the young and elderly subjects (Denda** et al. 2003). Loss of the epidermal calcium gradient may originate from a decreased number of ion pumps, ion channels, or ionotropic receptors in aged skin (**Denda** et al. 2001). Therefore, the alteration of epidermal calcium distribution in the aging skin negatively influences the **epidermal permeability barrier by impeding the delivery of LBs to the SC, which results in a decrease in the extracellular lipid bilayers.**

❑ Biochemical and Molecular Changes of Aging Skin Barrier

A report on the biochemical changes of epidermal lipids in the aged skin stated that the content of three major lipid species such as ceramide, cholesterol and fatty acids, was reduced (Ghadially et al. 1995). So, the structural abnormality of SC intercellular lipid membrane was best explained by a global reduction of SC lipids in the aged skin (about 1/3 less lipid weight % than in young SC). On the other hand, more profound decrease of cholesterol or ceramide species was reported (Rogers et al. 1996). Selective changes in specific SC ceramide species such as ceramide 2 (N-lingocerylsphingosine; NS), with concurrent increases in ceramide 3 (nonhydroxy N-acyl fatty acid and phytosphingosine; NP) relative to total ceramides content, have also been noted in aged epidermis (Denda et al. 1993). Alteration of SC lipid processing has been reported in epidermal aging. Acid sphingomyelinase (SM' ase) activity is reduced in aged human epidermis (8th decade) compared to young adults (2nd decade) (Yamamura and Tezuka 1990). SM' ase generates long (C24) and short (C16) chain-containing ceramide species. So, it is critical for epidermal barrier function (Schmuth et al. 2000; Jensen et al. 1999). The activities of acid-SM'ase and ceramide synthase were reduced only in the inner epidermis of aged (15-18 month-old) vs. young (2-3 month-old) hairless mouse epidermis, which correlated with reduced capacity for barrier repair in aging. Whereas, acid-SM' ase was normal in the outer epidermis, which correlates with normal barrier function under basal condition (Jensen et al. 2005).

The metabolic basis for barrier abnormality in the aged skin could be explained by the reduced activity of the rate limiting enzymes for each of these lipids such as serine palmitoyltransferase (SPT), 3-hydroxy-3-methylglutaryl-coenzyme A (HMG-CoA) reductase and acetyl coenzyme A carboxylase (ACC) (Ghadially et al. 1996). Collectively, the lipid synthesis and enzyme activity in the aged epidermis are not only reduced under basal condition, but also fail to upregulate sufficiently after acute barrier disruption. Thus, the lipid synthesis in the aged epidermis does not reach the level in the young epidermis after comparable insults.

The molecular basis for the epidermal lipid synthetic abnormality observed in the aged skin has been partially explored. One possible mechanism is that the content or activation of the sterol regulatory element binding proteins (SREBPs), which transcriptionally regulate several key enzymes of cholesterol, fatty acid syntheses is abnormal (Harris et al. 1998). The other mechanism is that autocrine or paracrine signaling responsible for the epidermal lipid metabolic pathway is partly abnormal (Gilhar et al. 1992). Treatment of IL-1α to cultured human keratinocytes stimulates epidermal lipid synthesis (Bastian et al. 1996). There are few studies on local cytokine levels in the skin during aging. IL-1α decreases in various tissues in the aged, including a decrease of cytokine production in the aged human cultured keratinocytes (Sauder et al. 1989) and lower mRNA levels in aged mice and humans (Gilchrest et al. 1994). There are not only age-dependent changes in cytokine expression, but also a decreased response to cytokines with aging (Barland et al. 2004; Ye et al. 2002). Aged transgenic mice with a knockout of the functional IL-1α receptor displayed a barrier abnormality versus age-matched, wild-type littermates (Ye et al. 2002). Topical treatment in the aged skin with an immunomodulator, imiguimod, normalizes barrier recovery rates in aged mice (Barland et al. 2004). Collectively, the reduction of cytokine production and/or downstream biological reactivity is a common feature of the aging tissues that could explain the functional abnormalities in the aging skin.

Among the specific mechanisms to impair the skin barrier with intrinsic aging or photoaging, reactive oxygen species (ROS) are the primary mediators of UV damage, while telomere shortening characterizes the process of intrinsic aging (Boukamp 2001). UV irradiation generates ROS including the superoxide anion, peroxide and singlet oxygen, which damage the epidermis. This ROS can modify the cellular components including DNA, proteins and lipid through chemical oxidation. In both intrinsic and photoaging, the oxidation of DNA contributes to the gene mutations, whereas the oxidation of proteins leads to reduced function (Levine and Stadtman 2001). Telomeres are repetitive DNA sequences that cap the ends of chromosomes. The terminal base pairs of these sequences are lost with each round of mitosis, resulting in progressive chromosome shortening with each somatic cell division, which is, therefore, more pronounced in aged cells (Yaar et al. 2002). There is a molecular connection between UV-induced DNA damage from photoaging and replication-induced telomere shortening from chronologic aging. Internal and external insults causing DNA damage can ultimately lead to cellular senescence and apoptosis through a common cellular pathway (Yaar et al. 2002).

Skin surface lipids are the first target of UV light. Especially squalene, as a major lipid originating from sebaceous glands, is changed to squalene hydroperoxide after both UVB and UVA irradiation (Saint-Leger et al. 1986). The fact that natural sebaceous gland-originated squalene is the substrate for squalene monohydroperoxides following UVA exposure was elucidated by the inverse correlation between squalene depletion and squalene monohydroperoxides (Ekanayake Mudiyanselage et al. 2003). The SC directly exposed to UVB and UVA light has oxidative tissue damage due to the peroxidation of lipids, which is inhibited by antioxidant such as vitamin E (Thiele 2001). SC antioxidant activity, including vitamin E, decline remarkably after exoposure to even physiological doses of UV (Lopez-Torres et al. 1998; Thiele et al. 1998). The SC, a mainly hydrophobic environment, would be expected to lack hydrophilic antioxidants, such as ascorbic acid and reduced glutathione. Therefore, vitamin E which is normally recycled, would be more important for antioxidant function in the SC (Stoyanovsky et al. 1995).

Several important metabolic enzymes, which are inactivated by mixed function oxidase during intrinsic aging, accumulate, but only after 60 years of age (Oliver et al. 1987). Photoaged skin shows high levels of different markers of oxidative stress, which include the accumulation of lipid peroxides, glycation end products and oxidized proteins (Jeanmaire et al. 2001; Sander et al. 2002). After chronic UV exposure, oxidatively modified proteins are significantly increased both in the papillary dermis and in the outermost layers of the SC, but less in nucleated epidermal cells (Sander et al. 2002; Thiele et al. 1999). In addition, catalase protein and activity are naturally higher in human SC and significantly depleted after UV exposure. It reflects that SC filters UV light and epidermal cells have more efficient antioxidant system (Sander et al. 2002; Hellemans et al. 2003).

❑ Functional Changes of Aging Skin Barrier

In humans, significant anatomic variability was noted for basal TEWL, SC hydration, skin surface pH and sebum content in aged skin as well as young skin. Among all measured factors, only basal TEWL was significantly lower in the aged group compared to the young. Comparing male and female volunteers, none of the four factors showed significant differences (Wilhelm et al. 1991). That is, the epidermal permeability barrier function, as assessed by TEWL rates, is normal or even supernormal under basal conditions in the aged skin, presumably due to a decrease in sweating and microcirculation or an increase of corneocyte cell surface area. But, its functional problems are revealed only after an insult. The time required to reconstitute competent SC is more than double in the elderly. That is, the aged skin barrier is disrupted more easily and repaired more slowly compared to young skin. These defects mainly originate from an overall deficiency in all key epidermal lipids (especially cholesterol), a focal decrease of SC intercellular lamellae and a diminished LB secretion (Ghadially et al. 1995, Choi et al. 2007).

Whereas these alterations are detectable in chronologically aged skin, they are further aggravated in human skin with superimposed photoaging (Reed et al. 1997). The effects of UVB on both epidermal barrier function and proliferation with chronological age showed that a single UVB exposure (7.5 MED) developed a barrier abnormality (increased TEWL) and DNA synthesis, which were significantly diminished in intrinsically aged versus young mouse epidermis. Therefore, the transient barrier abnormality at two to three days after UVB exposure is attenuated in aged skin compared to younger skin, presumably as a result of a decreased mitogenic response (Haratake et al. 1997).

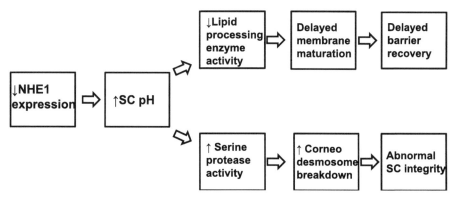

FIG. 3 *A proposed pathways leading to abnormal skin barrier function in moderately aged epidermis. Decreased NHE1 expression induces an increase of SC pH, in turn a decrease of lipid processing enzyme activity and delayed membrane maturation and finally delayed barrier recovery. Second branch of this pathway shows an increase of SP activity, in turn, increased CD breakdown and then abnormal SC integrity. (Cited from Choi et al. 2007).*

These functional changes occur incrementally with aging. In humans and mice of advanced age (>75 years in human or >18-24 months in mice), the skin barrier defects are linked to reduced epidermal lipid synthesis (Ghadially et al. 1995). In comparison, skin barrier defects in moderately aged humans (50-80 years) or mice (12-15 months) are linked instead to defective SC acidity. In moderately aged mouse epidermis, the abnormal acidification is linked to decreased NHE1 expression. Decreased NHE1 levels, in turn, lead to increased SC pH, which results in defective lipid processing and delayed maturation of SC lipid lamellar membranes, due to suboptimal activation of the pH-sensitive essential, lipid-processing enzyme, β-glucocerebrosidase. In moderately aged skin, the SC integrity is impaired due to increased pH-dependent activation of serine proteases, which contributes to premature degradation of CD (Choi et al. 2007) (Fig. 3).

Although various factors such as humidity, androgen excess and psychological stress, are known to impact barrier homeostasis negatively in young skin, it is not known whether these factors aggravate the barrier homeostasis in aged skin. A dry environment induces epidermal proliferation and scaling in both young and aged murine skin. However, no remarkable difference was found in the skin barrier recovery of aged mice in a dry environment (Choi et al. 2002). Important factors maintaining skin barrier function include SC hydration, SC pH, SC integrity/cohesion, antioxidant defense and antimicrobial properties. All of these are compromised to some degree in aged skin, in part as a result of the faulty lipid synthetic pathway (Fig. 4).

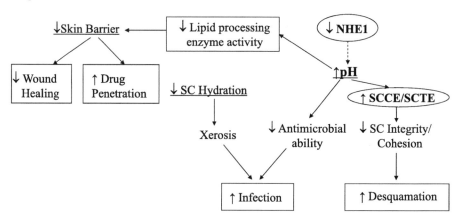

FIG. 4 *Important factors in maintaining skin barrier function include SC hydration, SC pH, SC integrity/cohesion, antioxidant defense and antimicrobial properties. All of these are compromised to some degree in aged skin, in part as a result of the faulty lipid synthetic pathway. Abnormal function of NHE1 is a specific underlying defect of pH elevation.*

Maintenance of optimal SC hydration is an important function of the epidermis and is dependent on several factors. These include the lamellar structure of SC intercellular lipids, which traps water within the corneocytes, the amount of natural moisturizing factors (NMFs), a complex mixture of low molecular weight produced within corneocytes by filaggrin degradation and the SC glycerol content (Verdier-Sévrain and Bonté 2007). In aged epidermis, all three of these factors are compromised. The decreased lipid content in the aged SC coupled with the disorganized lamellar structures and enlarged corneocytes, impair SC water retention. There is a significant age-related decline in the level of NMF. Electron microscope examination showed a decrease of keratohyalin granules in senile xerosis, which would lead to reduced synthesis of profilaggrin and subsequently low levels of NMF (Tezuka 1983). The NMF decrease in the aged SC likely results from reduced synthesis of profilaggrin (Takahashi and Tezuka 2004). The decline in NMF production may reflect the cumulative effects of actinic damage as it was observed only in photo-aged skin. The two possible mechanisms of low glycerol level in the aged SC could be explained as follows: First, the decrease in sebaceous lipid production in the aged skin could result in decreased glycerol generation from triglycerides. Second, the aged skin exhibits decreased levels of the epidermal water/glycerol transporter, aquaporin-3 (AQP3). AQP-3 deficient mice display defective skin hydration, elasticity and barrier function (Fluhr et al. 2003), which is corrected by glycerol replacement, suggesting that diminished glycerol transport to the SC generates the observed functional defects of the skin.

In the aged skin, an increased skin surface pH has been reported repeatedly. Zlotogorski reported that skin surface pH was significant higher in the advanced aged group (> 80 years) compare to the younger group (Zlotogorski 1987). A positive correlation between age and pH was also reported (Thune et al. 1988). In a large Chinese cohort, skin surface pH on the forehead of both males and females over the age of 70 years was higher than that in younger groups (Man et al. 2009).

Antimicrobial function of the SC does not solely depend on acidic pH. Antimicrobial peptides (AMPs) were demonstrated in the intercellular lipid domain of the SC which functions as the permeability barrier (Aberg et al. 2008; Elias and Choi 2005). Human β-defensin 2 (HBD-2) is stored in the LBs of epidermal keratinocytes as well as in the intercellular spaces, suggesting that HBD-2 is released along with the contents of LB to provide an antibiotic shield for the epidermis (Oren et al. 2003). As HBD-2 is under transcriptional control of IL-1α and IL-1β (Liu et al. 2002), alterations in IL-1α signaling with aging could decrease the upregulation of AMPs. Moreover, the decreased IL-1 signalling with aging reduces the inflammatory response exhibited by aging skin (Ye et al. 2002). Therefore, the defective IL-1α signaling in aged epidermis could increase the risk of infections by altering not only the antimicrobial properties of the barrier, but also by diminishing the inflammatory response to pathogens. Collectively, the aged skin is easily afflicted by inflammatory skin diseases, dry skin and eczema which could be triggered or exacerbated by impaired barrier homeostasis.

❑ Skin Barrier in the Diabetes Comparable to the Aging Skin

Diabetes mellitus (DM) showing a chronic hyperglycemic condition is clinically classified into type 1 and 2. Type 2 DM accounts for over 80% of all DM. Type 2 DM shows a complex pathophysiology such as insulin resistance and inadequate insulin production in typically old and obese individuals

(Ahmed and Goldstein 2006). Chronic uncontrolled hyperglycemia contributes to various complications. At least 30% of DM patients have some type of skin involvement related to DM (Perez and Kohn 1994). Dryness, pruritus, cutaneous infection and delayed wound healing are commonly observed problems in type 2 DM patients as well as people of advanced aged (Sakai et al. 2005). All of these skin problems result from an impaired skin barrier.

Park et al. proposed the hypothesis that long-standing hyperglycemic condition accelerates skin aging process, namely, the skin of chronic hyperglycemia showed a more advanced aged skin barrier using Otsuka Long-Evans Tohushima Fatty (OLETF) rat (Park et al. 2011). OLETF rats have typical characteristics of type 2 DM (Kawano et al. 1992). OLETF rats exhibited decreased epidermal lipid synthesis and AMP expression with increasing aging. Decreased epidermal lipid synthesis accounted for decreased LB production. In addition, there was significantly higher serum levels of AGEs and elevated AGE receptor in the epidermis. They concluded that long-standing hyperglycemia impairs skin barrier function including permeability and antimicrobial barriers by accelerating the skin aging process in proportion to the duration of hyperglycemica (Park et al. 2011). As diabetic skin also shows similar changes in the skin barrier as aged skin, both of them have very similar characteristics of the skin barrier compared to young skin (Table 1).

TABLE 1 Comparison of Skin Barrier between Young and Aged.

	Young	Aged
Basal TEWL	++	+~++
SC hydration	++	+
SC integrity/cohesion	++	+
SC pH	++	+++
Barrier recovery	++	+
Total epidermal lipids	++	+
Epidermal lipid synthesis	++	+
Epidermal cholesterol synthesis	++	+
LB number	++	+~++
LB secretion	++	+
SC intercellular lipid bilayer	++	+
IL-1α	++	+
IL-1 ra	++	+
Amphiregulin	++	+

++: basal, +: decreased, +++: increased

❏ Therapeutic Strategies in Aging Skin Barrier (Figure 5)

Equimolar mixtures of the three key lipids such as ceramide, cholesterol and fatty acids allow normal barrier recovery rates in young skin (Man et al. 1996). Moreover, the three component mixtures to 3:1:1 molar ratios as physiological lipid mixture significantly accelerate barrier recovery (Zettersten et al. 1997). In young skin, any of the three key species can predominate (Mao-Qiang et al. 1993). But, in aged epidermis, only topical cholesterol alone could accelerate barrier recovery (Ghadially et al. 1996). In addition, equimolar mixtures of the three key lipids could also accelerate barrier recovery if cholesterol is the predominant lipid (Zettersten et al. 1997). These reports emphasize the profound effect of a decrease in cholesterol synthesis in the aged epidermal permeability barrier (Barland et al. 2005).

Topical mevalonic acid has been demonstrated as having a role in acute barrier repair in aged skin but not young skin. Mevalonic acid is an intermediate substrate generated early in cholesterol biosynthesis. Similar to cholesterol, topical treatment with mevalonic acid to aged murine skin enhances the rate of barrier repair after acute disruption (Haratake et al. 2000).

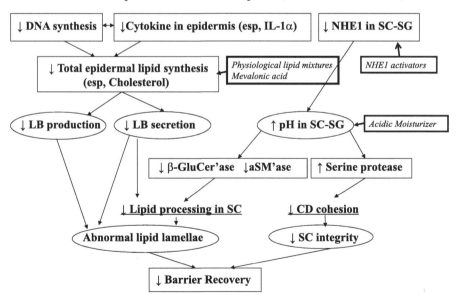

FIG. 5 *Therapeutic implications on altered skin barrier of aged skin. Mixtures of three key lipids such as ceramide, cholesterol and fatty acids at 3:1:1 molar ratios as physiological lipid mixture could be used for aged epidermis. Topical mevalonic acid also enhances the barrier repair after acute disruption. Considering a decreased skin surface acidity in the moderately aged skin as well as the advanced aged skin, the acidic moisturizer could be beneficial for the aged skin. In the future, a novel NHE1 activator will be used for aging skin barrier.*

Considering a decreased skin surface acidity in the moderately aged skin as well as the advanced aged skin, the acidic moisturizer could be beneficial for the aged skin. The barrier abnormalities in the aged skin were normalized by acidifying the SC exogenously, suggesting a basis for the well-known acidification therapies that are widely used to treat pathologic xerosis/eczema seen in moderately aged humans (Choi et al. 2007). A small size clinical study results showed that a 4-week treatment appling the pH 4.0 skin care products significantly improved the SC integrity of the elderly. The reduction of the increased baseline skin surface pH of elders is accompanied by improved SC integrity. So, the authors concluded that skin care products for elders have to be adjusted in the pH range of 3.5 to 4.0 (Blaak et al. 2011).

Restoring of the antioxidant barrier of the SC may be another therapeutic strategy for aging skin barrier. Topical antioxidants are recommended. Among lipid-soluble antioxidants, tocopherol has photoprotective properties (Thiele et al. 2000) and may stabilize SC lamellar membrane (Pelle et al. 1999). Theoretically, α-tocopherol (free vitamin E) may be more efficient for antioxidant production of skin surface lipids and skin barrier constituents compared to vitamin E esters. Photoprotection is also important as an antioxidant strategy to prevent damage to SC lipids and proteins.

The skin barrier in diabetic conditions exhibits many similar characteristics comparable to the aged skin. Therefore, therapeutic strategies for the aged skin barrier might be helpful to diabetic skin.

❏ References

Aberg, K.M., M.Q. Man, R.L. Gallo, T. Ganz, D. Crumrine, B.E. Brown, et al. 2008. Co-regulation and interdependence of the mammalian epidermal permeability and antimicrobial barriers. J Invest Dermatol 128: 917-25.

Ahmed, I. and B. Goldstein. 2006. Diabetes mellitus. Clin Dermatol 24: 237-46.

Baek, J.H., S.E. Lee, K.J. Choi, E.H. Choi and S.H. Lee. 2013. Acute modulations in stratum corneum permeability barrier function affect claudin expression and epidermal tight junction function via changes of epidermal calcium gradient. Yonsei Med J 54: 523-8.

Barland, C.O., E. Zettersten, B.S. Brown, J. Ye, P.M. Elias and R. Ghadially. 2004. Imiquimod-induced interleukin-1 alpha stimulation improves barrier homeostasis in aged murine epidermis. J Invest Dermatol 122: 330-6.

Barland, C.O., P.M. Elias and R. Ghadially. 2005. The aged epidermal permeability barrier: Basis for functional abnormalities. pp 535-552. *In*: Elias, P.M. and K.R. Feingold (ed.). Skin Barrier. Taylor & Francis, New York.

Bastian, B.C., R.J. Schacht, E. Kämpgen and E.B. Bröcker. 1996. Phospholipase A2 is secreted by murine keratinocytes after stimulation with IL-1 alpha and TNF-alpha. Arch Dermatol Res 288: 147-52.

Behne, M., Y. Uchida, T. Seki, P.O. de Montellano, P.M. Elias and W.M. Holleran. 2000. Omega-hydroxyceramides are required for corneocyte lipid envelope (CLE) formation and normal epidermal permeability barrier function. J Invest Dermatol 114: 185-92.

Behne, M.J., J.W. Meyer, K.M. Hanson, N.P. Barry, S. Murata, D. Crumrine, et al. 2002. NHE1 regulates the stratum corneum permeability barrier homeostasis. Microenvironment acidification assessed with fluorescence lifetime imaging. J Bio Chem 277: 47399-406.

Blaak, J., R. Wohlfart and N.Y. Schurer. 2011. Treatment of aged skin with a pH 4 skin care product normalizes increased skin surface pH and improves barrier function: Results of a pilot study. J Cosmetic Dermatol Sci Appl 1: 50-8.

Boukamp, P. 2001. Ageing mechanisms: the role of telomere loss. Clin Exp Dermatol 26: 562-5.

Braff, M.H., A. Di Nardo and R.L. Gallo. 2005. Keratinocytes store the antimicrobial peptide cathelicidin in lamellar bodies. J Invest Dermatol 124: 394-400.

Brandner, J.M. and E. Proksch. 2006. Epidermal barrier function: role of tight junctions. pp 191-210. *In*: Elias, P.M. and K.R. Feingold [eds.]. Skin Barrier. Taylor and Francis, New York.

Brandner, J.M., S. Kief, C. Grund, M. Rendl, P. Houdek, C. Kuhn, et al. 2002. Organization and formation of the tight junction system in human epidermis and cultured keratinocytes. Eur J Cell Biol 81: 253-263.

Briot, A., C. Deraison, M. Lacroix, C. Bonnart, A. Robin, C. Besson, et al. 2009. Kallikrein 5 induces atopic dermatitis-like lesions through PAR2-mediated thymic stromal lymphopoietin expression in Netherton syndrome. J Exp Med 206: 1135-47.

Choi, E.H., M.J. Kim, S.K. Ahn, W.S. Park, E.D. Son, G.W. Nam, et al. 2002. The skin barrier state of aged hairless mice in a dry environment. Br J Dermatol 147: 244-9.

Choi, E.H., M.J. Kim, B.I. Yeh, S.K. Ahn and S.H. Lee. 2003. Iontophoresis and sonophoresis stimulate epidermal cytokine expression at energies that do not provoke a barrier abnormality: lamellar body secretion and cytokine expression are linked to altered epidermal calcium levels. J Invest Dermatol 121: 1138-44.

Choi, E.H., M.Q. Man, P. Xu, S. Xin, Z. Liu, D.A. Crumrine, et al. 2007. Stratum corneum acidification is impaired in moderately aged human and murine skin. J Invest Dermatol 127: 2847-56.

Chung, J.H., V.N. Hanft and S. Kang. 2003. Aging and photoaging. J Am Acad Dermatol 49: 690-7.

Denda, M., J. Koyama, J. Hori, I. Horii, M. Takahashi, M. Hara, et al. 1993. Age- and sex-dependent change in stratum corneum sphingolipids. Arch Dermatol Res 285: 415-7.

Denda, M., Y. Ashida, K. Inoue and N. Kumazawa. 2001. Skin surface electric potential induced by ion-flux through epidermal cell layers. Biochem Biophys Res Commun 284: 112-117.

Denda, M., A. Tomitaka, H. Akamatsu and K. Matsunaga. 2003. Altered distribution of calcium in facial epidermis of aged adults. J Invest Dermatol 121: 1557-8.

Ekanayake Mudiyanselage, S., M. Hamburger, P. Elsner and J.J. Thiele. 2003. Ultraviolet A induces generation of squalene monohydroperoxide isomers in human sebum and skin surface lipids in vitro and in vivo. J Invest Dermatol 120: 915-22.

Elias, P.M. 2007. The skin barrier as an innate immune element. Semin Immunopathol 29: 3-14.

Elias, P.M. and E.H. Choi. 2005. Interactions among stratum corneum defensive functions. Exp Dermatol 14: 719-26.

Elias, P.M. and J.S. Wakefield. 2011. From saran wrap to current understanding of the cutaneous barrier. J Skin Barrier Res 13: 31-37.

Elias, P.M., S.K. Ahn, M. Denda, B.E. Brown, D. Crumrine, L.K. Kimutai, et al. 2002. Modulations in epidermal calcium regulate the expression of differentiation-specific markers. J Invest Dermatol 119: 1128-36.

Fisher, G.J., S. Kang, J. Varani, Z. Bata-Csorgo, Y. Wan, S. Datta, et al. 2002. Mechanisms of photoaging and chronological skin aging. Arch Dermatol 138: 1462-70.

Fluhr, J.W. and P.M. Elias. 2002. Stratum corneum pH: formation and function of the "acid mantle". Exog Dermatol 1: 163-175.

Fluhr, J.W., J. Kao, M. Jain, S.K. Ahn, K.R. Feingold and P.M. Elias. 2001. Generation of free fatty acids from phospholipids regulates stratum corneum acidification and integrity. J Invest Dermatol 117: 44-51.

Fluhr, J.W., M. Mao-Qiang, B.E. Brown, P.W. Wertz, D. Crumrine, J.P. Sundberg, et al. 2003. Glycerol regulates stratum corneum hydration in sebaceous gland deficient (asebia) mice. J Invest Dermatol 120: 728-37.

Fluhr, J.W., M.J. Behne, B.E. Brown, D.G. Moskowitz, C. Selden, M. Mao-Qiang, et al. 2004. Stratum corneum acidification in neonatal skin: secretory phospholipase A2 and the sodium/hydrogen antiporter-1 acidify neonatal rat stratum corneum. J Invest Dermatol 122: 320-9.

Forslind, B., Y. Werner-Linde, M. Lindberg and J. Pallon. 1999. Elemental analysis mirrors epidermal differentiation. Acta Derm Venereol (Stockh) 79: 12-17.

Furuse, M., M. Hata, K. Furuse, Y. Yoshida, A. Haratake, Y. Sugitani, et al. 2002. Claudin-based tight junctions are crucial for the mammalian epidermal barrier: a lesson from claudin-1-deficient mice. J Cell Biol 156: 1099-1111.

Ghadially, R., B.E. Brown, S.M. Sequeira-Martin, K.R. Feingold and P.M. Elias. 1995. The aged epidermal permeability barrier. Structural, functional and lipid biochemical abnormalities in humans and a senescent murine model. J Clin Invest 95: 2281-90.

Ghadially, R., B.E. Brown, K. Hanley, J.T. Reed, K.R. Feingold and P.M. Elias. 1996. Decreased epidermal lipid synthesis accounts for altered barrier function in aged mice. J Invest Dermatol 106: 1064-9.

Gilchrest, B.A., M. Garmyn and M. Yaar. 1994. Aging and photoaging affect gene expression in cultured human keratinocytes. Arch Dermatol 130: 82-6.

Gilhar, A., E. Aizen, T. Pillar and S. Eidelman. 1992. Response of aged versus young skin to intradermal administration of interferon gamma. J Am Acad Dermatol 27: 710-6.

Hachem, J.P., M. Behne, J. Fluhr, K.R. Feingold and P.M. Elias. 2002. Increased stratum corneum pH promotes activation and release of primary cytokine from the stratum corneum attributable to activation of serine proteases. J Invest Dermatol 119: 258.

Hachem, J.P., D. Crumrine, J. Fluhr, B.E. Brown, K.R. Feingold and P.M. Elias. 2003. pH directly regulates epidermal permeability barrier homeostasis and stratum corneum integrity/cohesion. J Invest Dermatol 121: 345-53.

Hachem, J.P., M.Q. Man, D. Crumrine, Y. Uchida, B.E. Brown, V. Rogiers, et al. 2005. Sustained serine proteases activity by prolonged increase in pH leads to degradation of lipid processing enzymes and profound alterations of barrier function and stratum corneum integrity. J Invest Dermatol 125: 510-20.

Hachem, J.P., E. Houben, D. Crumrine, M.Q. Man, N. Schurer, T. Roelandt, et al. 2006. Serine protease signaling of epidermal permeability barrier homeostasis. J Invest Dermatol 126: 2074-86.

Haratake, A., Y. Uchida, K. Mimura, P.M. Elias and W.M. Holleran. 1997. Intrinsically aged epidermis displays diminished UVB-induced alterations in barrier function associated with decreased proliferation. J Invest Dermatol 108: 319-23.

Haratake, A., K. Ikenaga, N. Katoh, H. Uchiwa, S. Hirano and H. Yasuno. 2000. Topical mevalonic acid stimulates de novo cholesterol synthesis and epidermal permeability barrier homeostasis in aged mice. J Invest Dermatol 114: 247-52.

Harris, I.R., A.M. Farrell, W.M. Holleran, S. Jackson, C. Grunfeld, P.M. Elias, et al. 1998. Parallel regulation of sterol regulatory element binding protein-2 and the enzymes of cholesterol and fatty acid synthesis but not ceramide synthesis in cultured human keratinocytes and murine epidermis. J Lipid Res 39: 412-22.

Hellemans, L., H. Corstjens, A. Neven, L. Declercq and D. Maes. 2003. Antioxidant enzyme activity in human stratum corneum shows seasonal variation with an age-dependent recovery. J Invest Dermatol 120: 434-9.

Holleran, W.M., Y. Takagi and Y. Uchida. 2006. Epidermal sphingolipids: metabolism, function and roles in skin disorders. FEBS letters 580: 5456-66.

Jeanmaire, C., L. Danoux and G. Pauly. 2001. Glycation during human dermal intrinsic and actinic ageing: an in vivo and in vitro model study. Br J Dermatol 145: 10-8.

Jensen, J.M., S. Schütze, M. Förl, M. Krönke and E. Proksch. 1999. Roles for tumor necrosis factor receptor p55 and sphingomyelinase in repairing the cutaneous permeability barrier. J Clin Invest 104: 1761-70.

Jensen, J.M., M. Förl, S. Winoto-Morbach, S. Seite, M. Schunck, E. Proksch, et al. 2005. Acid and neutral sphingomyelinase, ceramide synthase and acid ceramidase activities in cutaneous aging. Exp Dermatol 14: 609-18.

Kawano, K., T. Hirashima, S. Mori, Y. Saitoh, M. Kurosumi and Natori T. 1992. Spontaneous long-term hyperglycemic rat with diabetic complications. Otsuka Long-Evans Tokushima Fatty (OLETF) strain. Diabetes 41: 1422-8.

Korting, H.C., K. Hubner, K. Greiner, G. Hamm and O. Braun-Falco. 1990. Differences in the skin surface pH and bacterial microflora due to the long-term application of synthetic detergent preparations of pH 5.5 and pH 7.0. Results of a crossover trial in healthy volunteers. Acta Derm Venereol 70: 429-31.

Kubo, A., K. Nagao, M. Yokouchi, H. Sasaki and M. Amagai. 2009. External antigen uptake by Langerhans cells with reorganization of epidermal tight junction barriers. J Exp Med 206: 2937-46.

Lee, S.H., P.M. Elias, E. Proksch, G.K. Menon, M. Mao-Quiang and K.R. Feingold. 1992. Calcium and potassium are important regulators of barrier homeostasis in murine epidermis. J Clin Invest 89: 530-8.

Lee, S.H., E.H. Choi, K.R. Feingold, S. Jiang and S.K. Ahn. 1998. Iontophoresis itself on hairless mouse skin induces the loss of the epidermal calcium gradient without skin barrier impairment. J Invest Dermatol 111: 39-43.

Levine, R.L. and E.R. Stadtman. 2001. Oxidative modification of proteins during aging. Exp Gerontol 36: 1495-502.

Liu, A.Y., D. Destoumieux, A.V. Wong, C.H. Park, E.V. Valore, L. Liu, et al. 2002. Human beta-defensin-2 production in keratinocytes is regulated by interleukin-1, bacteria and the state of differentiation. J Invest Dermatol 118: 275-81.

Lopez-Torres, M., J.J. Thiele, Y. Shindo, D. Han and L. Packer. 1998. Topical application of alpha-tocopherol modulates the antioxidant network and diminishes ultraviolet-induced oxidative damage in murine skin. Br J Dermatol 138: 207-15.

Malminen, M., V. Koivukangas, J. Peltonen, S.L. Karvonen, A. Oikarinen and S. Peltonen. 2003. Immunohistological distribution of the tight junction components ZO-1 and occludin in regenerating human epidermis. Br J Dermatol 149: 255-260.

Man, M.Q. M., K.R. Feingold, C.R. Thornfeldt and P.M. Elias. 1996. Optimization of physiological lipid mixtures for barrier repair. J Invest Dermatol 106: 1096-101.

Man, M.Q., S.J. Xin, S.P. Song, S.Y. Cho, X.J. Zhang, C.X. Tu, et al. 2009. Variation of skin surface pH, sebum content and stratum corneum hydration with age and gender in a large Chinese population. Skin Pharmacol Physiol 22: 190-9.

Mao-Qiang, M., K.R. Feingold and P.M. Elias. 1993. Exogenous lipids influence permeability barrier recovery in acetone-treated murine skin. Arch Dermatol 129: 728-738.

Mao-Qiang, M., M. Jain, K.R. Feingold and P.M. Elias. 1996. Secretory phospholipase A2 activity is required for permeability barrier homeostasis. J Invest Dermatol 106: 57-63.

Mauro, T., W.M. Holleran, S. Grayson, W.N. Gao, M.Q. Man, E. Kriehuber, et al. 1998. Barrier recovery is impeded at neutral pH, independent of ionic effects: implications for extracellular lipid processing. Arch Dermatol Res 290 (4): 215-22.

Menon, G.K., S. Grayson and P.M. Elias. 1985. Ionic calcium reservoirs in mammalian epidermis: ultrastructural localization by ion-capture cytochemistry. J Invest Dermatol 84: 508-12.

Menon, G.K., L.F. Price, B. Bommannan, P.M. Elias and K.R. Feingold. 1994. Selective obliteration of the epidermal calcium gradient leads to enhanced lamellar body secretion. J Invest Dermatol 102: 789-95.

Ohnemus, U., K. Kohrmeyer, P. Houdek, H. Rohde, E. Wladykowski, S. Vidal, et al. 2008. Regulation of epidermal tight-junctions (TJ) during infection with exfoliative toxin-negative Staphylococcus strains. J Invest Dermatol 128: 906-916.

Oliver, C.N., B.W. Ahn, E.J. Moerman, S. Goldstein and E.R. Stadtman. 1987. Age-related changes in oxidized proteins. J Biol Chem 262: 5488-91.

Oren, A., T. Ganz, L. Liu and T. Meerloo. 2003. In human epidermis, beta-defensin 2 is packaged in lamellar bodies. Exp Mol Pathol 74: 180-182.

Park, H.Y., J.H. Kim, M. Jung, C.H. Chung, R. Hasham, C.S. Park, et al. 2011. A long-standing hyperglycaemic condition impairs skin barrier by accelerating skin ageing process. Exp Dermatol 20: 969-74.

Pelle, E., N. Muizzuddin, T. Mammone, K. Marenus and D. Maes. 1999. Protection against endogenous and UVB-induced oxidative damage in stratum corneum lipids by an antioxidant-containing cosmetic formulation. Photodermatol Photoimmunol Photomed 15: 115-9.

Perez, M.I and S.R. Kohn. 1994. Cutaneous manifestations of diabetes mellitus. J Am Acad Dermatol 30: 519-31.

Reed, J.T., P.M. Elias and R. Ghadially. 1997. Integrity and permeability barrier function of photoaged human epidermis. Arch Dermatol 133: 395-6.

Rogers, J., C. Harding, A. Mayo, J. Banks and A. Rawlings. 1996. Stratum corneum lipids: the effect of ageing and the seasons. Arch Dermatol Res 288: 765-70.

Saint-Leger, D., A. Bague, E. Lefebvre, E. Cohen and M. Chivot. 1986. A possible role for squalene in the pathogenesis of acne. II. In vivo study of squalene oxides in skin surface and intra-comedonal lipids of acne patients. Br J Dermatol 114: 543-52.

Sakai, S., K. Kikuchi, J. Satoh, H. Tagami and S. Inoue. 2005. Functional properties of the stratum corneum in patients with diabetes mellitus: similarities to senile xerosis. Br J Dermatol 153: 319-23.

Sander, C.S., H. Chang, S. Salzmann, C.S. Müller, S. Ekanayake-Mudiyanselage, P. Elsner, et al. 2002. Photoaging is associated with protein oxidation in human skin in vivo. J Invest Dermatol 118: 618-25.

Sauder, D.N., U. Ponnappan and B. Cinader. 1989. Effect of age on cutaneous interleukin 1 expression. Immunol Lett 20: 111-4.

Schmuth, M., M.Q. Man, F. Weber, W. Gao, K.R. Feingold, P. Fritsch, et al. 2000. Permeability barrier disorder in Niemann-Pick disease: sphingomyelin-ceramide processing required for normal barrier homeostasis. J Invest Dermatol 115: 459-66.

Schroder, J.M and J. Harder. 2006. Antimicrobial skin peptides and proteins. Cell Mol Life Sci 63: 469-86.

Schurer, N.Y. and P.M. Elias. 1991. The biochemistry and function of stratum corneum lipids. Adv Lipid Res 24: 27-56.

Stoyanovsky, D.A., A.N. Osipov, P.J. Quinn and V.E. Kagan. 1995. Ubiquinone-dependent recycling of vitamin E radicals by superoxide. Arch Biochem Biophys 323: 343-51.

Takahashi, M. and T. Tezuka. 2004. The content of free amino acids in the stratumcorneum is increased in senile xerosis. Arch Dermatol Res. 295: 448-52.

Tezuka, T. 1983. Electron-microscopic changes in xerosis senilis epidermis. Its abnormal membrane-coating granule formation. Dermatologica 166: 57-61.

Thiele, J.J. 2001. Oxidative targets in the stratum corneum. A new basis for antioxidative strategies. Skin Pharmacol Appl Skin Physiol 14 Suppl 1: 87-91.

Thiele, J.J., M.G. Traber and L. Packer. 1998. Depletion of human stratum corneum vitamin E: an early and sensitive in vivo marker of UV induced photo-oxidation. J Invest Dermatol 110: 756-61.

Thiele, J.J., S.N. Hsieh, K. Briviba and H. Sies. 1999. Protein oxidation in human stratum corneum: susceptibility of keratins to oxidation in vitro and presence of a keratin oxidation gradient in vivo. J Invest Dermatol 113: 335-9.

Thiele, J.J., F. Dreher and I. Packer. 2000. Antioxidant defense systems in skin. pp 145-188. *In*: Elsner, P. and H. Maibach [eds.]. Drugs vs. Cosmetics: Cosmeceuticals? Marcel Dekker, New York.

Thune. P., T. Nilsen, I.K. Hanstad, T. Gustavsen and H. Lövig Dahl. 1988. The water barrier function of the skin in relation to the water content of stratum corneum, pH and skin lipids. The effect of alkaline soap and syndet on dry skin in elderly, non-atopic patients. Acta DermVenereol 68: 277-83.

Verdier-Sévrain, S. and F. Bonté. 2007. Skin hydration: a review on its molecular mechanisms. J Cosmet Dermatol 6: 75-82.

Wertz, P.W. and K.C. Madison. 1989. Downing DT. Covalently bound lipids of human stratum corneum. J Invest Dermatol 92: 109-11.

Wilhelm, K.P., A.B. Cua and H.I. Maibach. 1991. Skin aging. Effect on transepidermal water loss, stratum corneum hydration, skin surface pH and casual sebum content. Arch Dermatol 127: 1806-9.

Wood, L.C., S.M. Jackson, P.M. Elias, C. Grunfeld and K.R. Feingold. 1992. Cutaneous barrier perturbation stimulates cytokine production in the epidermis of mice. J Clin Invest 90: 482-7.

Yaar, M., M.S. Eller and B.A. Gilchrest. 2002. Fifty years of skin aging. J Investig Dermatol Symp Proc 7: 51-8.

Yamamura, T. and T. Tezuka. 1990. Change in sphingomyelinase activity in human epidermis during aging. J Dermatol Sci 1: 79-83.

Ye, J., A. Garg, C. Calhoun, K.R. Feingold, P.M. Elias and R. Ghadially. 2002. Alterations in cytokine regulation in aged epidermis: implications for permeability barrier homeostasis and inflammation. I. IL-1 gene family. Exp Dermatol 11: 209-16.

Yuki, T., A. Hachiya, A. Kusaka, P. Sriwiriyanont, M.O. Visscher and K. Morita, et al. 2011. Characterization of tight junctions and their disruption by UVB in human epidermis and cultured keratinocytes. J Invest Dermatol 131: 744-752.

Zettersten, E.M., R. Ghadially, K.R. Feingold, D. Crumrine and P.M. Elias. 1997. Optimal ratios of topical stratum corneum lipids improve barrier recovery in chronologically aged skin. J Am Acad Dermatol 37: 403-8.

Zlotogorski, A. 1987. Distribution of skin surface pH on the forehead and cheek of adults. Arch Dermatol Res 279: 398-401.

4

Skin Dryness is a Factor that Accelerates Collagen Degradation and Results in Wrinkling

Hitoshi Masaki, Ph.D.

❑ Introduction

The appearance of the skin strongly affects the impression of human individuals. In particular, the facial appearance affects our perception of age, since age is perceived by wrinkling, sagging and an uneven color of the skin. In other words, aging is characterized by wrinkles and an uneven skin color, such as in solar lentigines. That concept is supported by an epidemiological survey.

A survey of female twins of Danish and British ancestry shows that the appearance of skin wrinkles significantly correlates with their perceived ages (Gunn et al. 2009). The facts indicate that differences in perceived ages are affected by life-style and environments, because those subjects had virtually identical genetic backgrounds.

On the other hand, skin dryness is a fundamental characteristic and is generally thought to be an initiation factor of several types of skin problems. Moisture in the skin is modulated by both the functions of barrier and water holding. The barrier function of the skin is achieved with three major components, epidermal lipids (ceramides, fatty acid and cholesterol) (Schürer et al. 1991), the manner of adherence (such as tight junctions localized in the granular layer) (Yamamoto et al. 2008) and by corneocytes (the top layer of

Tokyo University of Technology, School of Bioscience and Biotechnology, Advanced Cosmetic Course, Photoaging Research Laboratory, 1404-1, Katakura-cho, Hachioji, Tokyo 192-0982, Japan.
E-mail: masaki@stf.teu.ac.jp

the skin) (Hirao et al. 2003). The water holding function of the skin is regulated by natural moisturizing factors, such as filaggrin-derived free amino acids (Rawlings and Harding 2004), lactic acid and some ions (Nakagawa et al. 2004).

A dry environment can cause skin dryness and fine wrinkles can be formed on the skin surface, which are associated with shallow furrows and disarranged patterns in the surface texture (Sato et al. 2000). The appearance of wrinkles can be easily changed by hydration or by dehydration with acetone extraction. Hydration of the skin results in a shallower wrinkle depth, whereas dehydration gives the impression of deeper wrinkles (Fig. 1). A recent study in China showed that a dry environment induces early wrinkle formation (Kim et al. 2014). Wrinkles are thought to be formed by the reduction of water in the skin without any changes in the dermal matrix structure, because they can be improved by treatment with moisturizers (Hashizume 2004). However, there is little evidence that skin dryness contributes to deep wrinkle formation in spite of the general thinking that skin dryness develops deep wrinkle formation.

Thus, we discuss in this chapter the hypothesis that skin dryness is a trigger of wrinkle formation focusing on the status of collagen.

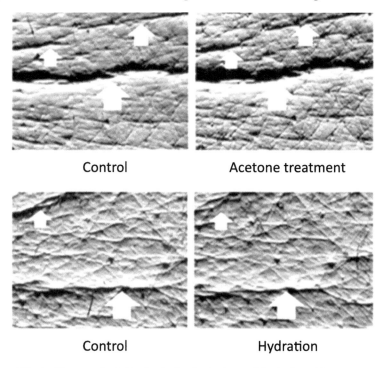

FIG. 1 *Changes of wrinkle depth after hydration or dehydration with acetone.*

❑ Hypothesis: From Skin Dryness to Wrinkles

A low humidity environment, such as in the winter season in Japan and reductions of moisture functions, including the barrier and water holding functions, lead to dry skin. In dry skin, the water distribution in the stratum corneum is altered compared with healthy skin. Especially, it is thought that the water content mostly decreases at the surface of the skin. When the uppermost layer of the stratum corneum is dehydrated by exposure to environmental dry conditions or by the reduction of moisture functions, the water needed is supplied from the deeper living cell layers of the epidermis to the stratum corneum to improve the dry state. For instance, skin exposed to a dry environment shows a reinforcement of its barrier function to improve skin dryness (Denda et al. 1998). Thus, the water flux in the skin could exert a signal that increases the secretion and/or synthesis of inflammatory cytokines from keratinocytes. Skin dryness is also caused by an excess usage of detergents such as sodium lauryl sulfate (SLS) (Okuda et al. 2002) and by the use of SLS-formulated creams (Tsang and Guy 2010).

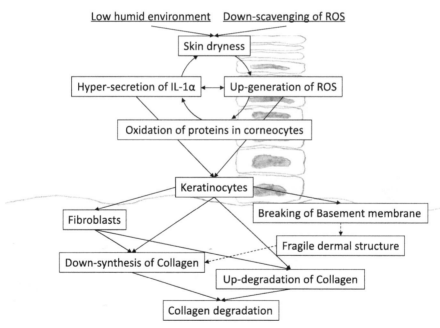

FIG. 2   *Hypothesis that skin dryness initiates collagen degradation.*

The process leading from skin dryness to wrinkle formation is hypothesized as follows (Fig. 2). Inflammatory cytokines that are hyper-secreted by signals of water flux alteration are a cause of oxidative stress. Inflammatory cytokines stimulate the production of reactive oxygen species

(ROS) in keratinocytes. ROS oxidize proteins to carbonylated proteins in keratinocytes. Carbonylated proteins appear in corneocytes during terminal differentiation. Carbonylated proteins also generate ROS following UVA irradiation (unpublished data). As a result, ROS enhances the synthesis of collagen degradation enzymes such as MMP (matrix metalloproteinase)-1 and MMP-9 and inflammatory cytokines, such as IL-1α and IL-8, in keratinocytes. Inflammatory cytokines secreted by keratinocytes can also penetrate into the dermis to affect fibroblasts and vascular endothelial cells. IL-1α also stimulates MMP-1 synthesis in keratinocytes and fibroblasts. MMP-1 produced by keratinocytes penetrates into the dermis through the basement membrane. MMP-1 from keratinocytes and fibroblasts results in the degradation of type I collagen in the papillary dermis. On the other hand, IL-8 enhances the infiltration of neutrophils into the papillary dermis. Of course, although neutrophil elastase decomposes elastin fibers, it also helps collagen degradation by MMP-1 through the digestion of decorin. MMP-9 cleaves the basement membrane structure due to its digestion of type IV collagen in that membrane, resulting in fragile scaffolds for the attachment of type VII, type I and III collagens.

In addition, carbonylated proteins in corneocytes reduce the moisture function and lead to skin dryness in an adverse loop. Repetition of that process leads to collagen degradation.

These events are triggered by alteration of the water flux in skin dryness and eventually lead to wrinkle formation. In the following sections, we introduce the precise mechanisms of collagen degradation and evidence that supports our hypothesis.

❏ Mechanisms of Collagen Degradation

ROS and IL-1α Regulate Collagen Degradation Through the Induction of MMP-1

Collagen fibers are replaced through a continual process of degradation and synthesis. The ROS-regulated collagen status with respect to the signal transductions involved is shown in Fig. 3. The pathway of collagen degradation can be summarized as follows: MMP-1 is responsible for the degradation of collagen (Pilcher et al. 1998). The pathway of MMP-1 synthesis in photoaged and in physiologically-aged skin has been well investigated. Elevations of intracellular ROS levels induce the transcription of MMP-1 (Brenneisen et al. 1997; Brenneisen et al. 1998; Zaw et al. 2006). For instance, fibroblasts isolated from donors of different ages have different levels of intracellular ROS. Fibroblasts from aged donors accumulate higher amounts of hydrogen peroxide compared with fibroblasts from young donors. This phenomenon is caused by levels of catalase enzyme that decrease with age. On the other hand, MMP-1 synthesis in aged fibroblasts is higher than in young fibroblasts (Shin et al. 2005). This negative correlation is demonstrated by the elevation of intracellular ROS levels. MMP-1 synthesis induced by ROS is elicited by an increase of activator protein-1 (AP-1), which is a heterodimer composed of c-jun and c-fos proteins and is a transcription factor that regulates MMP-1 and MMP-9 mRNA expression (Rittié and Fisher 2002). The synthesis of c-jun protein is initiated by the phosphorylation of epidermal growth factor receptor (EGF-R) (Wan et al. 2001). The phosphorylation of EGF-R is caused without ligand binding and is regulated by protein tyrosine phosphatase (PTP) (Bae et al. 1997). Excess ROS generated by UV irradiation or by physiological aging inactivates PTP by oxidation of an SH group in the active site. The inactivation of PTP continuously maintains the phosphorylation of EGF-R and results in the activation of c-jun N-terminal kinase (JNK), which is a member of the Mitogen-activated Protein Kinase (MAPK) family. The activation of JNK increases levels of c-jun protein in cells. On the other hand, c-fos protein is synthesized by activation of extracellular signal-regulated kinase (ERK1/2) due to signaling of NF-κB-IL-1-IL6 (Hwang et al. 2011; Wang and Bi 2006). ROS induces the translocation of NF-κB into the nucleus and up-regulates IL-1α mRNA expression. IL-1α activates ERK1/2 through IL-6 expression. As a result, AP-1 synthesis finally increases. AP-1 up-regulates the transcription of MMP-1 mRNA by binding to the AP-1 response element after translocation into the nucleus (Kida et al. 2005). This scheme suggests that ROS and IL-1α accelerate collagen decomposition through the induction of MMP-1.

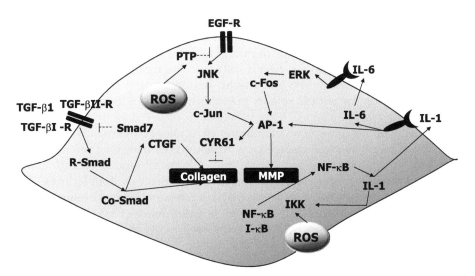

FIG. 3 *Pathway of ROS-induced collagen degradation.*

ROS and IL-1α Regulates Collagen Synthesis Through CCN1/CYR61 and CCN2/CTGF

As candidates that maintain collagen homeostasis, CYR61 and CTGF are proposed. Cysteine-rich protein-61 (CYR61) is a feedback protein of collagen synthesis and is also known as CCN1 (Brigstock 2003). By contrast, connective tissue growth factor (CTGF) accelerates collagen synthesis through the induction by TGF-β and is also known as CCN2. Both proteins are members of the CCN family of matricellular proteins. Over-expression of CCN1/CYR61 significantly inhibits the production of collagen type I at both the mRNA and protein levels (Borkham-Kamphorst et al. 2014). AP-1 also acts as a transcription factor for CCN1/CYR61 (Quan et al. 2010). IL-1α may induce the synthesis of CCN1/CYR61 through increases of AP-1. As described in the previous section, ROS and IL-1α increase AP-1 synthesis through the activation of two MAPKs, JNK and ERK1/2. On the other hand, the up-regulation of CCN2/CTGF caused by TGF-β is abolished by IL-1α (Nowinski et al. 2010). These facts suggest that ROS and IL-1α reduce the potential for collagen synthesis leading to an imbalance between CCN1/CYR61 and CCN2/CTGF (Fig. 2).

MMP-9 Disrupts the Basement Membrane Structure Through Digestion of Type IV Collagen

The basement membrane, which is composed of type IV collagen and laminin 5 (laminin-332), is located at the border between the epidermis and the dermis (Martin et al. 1983). Keratinocytes adhere to the basement membrane through integrin molecules and type VII collagen attaches to the basement membrane like a strap from the dermis side. Type I and type III collagens are held through the straps of type VII collagen. The tightly cohesive structure of the basement membrane leads to an understanding that the basement membrane plays a critical role in maintaining the epidermal and dermal structure.

Damage of the basement membrane in photoaged skin has also been identified using electron microscopy. Although the basement membrane in healthy skin is observed as a single line, that membrane in chronic UVB-exposed skin is fragmented and is sometimes seen as double lines. The alteration of the basement membrane by UVB irradiation can be suppressed by the application of CGS27023A, which is an inhibitor of MMP (Inomata et al. 2003). In that situation, MMP-9 is expressed in the epidermis intensively. On the other hand, mast cells and macrophages are frequently observed in photoaged skin. Matriptase originates from mast cells and activates MMP-9 via the processing of proMMP-9 (Iddamalgoda et al. 2008). These results indicate that damage of the basement membrane is caused by MMP-9.

Considering these facts, MMP-9 is a key enzyme in the degradation of the basement membrane and results in the fragile dermal structure and decreased cohesion of the epidermal-dermal junction.

IL-8 Accelerates the Fragility of the Dermal Structure by Recruiting Neutrophils

IL-8 is a chemokine which has the potential to recruit neutrophils (Smith et al. 1991). Neutrophils produce serine-type elastase and are highly observed in the infiltrations in the papillary region of photoaged skin (Yano et al. 2005). Healthy skin has fine elastin fibers, called oxytalan fibers, in the papillary region, however, photoaged and physiologically-aged skin completely lose their oxytalan fibers. The loss of oxytalan fibers is due to the contribution of elastases from fibroblasts, macrophages and neutrophils. Among elastases, a recent study proposed that neutrophil elastase is involved in the fragmentation of collagen fibers (Li et al. 2013). Although collagen fibers are not substrates for neutrophil elastase, the involvement of that elastase on collagen degradation has been demonstrated as follows: Decorin is a proteoglycan composed with of a core protein and a glycosaminoglycan. Decorin is bound to the surface of collagen fibers at sites susceptible to the protease activity of MMP-1 (Fig. 3). Since MMP-1 is not able to decompose decorin, decorin consequently interferes with collagen degradation by MMP-1. Neutrophil elastase helps collagen degradation by MMP-1 due to its degradation of decorin. The sum of these facts suggests that IL-8 initiates the degradation not only of elastin but also of collagen.

❑ Knowledge Supporting each Stage of the Hypothesis

Hyper-secretion of Inflammatory Cytokines under Dry Conditions

Advanced methodologies of non-invasive skin measurements have made it easy to evaluate skin conditions using biological parameters. Useful information on skin conditions can be determined by analyzing corneocytes collected by the tape-stripping method. Corneocytes from skin exposed to solar light show a higher ratio of IL-1 receptor antagonist (IL-1RA) and interleukin-1α (IL-1α) (IL-1RA/IL-1α), which is an inflammatory cytokine. That change is understood to result from inflammation in the epidermis involving IL-1α. IL-1α hyper-secreted following stimulation by solar light causes faint inflammation and IL-RA is produced to prevent the excess actions of IL-1α. In dry skin, the analysis of corneocytes gives similar results i.e. a higher ratio of IL-1RA/IL-1α, even in the absence of solar light exposure (Kikuchi et al. 2003). That result shows that the faint inflammation initiated by IL-1α occurs in the epidermis of dry skin. To identify experimentally the relationship between the hyper-secretion of IL-1α and skin dryness, sodium lauryl sulfate (SLS)< which is a typical anionic surfactant, is generally used to produce the roughened skin associated with skin dryness. SLS extracts intercellular lipids and natural moisturizing factors and thus reduces the moisture functions of the skin. A single application of 0.5% SLS or repeated applications of 0.1% SLS for 6 hours once a day for 4 days induced skin dryness and exhibited a lower skin water content and a higher level of trans-epidermal water loss (TEWL). In that condition, the stratum corneum showed a higher ratio of IL-1RA/IL-1α and the hyper-secretion of IL-8 and TNF-α (De Jongh et al. 2006). Those results indicate that skin dryness induces the hyper-secretion of inflammatory cytokines.

Evidence of ROS Generation in Dry Skin

It is well known that TNF-α stimulates ROS generation in cells and increases intracellular ROS levels. In addition, studies have shown that IL-1α also induces ROS generation in cells. Fibroblasts preloaded with 2′, 7′-dichlorodihydrofluorescein diacetate (DCFH-DA), which is a ROS-reactive fluorescent probe, showed intensive fluorescence following treatment with TNF-α orIL-1α (Fig. 4). On the other hand, corneocytes of dry skin have high levels of carbonylated proteins (Kobayashi et al. 2008) (Fig. 4). Those findings suggest that dry conditions increase oxidative stress in keratinocytes through the secretion of TNF-α and IL-1α and result in the oxidation of proteins in keratinocytes and corneocytes. Then, how docarbonylated proteins in the stratum corneum influence the skin homeostasis on moisture functions? An epidemiological assessment has reported that the level of carbonylated proteins in the stratum corneum show a negative correlation with skin surface water content and a positive correlation with TEWL (Fujita et al. 2007). Those facts suggest that protein oxidation in corneocytes affects the moisturization of the skin, which have been demonstrated by *ex vivo* and *in vitro* examinations. The skin surface water content of excised human skin treated with acrolein at various concentrations decreased in a dose-dependent manner of acrolein. Acrolein is a β-unsaturated small molecule that has an aldehyde group and is generated by lipid oxidation (Stevens and Maier 2008) (Fig. 5). In corneocytes, the existence of acrolein-derived carbonylated proteins is detected by immunostaining with an anti-acrolein antibody. Further, the water holding capacity of a gel prepared with keratin protein extracted from human hair decreased with acrolein treatment (Iwai and Hirao 2008). Furthermore, our preliminary examination also showed that carbonylated proteins in acrolein-treated porcine skin have an elevated TEWL (unpublished data).

The sum of these results supports the concept that once the skin develops dry conditions, it could be very hard to escape the adverse loop, since proteins in keratinocytes continue to be exposed to ROS and carbonylated proteins will continue to increase in the stratum corneum.

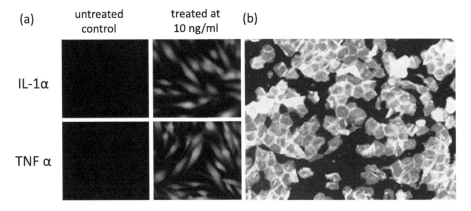

FIG. 4   Intracellular ROS and carbonylated proteins in corneocytes. *(a) Normal human dermal fibroblasts were treated with L-1α (10 ng/mL) or TNFα (10 ng/mL). (b) Intracellular ROS levels were visualized with 2', 7'-dichlorodihydrofluorescein diacetate. Carbonylated proteins were fluorescence-labeled with fluorescein-5-thiosemicarbazide.*

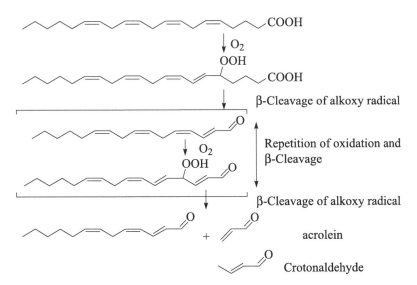

FIG. 5   *β–unsaturated aldehyde compounds by lipid peroxidation chain reaction.*

Verification of the Hypothesis Using a Dry Skin Model of a Reconstructed Epidermis

In order to verify the hypothesis that skin dryness is an initiator of wrinkling, a dry skin model was developed using a reconstructed epidermal model

(REM) (Yokota et al. 2014). To generate dry conditions on the surface of REMs, an ampoule tube filled with calcium chloride was attached to each REM and was cultured for 7 days (Fig. 6). To identify secreted substances, the conditioned medium was then analyzed using a protein array system. As a result, the hyper-secretion of IL-1α, IL-1ra, IL-8 and MMP-9 was detected in the conditioned medium of REMs cultured in dry conditions (Fig. 7). In a histological study, the existence of carbonylated proteins in the stratum corneum of REMs cultured in dry conditions was observed (Fig. 8).

(a)   **(b)**

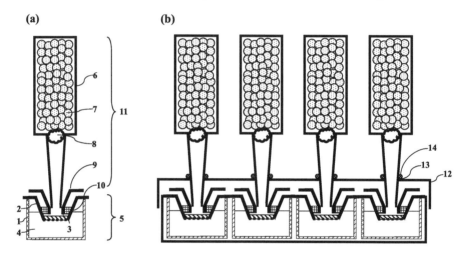

FIG. 6   CaCl₂-filled ampoules to generate dry conditions at the surface of REMs. *These images show the CaCl₂-filled ampoule used in the study. (a) Details about each part of the CaCl₂-filled ampoule loaded on a REM. (b) REMs with the CaCl₂-filled ampoule cultivated in 12 well plates. The name of each part is as follows, 1: culture well, 2: culture insert, 3: REM, 4: medium, 5: REM culture kit (1-4), 6: ampoule, 7: CaCl₂ (desiccant), 8: cotton plug, 9: small culture insert, 10: silicon tube, 11: CaCl₂-filled ampoule (6-10), 12: culture plate cover, 13: through-hole, 14: vaseline.*

As described in the previous section, IL-1RA/IL-1α in the stratum corneum of dry skin shows a higher ratio than that from healthy skin. The elevation of that ratio has been explained by the fact that IL-1RA is induced due to the hyper-secretion of IL-1α. The dry skin model also secreted high levels of IL-1α and IL-1RA. Thus, the *in vitro* results are consistent with the *in vivo* results, which supports the validity of the dry skin model to characterize phenomena causing dry skin *in vivo*. Furthermore, the conditioned medium of the dry skin model increases the production of MMP-1 by human dermal fibroblasts.

The results of this *in vitro* study support the hypothesis that skin dryness initiates wrinkling due to the hyper-secretion of IL-1α, IL-8 and MMP-9.

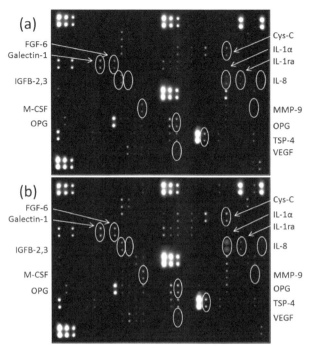

FIG. 7   **Secretion profiles of cytokines and proteins.** *REMs were cultured under the following conditions; (a) REM without a CaCl$_2$-filled ampoule and (b) REM with a CaCl$_2$-filled ampoule. After 24 h, culture media were examined using a Biotin Label-based Human Obesity Antibody Array 1 kit.*

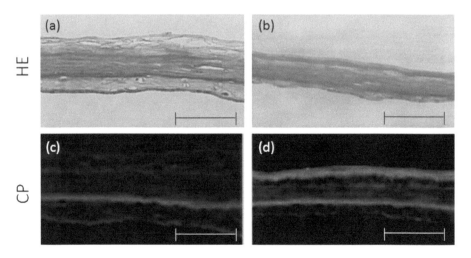

FIG. 8   **Histology of REMs after cultivation under dry conditions.** *Representative histologies of REMs without (a, c) or with (b, d) a CaCl$_2$-filled ampoule. A representative image of each condition is shown (a,b: HE, c, d: carbonylated protein). Scale bar: 50 µm.*

❏ Conclusion

In general, reduction of the skin surface water content causes fine wrinkling, known as epidermal wrinkling. Since the fine wrinkling can be restored by treatment with a moisturizer, the cause of wrinkles is understood to result from alterations of the epidermis, especially the stratum corneum, due to reductions of its water holding capacity. However, deep wrinkles are caused by dermal structural alterations in the papillary region induced by collagen degradation. This chapter developed the hypothesis that skin dryness accelerates wrinkling by enhancing collagen degradation. To obtain data to support that hypothesis, we developed an *in vitro* dry skin model and clarified parameters caused by dry conditions. Parameters detected from the *in vitro* dry skin model were consistent with results obtained from the stratum corneum of dry skin *in vivo*. IL-1α, IL-8 and MMP-9 secreted from keratinocytes in the *in vitro* dry skin model play critical roles in collagen degradation and wrinkling. The cascade of events of our hypothesis is summarized in Fig. 9 and available experimental evidence supports that mechanism. We expect that this new concept will provide important clues to develop new formulations to prevent skin wrinkling.

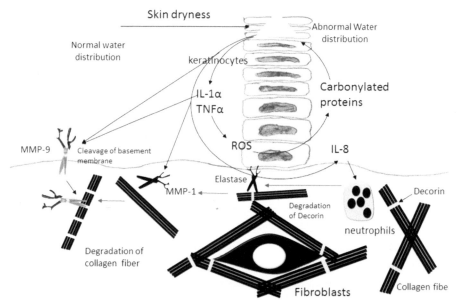

FIG. 9 *Scheme summarizing the hypothesis of skin dryness initiating collagen degradation resulting in wrinkles.*

❏ References

Bae, Y.S., S.W. Kang, M.S. Seo, I.C. Baines, E. Tekle, P.B. Chock, et al. 1997. Epidermal growth factor (EGF)-induced generation of hydrogen peroxide. Role in EGF receptor-mediated tyrosine phosphorylation. J Biol Chem 272: 217-221.

Borkham-Kamphorst, E., C. Schaffrath, E. Van de Leur, U. Haas, L. Tihaa, S.K. Meurer, et al. 2014. The anti-fibrotic effects of CCN1/CYR61 in primary portal myofibroblasts are mediated through induction of reactive oxygen species resulting in cellular senescence, apoptosis and attenuated TGF-β signaling. Biochim Biophys Acta 1843: 902-914.

Brenneisen, P., K. Briviba, M. Wlaschek, J. Wenk and K. Scharffetter-Kochanek. 1997. Hydrogen peroxide (H_2O_2) increases the steady-state mRNA levels of collagenase/MMP-1 in human dermal fibroblasts. Free Radic Biol Med 22: 515-524.

Brenneisen, P., J. Wenk, L.O. Klotz, M. Wlaschek, K. Briviba, T. Krieg, et al. 1998. Central role of ferrous/ferric iron in the ultraviolet B irradiation-mediated signaling pathway leading to increased interstitial collagenase (matrix-degrading metalloprotease (MMP-1) and stromelysin-1 (MMP-3) mRNA levels in cultured human dermal fibroblasts. J Biol Chem 273: 5279-5287.

Brigstock, D.R. 2003. The CCN family: a new stimulus package. J Endocrinol 178: 169-175.

De Jongh, C.M., M.M. Verberk, C.E. Withagen, J.J. Jacobs, T. Rustemeyer and S. Kezic. 2006. Stratum corneum cytokines and skin irritation response to sodium lauryl sulfate. Contact Dermatitis 54: 325-333.

Denda, M., J. Sato, Y. Masuda, T. Tsuchiya, J. Koyama, M. Kuramoto, et al. 1998. Exposure to a dry environment enhances epidermal permeability barrier function. J Invest Dermatol 111: 858-863.

Fujita, H., T. Hirao and M. Takahashi. 2007. A simple and non-invasive visualization for assessment of carbonylated protein in the stratum corneum. Skin Res Technol 13: 84-90.

Gunn, D.A., H. Rexbye, C.E. Griffiths, P.G. Murray, A. Fereday, S.D. Catt, et al. 2009. Why some women look young for their age. PLoS One 1; 4 (12): e8021.

Hashizume, H. 2004. Skin aging and dry skin. J Dermatol 31: 603-609.

Hirao, T., T. Terui, I. Takeuchi I, H. Kobayashi, M. Okada, M. Takahashi, et al. 2003. Ratio of immature cornified envelopes does not correlate with parakeratosis in inflammatory skin disorders. Exp Dermatol 12: 591-601.

Hwang, Y.P., H.G. Kim, J.H. Choi, E.H. Han, K.I. Kwon, Y.C. Lee, et al. 2011. Saponins from the roots of Platycodon grandiflorum suppress ultraviolet A-induced matrix metalloproteinase-1 expression via MAPKs and NF-κB/AP-1-dependent signaling in HaCaT cells. Food Chem Toxicol 49: 3374-3382.

Iddamalgoda, A., Q.T. Le, K. Ito, K. Tanaka, H. Kojima and H. Kido. 2008. Mast cell tryptase and photoaging: possible involvement in the degradation of extracellular matrix and basement membrane proteins. Arch Dermatol Res 300 Suppl 1: S69-S76.

Inomata, S., Y. Matsunaga, S. Amano, K. Takada, K. Kobayashi, M. Tsunenaga, et al. 2003. Possible involvement of gelatinases in basement membrane damage and wrinkle formation in chronically ultraviolet B-exposed hairless mouse. J Invest Dermatol 120: 128-134.

Iwai, I. and T. Hirao. 2008. Protein carbonyls damage the water-holding capacity of the stratum corneum. Skin Pharmacol Physiol 21: 269-273.

Kida, Y., M. Kobayashi, T. Suzuki, A. Takeshita, Y. Okamatsu, S. Hanazawa, et al. 2005. Interleukin-1 stimulates cytokines, prostaglandin E2 and matrix metalloproteinase-1 production via activation of MAPK/AP-1 and NF-kappaB in human gingival fibroblasts. Cytokine 29: 159-168.

Kikuchi, K., H. Kobayashi, T. Hirao, A. Ito, H. Takahashi and H. Tagami. 2003. Improvement of mild inflammatory changes of the facial skin induced by winter environment with daily applications of a moisturizing cream. A half-side test of biophysical skin parameters, cytokine expression pattern and the formation of cornified envelope. Dermatology 207: 269-275.

Kim, E.J., J.Y. Han, H.K. Lee, Q.Q. He, J.C. Cho, L. Wei, et al. 2014. Effect of the regional environment on the skin properties and the early wrinkles in young Chinese women. Skin Res Technol 20: 498-502.

Kobayashi, Y., I. Iwai, N. Akutsu and T. Hirao. 2008. Increased carbonyl protein levels in the stratum corneum of the face during winter. Int J Cosmet Sci 30: 35-40.

Li, Y., W. Xia, Y. Liu, H.A. Remmer, J. Voorhees and G.J. Fisher. 2013. Solar ultraviolet irradiation induces decorin degradation in human skin likely via neutrophil elastase. PLoS One 30; 8(8): e72563.

Martin, G.R., D.H. Rohrbach, V.P. Terranova and L.A. Liotta. 1983. Structure, function and pathology of basement membranes. Monogr Pathol 24: 16-30.

Nakagawa, N., S. Sakai, M. Matsumoto, K. Yamada, M. Nagano, T. Yuki, et al. 2004. Relationship between NMF (lactate and potassium) content and the physical properties of the stratum corneum in healthy subjects. J Invest Dermatol 122: 755-763.

Nowinski, D., A. Koskela, E. Kiwanuka, M. Boström, B. Gerdin and M. Ivarsson. 2010. Inhibition of connective tissue growth factor/CCN2 expression in human dermal fibroblasts by interleukin-1alpha and beta. J Cell Biochem 110: 1226-1233.

Okuda, M., T. Yoshiike and H. Ogawa. 2002. Detergent-induced epidermal barrier dysfunction and its prevention. J Dermatol Sci 30: 173-179.

Pilcher, B.K., B.D. Sudbeck, J.A. Dumin, H.G. Welgus and W.C. Parks. 1998. Collagenase-1 and collagen in epidermal repair. Arch Dermatol Res 290 Suppl: S37-S46.

Quan, T., Z. Qin, Y. Xu, T. He, S. Kang, J.J. Voorhees, et al. 2010. Ultraviolet irradiation induces CYR61/CCN1, a mediator of collagen homeostasis, through activation of transcription factor AP-1 in human skin fibroblasts. J Invest Dermatol 130: 1697-1706.

Rawlings, A.V. and C.R. Harding. 2004. Moisturization and skin barrier function. Dermatol Ther 17 Suppl 1: 43-48.

Rittié, L. and G.J. Fisher. 2002. UV-light-induced signal cascades and skin aging. Ageing Res Rev 1: 705-720.

Sato, J., M. Yanai M, T. Hirao and M. Denda. 2000. Water content and thickness of the stratum corneum contribute to skin surface morphology. Arch Dermatol Res 292: 412-417.

Schürer, N.Y., G. Plewig and P.M. Elias. 1991. Stratum corneum lipid function. Dermatologica 183: 77-94.

Shin, M.H., G.E. Rhie, Y.K. Kim, C.H. Park, K.H. Cho, K.H. Kim, et al. 2005. H_2O_2 accumulation by catalase reduction changes MAP kinase signaling in aged human skin in vivo. J Invest Dermatol 125: 221-229.

Smith, W.B., J.R. Gamble, I. Clark-Lewis and M.A. Vadas. 1991. Interleukin-8 induces neutrophil transendothelial migration. Immunology 72: 65-72.

Stevens, J.F. and C.S. Maier. 2008. Acrolein: sources, metabolism and biomolecular interactions relevant to human health and disease. Mol Nutr Food Res 52: 7-25.

Tsang, M. and R.H. Guy. 2010. Effect of Aqueous Cream BP on human stratum corneum in vivo. Br. J Dermatol 163: 954-958.

Wan, Y., A. Belt, Z. Wang, J. Voorhees and G. Fisher. 2001. Transmodulation of epidermal growth factor receptor mediates IL-1 beta-induced MMP-1 expression in cultured human keratinocytes. Int J Mol Med 7: 329-334.

Wang, X.Y. and Z.G. Bi. 2006. UVB-irradiated human keratinocytes and interleukin-1alpha indirectly increase MAP kinase/AP-1 activation and MMP-1 production in UVA-irradiated dermal fibroblasts. Chin Med J (Engl) 119: 827-831.

Yamamoto, T., M. Kurasawa, T. Hattori, T. Maeda, H. Nakano and H. Sasaki. 2008. Relationship between expression of tight junction-related molecules and perturbed epidermal barrier function in UVB-irradiated hairless mice. Arch Dermatol Res 300: 61-68.

Yano, K., K. Kadoya, K. Kajiya, Y.K. Hong and M. Detmar. 2005. Ultraviolet B irradiation of human skin induces an angiogenic switch that is mediated by upregulation of vascular endothelial growth factor and by downregulation of thrombospondin-1. Br J Dermatol 152: 115-121.

Yokota, M., K. Shimizu, D. Kyotani, S. Yahagi, S. Hashimoto and H. Masaki. 2014. The possible involvement of skin dryness on alterations of the dermal matrix. Exp Dermatol 23 Suppl 1: 27-31.

Zaw, K.K., Y. Yokoyama, M. Abe and O. Ishikawa. 2006. Catalase restores the altered mRNA expression of collagen and matrix metalloproteinases by dermal fibroblasts exposed to reactive oxygen species. Eur J Dermatol 16: 375-379.

5

CHAPTER

CCN Family Proteins in Skin Connective Tissue Aging

Taihao Quan

❑ Introduction

Emerging evidence indicates that members of the CCN (CYR61/CTGF/NOV) family proteins mediate aberrant collagen homeostasis in dermal fibroblasts and contributes to human skin connective tissue aging (Quan et al. 2002; Quan et al. 2006; Quan et al. 2011a; Quan et al. 2012b; Quan et al. 2010c). The CCN family comprises six distinct members: cysteine-rich protein 61 (CCN1), connective tissue growth factor (CCN2), nephroblastoma overexpressed (CCN3), Wnt-inducted secreted protein-1 (CCN4), Wnt-inducted secreted protein-2 (CCN5) and Wnt-inducted secreted protein-3 (CCN6) (Leask and Abraham 2006; Perbal 2004; Perbal et al. 2003). The CCN acronym is taken from the names of the first three members of the family to be discovered: Cyr61/CCN1, CTGF/CCN2 and NOV/CCN3. CCN proteins are secreted, ECM-associated matricellular proteins and are involved in a variety of cellular functions such as regulation of cell adhesion, proliferation, migration, chemotaxis, apoptosis, motility and ECM remodeling in wound healing (Chen and Lau 2009; Lau and Lam 1999; Perumal et al. 2008). Like other matricellular proteins such as thrombospondins, APARC, steopontin and tenascinC/X, the members of CCN family are nonstructural matricellular proteins and serve as signaling modulators. CCN proteins interact with various types of ECM proteins, growth factors, cytokines and cell surface proteins, typically integrins. Altered expression of CCN family members is associated with several pathological states, including tissue

Department of Dermatology, University of Michigan Medical School, Ann Arbor, Michigan, USA.
E-mail: thquan@umich.edu

fibrosis, inflammation and cancer. Although the first CCN family member was discovered over two decades ago, expression and potential functions of these proteins in normal human skin *in vivo* has received little attention. This chapter describes the role of CCN proteins in skin connective tissue aging and in age-related skin diseases.

❏ Expression of CCN Family Members in Young and Aged Human Skin *In vivo*

The localization and expression of the six CCN family proteins in human skin *in vivo* has been investigated (Quan 2013; Quan et al. 2009; Quan et al. 2010d; Rittie et al. 2011). The transcripts of all six CCN genes are expressed in human skin *in vivo* (Quan et al. 2010d). Of all six CCN genes, CCN5 was most highly expressed followed by CCN2>CCN3>CCN1>CCN4>CCN6 in human skin *in vivo*. The localization of CCN family proteins in human skin demonstrates that CCN3 and CCN5 proteins are prominently expressed in epidermal keratinocytes, while CCN2 is primarily expressed in epidermal melanocytes (Rittie et al. 2011). Among all CCN family members, transcriptions of CCN2, CCN3 and CCN5 are most highly expressed in the dermis. Although the expression of CCN1 is relatively low in full-thickness human skin, CCN1 is predominantly expressed in dermal fibroblasts (Quan et al. 2006). Interestingly, mRNA levels of all four of these growth arrest-associated CCN members, CCN3, CCN3, CCN5 and CCN6, are significantly elevated in aged, compared to young human skin *in vivo* (Quan et al. 2010d). Additionally, CCN1, the predominant CCN in dermal fibroblasts, is also elevated in aged human skin (Quan et al. 2006).

CCN family members are also temporally and specifically regulated during different phases (inflammation, proliferation and remodeling) of the wound healing (Rittie et al. 2011) and UV irradiation in human skin *in vivo* (Quan et al. 2010a; Quan et al. 2009). Solar-simulated UV irradiation time dependently increases mRNA expression of growth stimulation-associated CCN genes, CCN1 and CCN2, in human skin *in vivo*. In contrast, mRNA levels of growth arrest-associated CCN genes, CCN3, CCN4, CCN5 and CCN6, are reduced by solar-simulated UV irradiation in human skin *in vivo*. The knowledge gained from these studies provides a foundation for investigating the functional roles of CCN proteins in cutaneous biology and human skin aging.

❏ CCN1 and Skin Connective Tissue Aging

CCN1 is originally identified as a growth factor and serum-inducible immediate early gene in mouse 3T3 fibroblasts (Brunner et al. 1991; O'Brien et al. 1990). Human CCN1 is identified from a human embryo library (Jay et al., 1997) and found to be highly conserved to the mouse homologue. CCN1 has been reported to regulate cell adhesion and migration, chemotaxis, inflammation, cell-matrix interactions, synthesis of ECM proteins and wound healing, in a variety of cells in culture (Chen et al. 2001b; Kireeva et al. 1997; Kular et al. 2011). CNN1 exhibits a distinct expression profile during embryonic development with highest expression in the developing circulatory and skeletal systems. Disruption of CNN1 is embryonic lethal primarily due to failure of placenta vascular development (Mo et al. 2002).

In human skin *in vivo*, CCN1 is predominantly expressed in dermal fibroblasts (Qin et al. 2013; Quan et al. 2006), the primary cells responsible for ECM homeostasis. Interestingly, CCN1 is substantially elevated in dermal fibroblasts in naturally-aged and photoaged human skin *in vivo* (Quan et al. 2006; Quan et al. 2010a; Quan et al. 2009). In cultured human skin dermal fibroblasts, elevated expression of CCN1 markedly reduces type I procollagen and concurrently increases MMP-1 (Qin et al. 2013; Quan et al. 2006; Quan et al. 2013). Elevated CCN1 in human dermal fibroblasts alters expression of numerous secreted proteins and that the pattern of CCN-induced alterations closely resemble those observed in aged dermis (Quan et al. 2006; Quan et al. 2013; Quan et al. 2011a; Quan et al. 2010a). CCN1-induced secreted proteins are referred to as "Age-Associated Dermal Microenvironment (AADM)" (Quan and Fisher 2015; Quan et al. 2011a). CCN1-induced AADM promotes skin connective tissue aging through following major mechanisms: 1) reduced production of dermal ECM components, such as type I and type III collagens, which contributes to dermal thinning; 2) induction of multiple MMPs (MMP-1, MMP-3, MMP-9, MMP-10 and MMP-23), which promote fragmentation of ECM proteins; and 3) increased expression of pro-inflammatory cytokines (IL-1β, IL-6 and IL-8), which promotes inflammatory microenvironment (inflammaging). CCN1-induced AADM accounts for many of the characteristic features of aged human skin dermis, including alterations of collagen homeostasis and aberrant skin functions.

❑ CCN1 Inhibits Collagen Production Through Impairment of TGF-β Signaling

Since TGF-β pathway functions as a major regulator of collagen production and CCN1 inhibits collagen expression, the effect of elevated CCN1 on collagen has been investigated (Quan et al. 2006). Elevated CCN1 has no effect on the expression levels of TGF-β type I receptor, TGF-β1, β2, β3 or TGF-β signal transducers, Smad2, Smad3 and Smad4. However, elevated CCN1 specifically down-regulates the expression of TGF-β type II receptor (TβRII), which is also reduced in aged human skin (Quan et al. 2006). Elevated CCN1 reduces TβRII mRNA and protein levels by 51% and 59%, respectively. Furthermore, elevated CCN1 inhibits basal and TGF-β1-induced TGF-β reporter (p3TP-Luc) activity, indicating elevated CCN1 impairs the expression of TGF-β target genes. The reduction of TβRII in aged human skin *in vivo* is consistent with the observed down regulation of TβRII in response to CCN1 overexpression in cultured human skin fibroblasts (Quan et al. 2006). These data demonstrate that elevated CCN1 inhibits collagen production by impairment of TGF-β signaling. These results also partially explain underlying mechanism of reduced TβRII in aged and photoaged human skin by providing the evidence that CCN1-mediated inhibition of TβRII in human dermal fibroblasts.

❏ CCN1 Upregulates MMPs Through Functional Interaction with αVβ3 Integrin and Up-regulation of AP-1

CCN1 and other CCN family proteins are composed of an N-terminal signal peptide followed by four conserved structural/functional domains (Lau and Lam 1999; Perbal 2004). These domains share a high degree of sequence homology with 1) insulin-like growth factor binding proteins (IGFBP), 2) Von Willebrand factor type C repeat (VWC), 3) thrombospondin type I repeat (TSP1) and 4) C-terminal cysteine knots (CT). Interestingly, these four distinct structural domains are separated by proteases-sensitive residues and each of these domains is encoded by a separate exon. The multi-modular structural organization of CCN1 protein suggests that its diverse biological functions are programmed by the combinatorial actions of individual domains, either acting independently or interdependently (Chen and Lau 2009; Grzeszkiewicz et al. 2001; Kireeva et al. 1998).

CCN1 exerts a range of diverse functions by interacting with numerous integrins, in a cell type and function-specific manner (Chen and Lau 2009; Leu et al. 2002). As CCN1 can stimulate MMP-1 in human dermal fibroblasts, an important question is the identity of a cell surface CCN1-binding integrin that mediates CCN1 stimulation of MMP-1. Screening of integrins by antibody neutralization reveals that integrin αVβ3 acts as a cell surface receptor for CCN1; CCN1 physically interacts with integrin αVβ3 to mediate MMP-1 induction (Qin et al. 2013). Integrin αVβ3 is implicated in the pathophysiological of wound healing, angiogenesis and tumor metastasis (Jin and Varner 2004; Menendez et al. 2003). These data provide evidence that integrin aVβ3 contributes to human skin connective tissue aging by stimulating MMP-1 expression through functional interaction with CCN1. It has been reported that CCN1 interacts with integrin αVβ3 through VWC domain (Chen and Lau 2009; Grzeszkiewicz et al. 2001). As VWC domain is able to interact with integrin αVβ3, however, the VWC domain alone is unable to stimulate MMP-1 expression. Interestingly, combined expression of VWC domain with domains adjacent to VWC can stimulate MMP-1 expression. These data indicate that the interaction of VWC domain with integrin αVβ3 requires, functional cooperation with adjacent IGFBP and TSP1 domains. It appears that while the interaction of VWC domain with integrin αVβ3 is necessary, this interaction alone is not sufficient to stimulate MMP-1 expression. The complex interaction between CCN1 domains and integrins, including the possibility that the adjacent IGFBP and TSP1 domains may interact with other integrins, which may be together with integrin αVβ3 to mediate CCN1 stimulation of MMP-1. The nature of this co-operative regulation of these CCN1 domains is unknown.

Overexpression of CCN1 in human skin fibroblasts reveals that CCN1 is not detected as a soluble protein in conditioned culture medium, suggesting that CCN1 preferentially associates with extracellular matrix following secretion. CCN1-binding to the ECM may alter fibroblasts interactions with the ECM and with associated integrins. ECM-bound CCN1 may function as a "docking" protein that coordinates interactions between ECM proteins and cell surface integrins, ultimately orchestrating the cell response to the ECM microenvironment. Consistent with this notion, CCN1 activates integrin outside-in signaling resulting in activation of focal adhesion kinase (FAK), a key effector of the integrin signaling pathway and its downstream target paxillin, in human dermal fibroblasts (Qin et al. 2013). This finding suggests that signaling downstream of CCN1/integrin αVβ3 may drive MMP-1 expression through FAK-dependent pathway. In addition, CCN1 also activates Erk1/Erk2 and AP-1 transcription factor, the major regulators of MMP-1 expression (Quan et al. 2006). It is well-documented that integrin signaling activates the MAPK/Erk/AP-1 pathway (Cabodi et al. 2010; Giancotti and Ruoslahti 1999). These data suggest that CCN1/integrin αVβ3 signaling may stimulate MMP-1 through FAK and MAPK pathways.

Dermal fibroblasts reside in collagen-rich ECM microenvironment in human skin. CCN1 structural domains (IGFBP, VWC and TSP1) can alter collagen ECM environment. CCN1 functional domains can degrade type I collagen, the major structural protein in skin dermis and cause disorganized collagen fibrils in three-dimensional collagen lattices. Furthermore, CCN1 domains can alter collagen gel contraction which is a visible readout of changes in ECM integrity and cell-matrix interactions. These data further suggest that elevated CCN1 in aged dermal fibroblasts causes type I collagen fragmentation and altered dermal structural integrity, the most prominent feature of aged human skin. Together, these data strongly suggest that CCN1 contributes to skin aging by stimulating MMP-1 expression through domain-specific interactions with integrin αVβ3. CCN1 is elevated in aged human dermal fibroblasts *in vivo*, the major cells responsible for collagen homeostasis in skin. Upon secretion, CCN1 binds to ECM and through its IGFBP, VWC and TSP1 domains interacts with integrin αVβ3. Interaction of CCN1 domains with integrin αVβ3 triggers FAK and MAPK/AP-1 pathways and thus stimulates MMP1 expression. CCN1-associated up-regulation of MMP-1 causes dermal collagen fragmentation and thus contributes to skin aging. Targeting the CCN1/integrin αVβ3 pathway may be an effective therapeutic strategy to reduce collagen loss and thereby lessen the deleterious impact of aging on the health of human skin.

Additionally, elevated CCN1 activates transcription factor AP-1, the major driving force of MMP-1 expression in human skin fibroblasts (Quan et al. 2006). Elevated CCN1 significantly increases AP-1 reporter activity, compared to empty vector control. Transcription factor AP-1 not only functions as a primary inducer of MMP-1 transcription (Birkedal-Hansen et al. 1993; Matrisian 1994; Mauviel 1993), but also negatively regulates type I procollagen expression (Fisher et al. 2000a; Verrecchia et al. 2000). This inhibition of procollagen may be mediated by transrepression of Smad3 by AP-1 (Dennler et al. 2000; Verrecchia et al. 2000). Therefore, elevated CCN1 impairs type I procollagen production by down-regulating TβRII and inducing transcription factor AP-1. Similarly, elevated CCN1 induces MMP-1 expression by both increasing transcription factor AP-1 and impairing TGF-β signaling, which has been shown to negatively regulates MMP-1. These data indicate that elevated CCN1 induces MMP-1 by both reducing TGF-β responsiveness and increasing AP-1 activity.

❑ CCN1 and Pro-inflammatory Cytokines

CCN1-induced pro-inflammatory cytokines may have a significant impact on the development of AADM. For example, IL-1β, an AADM-associated cytokines, not only up-regulate multiple MMPs but also down-regulates type I collagen synthesis (Qin et al. 2014b). IL-1β is elevated in the dermis of naturally-aged and photoaged human skin (Qin et al. 2014b). CCN1 markedly induces IL-1β, which in turn contributes to CCN1-mediated reduction of type I collagen expression and induction of MMP-1 expression.

Skin is the outermost tissue and a first line of defense against the threats of solar UV radiation, which alters skin connective tissue and causes premature skin aging (photoaging). Solar UV radiation is a potent environmental hazard and skin is its primary target in humans. Acute exposure to UV light leads to sunburn, pigmentation and inflammation, whereas repeated chronic exposure leads to the accumulation of connective tissue damage (photoaging) and skin cancer (Bernstein and Uitto 1996; Fisher et al. 1996; Fisher et al. 1997; Gilchrest and Yaar 1992; Ichihashi et al. 2003; Kripke 1984; Narayanan et al. 2010; Uitto and Bernstein 1998). One important mechanism by which UV irradiation initiates such deleterious alterations in human skin involves proinflammatory cytokines (Clydesdale et al. 2001; Kondo 2000; Kondo and Sauder 1995; Krutmann 2000; Urbanski et al. 1990). UV-inducible proinflammatory cytokines not only orchestrate skin defense responses but also cause dermal connective tissue damage. Proinflammatory cytokines such as IL-1β negatively regulate collagen homeostasis by inhibiting collagen production and stimulating collagen degradation and therefore contribute to skin connective tissue damage in photoaged human skin (Bauge et al. 2007; Fisher et al. 2002; Fisher and Voorhees 1998; Honda et al. 2008). Although epidermal keratinocytes and leukocytes are a rich source of proinflammatory cytokines, it remains unclear whether other cell types such as dermal fibroblasts, the primary cells responsible for collagen homeostasis, produce IL-1β in response to UV irradiation in human skin. Moreover, little is known about the underlying mechanism of chronic inflammation in photoaged human skin.

UV radiation-induced proinflammatory cytokines are not only play a significant role in skin inflammation but also connective tissue alterations (photoaging). CCN1 contributes to skin connective tissue alteration through up-regulation of IL-1β in UV irradiation-induced photoaged human skin (Qin et al. 2014a). Both CCN1 and IL-1β are markedly induced by acute UV irradiation and constitutively elevated in chronic photoaged human skin *in vivo*. IL-1β is one of the primary cytokines induced by UV irradiation in human skin (Faustin and Reed 2008; Feldmeyer et al. 2007; Kondo et al. 1994; Vicentini et al. 2011). The basal level of IL-1β in normal human skin is extremely low, but markedly increased following acute UV irradiation. Both CCN1 and IL-1β mRNA are rapidly and potently induced by UV irradiation in human skin *in vivo*. Interestingly, both CCN1 and IL-1β are also constitutively elevated in chronic photoaged forearm skin, suggesting that persistent elevation of CCN1 may drive IL-1β induction in chronic photoaged human skin *in vivo*. Indeed, overexpression of CCN1 in dermal fibroblasts significantly up-regulates IL-1β at both the mRNA and protein levels. In contrast, no significant change in CCN1 expression is observed following IL-1β treatment, indicating that CCN1 upregulates IL-1β expression but not vice versa. Importantly, blocking IL-1β signaling by a well-known naturally occurring inhibitor, IL-1rα, partially prevented CCN1-induced inhibition of type I collagen and up-regulation of MMP-1, suggesting that IL-1β mediates CCN1-induced aberrant collagen homeostasis. Furthermore, knockdown of CCN1 significantly reduces UV-induced IL-1β and therefore partially prevents UV-induced aberrant collagen homeostasis. These data demonstrate that induction of CCN1 by UV irradiation drives the up-regulation of IL-1β, which in turn mediates UV-induced aberrant collagen homeostasis. Elevated expression of CCN1 is likely an important mediator of UV irradiation-induced skin inflammation and connective tissue alterations.

Although proinflammatory cytokines are known to mediate UV irradiation-induced skin connective tissue alterations, little is known about the induction of proinflammatory cytokines in stromal dermal fibroblasts and chronic inflammation in photoaged human skin. Induction of CCN1 in dermal fibroblasts upon UV irradiation drives the up-regulation of IL-1β, which mediates CCN1-induced aberrant collagen homeostasis in human skin dermis. Solar UV radiation readily penetrates the reticular dermis, rendering dermal fibroblasts accessible targets (Herrmann et al. 1993; Wlaschek et al. 2001). As dermal fibroblasts are the major cell type of the dermal compartment, these cells may function as immunocompetent cells in acute inflammatory reactions caused by UV irradiation in human skin through a

CCN1-mediated elevation of IL-1β. Furthermore, elevated CCN1 in dermal fibroblasts may play a pivotal role in the sustained elevation of IL-1β and chronic inflammation in photoaged human skin. Recent evidence indicates that CCN proteins could represent a new class of modulators of inflammation (Chen et al. 2007; Jun and Lau 2010; Kular et al. 2011). Consistent with this notion, CCN1 induced by wound healing activates a proinflammatory genetic programme in human skin fibroblasts and marine macrophages (Bai et al. 2010; Chen et al. 2001c). Evidence also indicates a potential role for CCN1 in chronic inflammatory diseases such as atherosclerosis, rheumatoid arthritis, inflammatory kidney diseases and neuroinflammatory diseases (Kular et al. 2011). CCN1 could therefore represent a potential therapeutic target for treating solar UV-induced sunburn, inflammation and skin damage.

CCN1 is rapidly and potently induced by UV irradiation and continuously elevated in chronic photoaged human skin *in vivo*. Elevated CCN1 is known to trigger the generation of reactive oxygen species (ROS) and functions as an activator of the AP-1 transcription factor (Chen et al. 2007; Quan et al. 2006). CCN1 has also been shown to activate NF-κb signaling, leading to the up-regulation of multiple proinflammatory cytokines including IL-1β (Bai et al. 2010). UV irradiation leads to the activation of two major signaling pathways, namely AP-1 and NF-κB (Fisher et al. 2000b; Fisher et al. 1996; Fisher et al. 1997). AP-1 transcription factor and NF-κb signaling are two primary inducers of many proinflammatory cytokines including IL-1β. It is also well documented that there is functional cooperation between AP-1 and NF-κb in IL-1β production (Kang et al. 2005). Therefore, it is conceivable that elevated CCN1 up-regulates IL-1β through ROS-mediated activation of AP-1 transcription factor and NF-κb signaling in UV-irradiated and chronic photoaged human skin *in vivo*.

Elevated CCN1 not only inhibits type I collagen but also induces MMP-1 and thus contributes to aberrant collagen homeostasis in aged human skin. One important question is that how CCN1 exert such dual effects on collagen homeostasis. It has been reported that IL-1β impairs TGF-β signaling by down-regulating the TGF-β type II receptor, resulting in the development of degenerative and inflammatory diseases in osteoarthritis (Bauge et al. 2007). TGF-β signaling is the primary regulator of collagen homeostasis, regulating both collagen biosynthesis and degradation (Chen et al. 2000; Hall et al. 2003; Varga et al. 1987; White et al. 2000). Consistent with this notion, CCN1 impairs TGF-β signaling as a result of down-regulation of the TGF-β type II receptor (Quan et al. 2006). Therefore, it is conceivable that elevated CCN1 impairs TGF-β signaling through the up-regulation of IL-1β and thereby contributes to aberrant collagen homeostasis. Indeed, TGF-β pathway is impaired in UV-irradiated and photoaged human skin *in vivo*, largely due to down-regulation of the TGF-β type II receptor (Quan et al. 2004; Quan et al. 2006; Quan et al. 2001b). These data suggest that elevated CCN1 negatively regulates collagen homeostasis through IL-1β-mediated impairment of TGF-β signaling. In addition, cytokine-mediated AP-1 and NF-κb signaling, which are activated by CCN1, negatively regulate collagen gene expression in human dermal fibroblasts (Fisher et al. 2000b; Kouba et al. 1999; Rippe et al. 1999).

There is strong association of aging with chronic low grade inflammatory activity which may progress to long term tissue damage and systemic chronic inflammation (Daynes et al. 1993). Accumulating evidence supports the concept of "inflammaging", which posits that low grade chronic elevation of proinflammatory mediators can be a driving force for the aging progress (Franceschi et al. 2007). Central to this concept is that healthy aging is not an inflammatory disease, but rather sub-clinical inflammation contributes to the gradual decline of organ function, which occurs during the aging process. For example, IL-6 is increased in the aged and has been suggested to be a marker of health status in the elderly (Maggio et al. 2006). Interestingly, IL-6 is markedly induced by CCN1 in human skin dermal fibroblasts and constitutively elevated in aged skin (Quan et al. 2009). Although aged skin does not display overt inflammation, the possibility that AADM-associated cytokines contribute to human skin connective tissue aging deserves further investigation.

CCN proteins functions primarily through interactions with integrins in a cell-type, function-specific manner (Chen and Lau 2009). CCN1 has been reported to interact with integrins to increase intracellular levels of ROS, which function as important effectors of CCN1 actions (Jun and Lau 2010; Lau 2011). The ability of CCN1 to induce AADM in dermal fibroblasts may be mediated by integrin-coupled generation of ROS. It is well-documented that the integrin pathway and ROS lead to activation of transcription factor AP-1, which up-regulates MMPs and proinflammatory cytokines, including IL-1β and IL-6 (Jun and Lau 2010; Qin et al. 2014b). Therefore, it is conceivable that elevated CCN1 up-regulates MMPs and cytokines through activation of integrin and/or ROS-mediated activation of AP-1 in aged human skin dermal fibroblasts. CCN1 is not only induced by oxidative stress, but also increases intracellular levels of ROS, suggesting a positive feedback loop involving CCN1 and ROS/AP-1 may result in sustained elevation of ROS and CCN1 in fibroblasts in aged human skin.

❑ UV Irradiation Negatively Regulates Collagen Homeostasis by Induction of CCN1

CCN1 is elevated in the dermis of photoaged human skin. In addition, CCN1 is rapidly and markedly induced by acute UV-irradiation in human skin *in vivo* and UV-irradiated cultured human skin fibroblasts (Quan et al. 2010a). Inhibition of UV irradiation-induced CCN1 by siRNA significantly attenuates UV irradiation-induced inhibition of type I procollagen and up-regulation of MMP-1, indicating CCN1 functions as a key mediator of

UV-induced aberrant collagen homeostasis. UV irradiation significantly activates CCN1 promoter without changing the stability of CCN1 mRNA and protein, indicating the primary mechanism of CCN1 induction by UV irradiation is transcriptional. Analysis of CCN1 promoter reveals that CCN1 proximal promoter contains functional AP-1 binding site. Analysis of proteins bound to the AP-1 site reveals that UV irradiation increased binding of AP-1 family members, c-Jun and c-Fosto CCN1 AP-1 binding site. Deletion or mutation of AP-1 binding site in the CCN1 promoter substantially reduces UV activation of CCN1 promoter. Furthermore, functional blockade of c-Jun by expression of dominant negative mutant, or siRNA-mediated knockdown of c-Jun substantially reduces UV irradiation irradiation-induced activation of CCN1 promoter and CCN1 expression. These data demonstrate that CCN1 is transcriptionally regulated by UV irradiation via induction of transcription factor AP-1 and that CCN1 is a novel mediator of solar UV irradiation-induced dermal connective tissue damage.

CCN1 has been shown to be transcriptionally activated by a variety of extracellular stimuli and human CCN1 promoter contains several potential transcription factor-binding sites (Han et al. 2003; Kunz et al. 2003). Among them, HIF-1α (Kunz et al. 2003) and CREB (Han et al. 2003) have been shown to positively regulate CCN1 promoter. FOXO3a functions as a negative regulator of CCN1 transcription (Lee et al. 2007). Despite the presence of several functional transcription factor binding sites in the CCN1 promoter, transcriptional regulation of CCN1 in response to UV irradiation is primarily controlled by c-Jun/AP-1, in primary human dermal fibroblasts. Interestingly, elevated CCN1 activates transcription factor AP-1, (Quan et al. 2006), suggesting that a positive feedback mechanism may contribute to sustained elevation of CCN1 in photoaged and UV-irradiated human skin. Taken together, these data indicate that c-Jun/AP-1 functions as an important regulator in up-regulation of CCN1 transcription and requires for elevated CCN1 gene expression by UV irradiation.

❑ Oxidant Exposure Induces CCN1 via c-Jun/ AP-1 to Reduce Collagen Expression

The oxidative stress theory of aging is a widely accepted hypothesis for the molecular basis of aging (Harman 1981, 1992) and considers an important pathogenic factor involved in age-related diseases (Droge 2002; Harman 1981). Human skin is a primary target of oxidative stress from reactive oxygen species (ROS) generated from both extrinsic sources like ultraviolet irradiation (UV) (photoaging) (Scharffetter-Kochanek et al. 2000; Yaar and Gilchrest 2007) and endogenous oxidative metabolism (natural aging) (Fisher et al. 2009). ROS has been shown to inhibit collagen synthesis and stimulate collagen degradation and thus contributes to connective tissue aging (Fisher et al. 2002; Fisher et al. 2009).

CCN1, a negative regulator of collagen production, is markedly induced by ROS and mediates loss of type I collagen in human dermal fibroblasts (Qin et al. 2014c). Knockdown of CCN1 by CCN1 siRNA significantly attenuates ROS-mediated reduction of type I procollagen mRNA and protein. These data indicate that elevated CCN1 mediates loss of type I procollagen caused by ROS in human dermal fibroblasts. Furthermore, antioxidant N-acetyl-L-cysteine significantly reduces CCN1 expression and prevented ROS-induced loss of type I collagen in both human dermal fibroblasts and human skin *in vivo* (Qin et al. 2014c). ROS increases c-Jun, a critical member of transcription factor AP-1 complex and increased c-Jun binding to the AP-1 site of the CCN1 promoter. Functional blocking of c-Jun significantly reduces CCN1 promoter and gene expression and thus prevents ROS-induced loss of type I collagen. Therefore, targeting the c-Jun/CCN1 axis may provide clinical benefit for connective tissue aging in human skin. The protective effects of antioxidants have been well-studied in cell culture systems and in animal models (Firuzi et al. 2011). However, in humans, antioxidant based therapies have been generally disappointing (Pashkow 2011). Human skin is an excellent and accessible model organ to study the protective effects of antioxidants. NAC, a well-known antioxidant, effectively prevents UV/ROS induction of c-Jun and its downstream effector CCN1. NAC is a metabolic precursor of glutathione, a co-factor for the enzyme glutathione peroxidase, which reduces hydrogen peroxide to water and is among the most abundant endogenous antioxidants. NAC is safe for human use and we previously demonstrated that NAC penetrates human skin and effectively mitigates ROS-driven responses to acute UV in human skin *in vivo* (Kang et al. 2003).

Interestingly, CCN1 is not only induced by oxidative exposure, but also increases intracellular ROS levels (Jun and Lau 2010; Juric et al. 2012), suggesting that a positive feedback loop involving CCN1 and ROS may cause sustained elevation of ROS and CCN1 in fibroblasts in aged human skin. Investigating this possibility is a worthwhile goal for future research. Secreted CCN1 may function as "docking" protein to facilitate interactions between cell surface receptors and ECM proteins. CCN1 has been shown to exert a range of diverse functions through interaction with multiple integrins in a cell-type, function-specific manner (Chen and Lau 2009). In human skin dermal fibroblasts CCN1 interacts with $\alpha V \beta 3$ integrin to mediate up-regulation of MMP-1 (Qin et al. 2013). Further investigation will be required to determine the role of integrin (s) in CCN1-dependent inhibition of type I collagen in response to ROS.

❑ CCN1 and Senescent Cells

Studies in a mouse model have demonstrated that CCN1 exerts potent anti-fibrotic activity via induction of myofibroblast senescence during cutaneous wound healing (Jun and Lau 2010). The myofibroblasts play an important role in wound healing through ECM production and wound contraction.

Upon wound healing completion, the myofibroblasts become programmed senescence in order to prevent excess fibrosis. The central finding from Jun et al. demonstrate that the programed myofibroblasts senescence is regulated by CCN1 and thus CCN1 modulates wound healing (Jun and Lau 2010). Interestingly, as replicative senescence is a form of cellular aging, CCN1 mRNA and protein levels are significantly elevated in replicative senescent dermal fibroblasts (Quan et al. 2012b). Replicative senescent dermal fibroblasts also express reduced levels of type I procollagen and increased levels of MMP-1, as observed in aged human skin. Knockdown of elevated CCN1 in senescent dermal fibroblasts normalizes both type I procollagen and MMP-1 expression, indicating CCN1 mediates senescence-associated aberrant collagen homeostasis. Interestingly, elevated expression of CCN1 markedly stimulates collagen fibrils fragmentation caused by replicative senescent dermal fibroblasts. Atomic force microscopy (AFM) further revealed collagen fibril fragmentation and disorganization are largely prevented by knockdown of CCN1 in replicative senescent dermal fibroblasts, suggesting CCN1 mediates MMP-1-induced alterations of collagen fibrils by replicative senescent dermal fibroblasts. Given the ability of CCN1 to regulate both production and degradation of type I collagen in senescent cells, it is likely that elevated-CCN1 functions as an important mediator of collagen loss, which is observed in aged human skin. Molecular mechanisms that are responsible for the elevated expression of CCN1 in replicative senescent dermal fibroblasts remain to be determined. One possibility is that replicative senescence is often associated with increased oxidative stress (Brandl et al. 2011; Campisi 2003), which in turn functions as a positive regulator for CCN1 induction (Qin et al. 2014c). These data suggest that CCN1 might be induced by oxidative stress in replicative senescent dermal fibroblasts and mediates aberrant alteration of collagen homeostasis.

❑ Retinoid Suppression of CCN1

Vitamin A and its metabolites have been shown to improve aged human skin by promoting deposition of new collagen and preventing its degradation (Kafi et al. 2007). In skin equivalent cultures, all-*trans* retinoic acid (RA), the major bioactive form of vitamin A, significantly increases type I procollagen and reduces MMP-1 (Quan et al. 2012b). Treatment of recombinant human CCN1 to skin equivalent cultures, markedly reduces type I procollagen and increases MMP-1 (Quan et al. 2012b). Interestingly, all-*trans* retinoic acid significantly inhibits CCN1 expression in skin equivalent cultures (Quan et al. 2012b). Human skin has the capacity to convert vitamin A (all-*trans* retinol, ROL) to its biologically active metabolite all-*trans* retinoic acid. Topical treatment with retinol (vitamin A, 0.4%) for seven days significantly reduces CCN1 gene expression, compared to vehicle-treated skin, in both naturally-aged and photoaged human skin *in vivo* (Quan et al. 2012b). These studies demonstrate the mechanism by which retinoids improve aged skin, through increased collagen production, may involve down-regulation CCN1.

The mechanism (s) by which retinoid inhibits CCN1 expression in naturally aged or photoaged human skin remains to be determined. One possibility is that retinoid reduces CCN1 through inhibition of AP-1 transcription factor. Transcriptional regulation of CCN1 in response to UV irradiation is primarily controlled by AP-1 transcription factor, in primary human dermal fibroblasts (Quan et al. 2010a). AP-1 transcriptional activity is elevated in both chronologically aged and photoaged human skin (Fisher et al. 2002; Fisher and Voorhees 1998; Fisher et al. 1997) and is critically important in mediating skin connective tissue damage. Importantly, elevated AP-1 is suppressed by applications of retinoid in aged and photoaged human skin *in vivo* (Varani et al. 2000), suggesting that retinoid down-regulates CCN1 expression by inhibiting AP-1 transcription factor. Interestingly, elevated CCN1 also activates transcription factor AP-1, (Quan et al. 2006), suggesting that a positive feedback mechanism may contribute to sustained elevation of CCN1 in aged and photoaged human skin.

Treatment of skin equivalent cultures with RA resulted in increased epidermal cells layers and CRABPII expression, which are characteristic responses of human epidermis to retinoid treatment *in vivo*. Skin equivalent cultures have been shown to be a useful model to study functional interactions between epidermis and dermis (Afaq et al. 2009; Martin et al. 2008). Neither CCN1 nor type I collagen is regulated by retinoid in primary fibroblasts cultured in monolayer or three dimensional collagen lattices. An increasing body of evidence indicates that interactions between epidermal keratinocytes and dermal fibroblasts play a pivotal role in dermal fibroblasts behavior and functions (Ghaffari et al. 2009; Harrison et al. 2006; Nowinski et al. 2002). The interaction between epidermal keratinocytes and dermal fibroblasts may be involved in regulation of CCN1 expression by retinoid, in dermal fibroblasts. Skin equivalent cultures appear to be a useful model to investigate the nature of these interactions.

Figure 1 depicts a model in which elevated CCN1 in aged dermal fibroblasts contributes to human skin connective tissue aging through creating age-associated dermal microenvironment (AADM). Like other organs, human skin is exposed to reactive oxygen species (ROS) generated from both environmental sources such as solar ultraviolet irradiation and endogenous oxidative metabolism. Chronic exposure to ROS up-regulates CCN1 expression. Through interaction with integrins elevated CCN1 impairs dermal fibroblast production of collagen by inhibiting TGF-β signaling and promoting production of MMPs and proinflammatory cytokines. These alterations lead to thin and fragmented dermal collagenous ECM, characteristic features of aged human skin. Elevated expression of CCN1 in human dermal fibroblasts acts through multiple pathways to promote AADM: 1) impairment of TGF-β signaling by down-regulation of TβRII and thus contributes to age-associated thinning of the dermis (Quan et al. 2006);

2) induction of multiple MMPs via up-regulation of transcription factor AP-1, a major regulator of multiple MMPs and thus contributes to age-associated ECM fragmentation (Qin et al. 2013; Quan et al. 2006; Quan et al. 2011a); and 3) elevation of multiple pro-inflammatory cytokines and thus contributes to age-associated inflammatory microenvironment (inflammaging) (Qin et al. 2014b; Quan et al. 2011a).

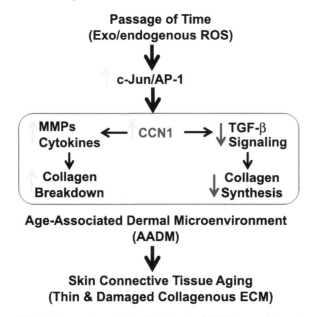

FIG. 1 *Proposed model in which elevated CCN1 in aged dermal fibroblasts contributes to human skin connective tissue aging through creating age-associated dermal microenvironment (AADM) (see text for details).*

❑ CCN2 in Human Skin Connective Tissue Aging

Connective tissue growth factor (CCN2/CTGF) is another member of the CCN (CCN1-6) family of proteins. CCN2 exhibits diverse biological activities *in vitro*, such as cell proliferation, adhesion, migration and ECM production (Babic et al. 1999; Brigstock 1999a; Chen et al. 2001a; Duncan et al. 1999a; Grotendorst 1997a; Gupta et al. 2000a). It has been reported that CCN2 plays an important role in regulating procollagen synthesis (Brigstock 1999b; Duncan et al. 1999b; Grotendorst 1997b; Gupta et al. 2000b). CCN2 is rapidly induced by TGF-β and appears to function as a downstream mediator of TGF-β actions (Quan et al. 2010c). CCN2 is markedly elevated in numerous fibrotic human disorders that involve skin, lungs and kidneys (Abraham et al. 2000; Bradham et al. 1991; Grotendorst et al. 1996; Shi-Wen et al. 2008; Underhill et al. 2012). CCN2 stimulates collagen synthesis when injected into mouse skin or added to cultured renal fibroblasts (Duncan et al. 1999a). CCN2, in conjunction with TGF-β, is believed to stimulate excessive deposition of collagen, the hallmark of fibrotic diseases. These findings have generated interest in development of new drugs that interfere with CCN2 function to combat fibrotic disorders. Although the role of CCN2 in the pathophysiology of fibrotic diseases has received considerable attention; the physiological role of CCN2 in the regulation of collagen expression in normal human skin has been only recently studied. Initially, CCN2 is detected in fibrotic skin diseases, such as scleroderma, but not in normal skin or cultured normal human dermal fibroblasts. However, CCN2 is later found to be readily detectable and constitutively expressed in normal human skin *in vivo* and normal human dermal fibroblasts (Quan et al. 2002), suggesting that CCN2 might be a physiological regulator of collagen expression. In human dermal fibroblasts, CCN2 functions as a downstream mediator of TGF-β/Smad pathway and is necessary for optimal TGF-β-dependent regulation of type I procollagen synthesis (Quan et al. 2010c). In primary human skin fibroblasts, neutralization of endogenous TGF-β or knockdown of CCN2 substantially reduces expression of type I procollagen mRNA, protein and promoter activity.

In contrast, overexpression of CCN2 stimulates type I procollagen expression and increases type I procollagen promoter activity. Inhibition of TGF-β receptor kinase, knockdown of Smad4, or overexpression of inhibitory Smad7 abolishes CCN2 stimulation of type I procollagen expression. Importantly, CCN2 is significantly reduced in fibroblasts in naturally-aged human skin *in vivo* (Quan et al. 2010c). Both TβRII and CCN2 expression are reduced in aged human skin. This similarity is consistent with TGF-β signaling being the major regulator of CCN2 expression. In addition, acute UV irradiation reduces CCN2 expression in human skin *in vivo* and dermal fibroblast in culture (Quan et al. 2002), suggesting that reduced CCN2 likely contributes to UV-induced photoaging in human skin. These data provide evidence that CCN2 functions as an intrinsic, physiological mediator of type I procollagen expression and that reduced expression of CCN2 contributes to age-dependent reduction of type I procollagen production observed in human skin. Reduced expression of CCN2 in dermal fibroblasts in aged human skin *in vivo* mirrors reduced expression of type I procollagen. These data suggest that reduced CCN2 levels likely contribute to aberrant collagen homeostasis observed in naturally-aged and photodamaged human skin.

TGF-β is the most potent stimulator of CCN2 gene expression (Holmes et al. 2001; Leask et al. 2003). Therefore, impaired TGF-β signaling due to reduced expression of type II TGF-β receptor in aged human skin is likely a major contributing factor to the observed reduction of CCN2. UV irradiation down-regulates type II TGF-β receptor and thereby substantially reduces cellular responsiveness to TGF-β (Quan et al. 2001a). Interestingly, type II TGF-β receptor expression is reduced in dermal fibroblasts in aged human skin *in vivo* (Quan et al. 2006). These data indicate that down-regulation of type II TGF-β receptor may contribute to reduced expression of CCN2 in aged human skin. Additionally, it has been shown that JNK/c-Jun/MAPK pathway antagonizes TGF-β induction of CCN2 transcription (Leask et al. 2003; Leivonen et al. 2001). JNK/c-Jun/MAPK pathway is upregulated in aged compared to young human skin *in vivo* (Chung et al. 2000), suggesting that activated JNK/c-Jun/MAPK pathway may contribute to reduced expression of CCN2 in aged human skin. c-Jun directly interacts with activated Smad proteins in the nucleus to prevent their binding to target genes (Verrecchia et al. 2000). c-Jun also competes with Smad proteins for the common transcription co-activator p300. Both mechanisms can simultaneously contribute to the c-Jun-mediated inhibition of TGF-β/Smad signaling pathway. Therefore, elevated c-Jun may impair TGF-β/Smad signaling, which may in turn contribute to reduced expression of CCN2 observed in aged human skin.

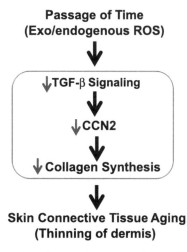

FIG. 2 *Proposed model in which TGF-β-related reduction of CCN2 in aged dermal fibroblasts contributes to human skin connective tissue aging through inhibition of type I collagen (see text for details).*

In contract to CCN1, ROS significantly reduced expression of CCN2 (Qin et al. 2014c). CCN1 and CCN2 are functionally distinct. These data suggest that ROS-mediated inhibition of collagen production involves not only elevated CCN1 expression but also reduced CCN2 expression. ROS also significantly reduced expression of CCN4 and CCN5 (Qin et al. 2014c). As the functions of CCN4 and CCN5 in collagen are unknown, further investigation will be required to determine the role of these proteins in ROS-mediated inhibition of type I collagen. Figure 2 depicts a model in which TGF-β-related reduction of CCN2 in aged dermal fibroblasts contributes to human skin connective tissue aging through inhibition of type I collagen. Like other organs, human skin is exposed to reactive oxygen species (ROS) generated from both environmental sources such as solar ultraviolet irradiation and endogenous oxidative metabolism. Chronic exposure to ROS down-regulates TGF-β type II receptor and thus impairs TGF-β signaling, the primary regulator of CCN2. Reduced CCN2 contributes to thinning of the dermis by inhibition of type I procollagen synthesis in aged human skin.

❑ Acknowledgments

This study is supported by the National Institutes of Health (Bethesda, MD) Grants: ES014697 and ES014697 30S1 to Taihao Quan, AG019364 to Gary J. Fisher and Taihao Quan, AG031452 and AG025186 to Gary J. Fisher. The author would like to thank Drs Gary J. Fisher and John J. Voorhees for their help and support. The authors also thank Drs Zhaoping Qin, Tianyuan He, Yuan Shao, Patrick Robichaud and Trupta Purohit for technical assistance.

❑ References

Abraham, D.J., X. Shiwen, C.M. Black, S. Sa, Y. Xu and A. Leask. 2000. Tumor necrosis factor alpha suppresses the induction of connective tissue growth factor by transforming growth factor-beta in normal and scleroderma fibroblasts. J Biol Chem 275: 15220-15225.

Afaq, F., M.A. Zaid, N. Khan, M. Dreher and H. Mukhtar. 2009. Protective effect of pomegranate-derived products on UVB-mediated damage in human reconstituted skin. Exp Dermatol 18: 553-561.

Babic, A., C. Chen and F. Lau. 1999. Fisp12/mouse connective tissue growth factor mediates endothelial cell adhesion and migration through integrin αvβ3, promotes endothelial cell survival and induces angiogenesis *in vivo*. Mol Cell Biol 19: 2958-2966.

Bai, T., C.C. Chen and L.F. Lau. 2010. Matricellular protein CCN1 activates a proinflammatory genetic program in murine macrophages. J Immunol 184: 3223-3232.

Bauge, C., F. Legendre, S. Leclercq, J.M. Elissalde, J.P. Pujol, P. Galera, et al. 2007. Interleukin-1beta impairment of transforming growth factor beta1 signaling by down-regulation of transforming growth factor beta receptor type II and up-regulation of Smad7 in human articular chondrocytes. Arthritis Rheum 56: 3020-3032.

Bernstein, E.F. and J. Uitto. 1996. The effect of photodamage on dermal extracellular matrix. Clin Dermatol 14: 143-151.

Birkedal-Hansen, H., W. Moore, M. Bodden, L. Windsor, B. Birkedal-Hansen, A. DeCarlo, et al. 1993. Matrix metalloproteinases: a review. Crit Rev Oral Bio Med 4: 197-250.

Bradham, D.M., A. Igarashi, R.L. Potter and G.R. Grotendorst. 1991. Connective tissue growth factor: a cysteine-rich mitogen secreted by human vascular endothelial cells is related to the SRC-induced immediate early gene product CEF-10. J Cell Biol 114: 1285-1294.

Brandl, A., M. Meyer, V. Bechmann, M. Nerlich and P. Angele. 2011. Oxidative stress induces senescence in human mesenchymal stem cells. Exp Cell Res 317: 1541-1547.

Brigstock, D. 1999a. The connective tissue growth factor/Cysteine-rich 61/nephroblastoma overexpressed (CCN) family. Endocrine Rev 20: 189-206.

Brigstock, D.R. 1999b. The connective tissue growth factor/cysteine-rich 61/nephroblastoma overexpressed (CCN) family. Endocr Rev 20: 189-206.

Brunner, A., J. Chinn, M. Neubauer and A. Purchio. 1991. Identification of a gene family regulated by transforming growth factor-beta. DNA Cell Biol 10: 293-300.

Cabodi, S., M. del Pilar Camacho-Leal, P. Di Stefano and P. Defilippi. 2010. Integrin signalling adaptors: not only figurants in the cancer story. Nat Rev Cancer 10: 858-870.

Campisi, J. 2003. Cancer and ageing: rival demons? Nat Rev Cancer 3: 339-349.

Chen, C.C. and L.F. Lau. 2009. Functions and mechanisms of action of CCN matricellular proteins. Int J Biochem Cell Biol 41: 771-783.

Chen, C.-C., N. Chen and L. Lau. 2001a. The angiogenic factors Cyr61 and connective tissue growth factor induce adhesive signaling in primary human skin fibroblasts. J Biol Chem 276: 10443-10452.

Chen, C.C., N. Chen and L.F. Lau. 2001b. The angiogenic factors Cyr61 and connective tissue growth factor induce adhesive signaling in primary human skin fibroblasts. J Biol Chem 276: 10443-10452.

Chen, C.C., F.E. Mo and L.F. Lau. 2001c. The angiogenic factor Cyr61 activates a genetic program for wound healing in human skin fibroblasts. J Biol Chem 276: 47329-47337.

Chen, C.C., J.L. Young, R.I. Monzon, N. Chen, V. Todorovic and L.F. Lau. 2007. Cytotoxicity of TNFalpha is regulated by integrin-mediated matrix signaling. EMBO J 26: 1257-1267.

Chen, S.J., W. Yuan, S. Lo, M. Trojanowska and J. Varga. 2000. Interaction of smad3 with a proximal smad-binding element of the human alpha2(I) procollagen gene promoter required for transcriptional activation by TGF-beta. J Cell Physiol 183: 381-392.

Chung, J., S. Kang, J. Varani, J. Lin, G. Fisher and J. Voorhees. 2000. Decreased extracellular-signal-regulated kinase and increased stress-activated MAP kinase activities in aged human skin *in vivo*. J Invest Dermatol 114: 177-182.

Clydesdale, G.J., G.W. Dandie and H.K. Muller. 2001. Ultraviolet light induced injury: immunological and inflammatory effects. Immunol Cell Biol 79: 547-568.

Daynes, R.A., B.A. Araneo, W.B. Ershler, C. Maloney, G.Z. Li and S.Y. Ryu. 1993. Altered regulation of IL-6 production with normal aging. Possible linkage to the age-associated decline in dehydroepiandrosterone and its sulfated derivative. J Immunol 150: 5219-5230.

Dennler, S., C. Prunier, N. Ferrand, J. Gauthier and A. Atfi. 2000. c-Jun inhibits transforming growth factor beta-mediated transcription by repressing Smad3 transcriptional activity. J Biol Chem 275: 28858-28865.

Droge, W. 2002. Free radicals in the physiological control of cell function. Physiol Rev 82: 47-95.

Duncan, M., K. Frazier, S. Abramson, S. Williams, H. Klapper, X. Huang, et al. 1999a. Connective tissue growth factor mediates transforming growth factor β-induced collagen synthesis: down-regulation by cAMP. FASEB J 13: 1774-1786.

Duncan, M.R., K.S. Frazier, S. Abramson, S. Williams, H. Klapper, X. Huang, et al. 1999b. Connective tissue growth factor mediates transforming growth factor beta-induced collagen synthesis: down-regulation by cAMP. FASEB J 13: 1774-1786.

Faustin, B. and J.C. Reed. 2008. Sunburned skin activates inflammasomes. Trends Cell Biol 18: 4-8.

Feldmeyer, L., M. Keller, G. Niklaus, D. Hohl, S. Werner and H.D. Beer. 2007. The inflammasome mediates UVB-induced activation and secretion of interleukin-1beta by keratinocytes. Curr Biol 17: 1140-1145.

Firuzi, O., R. Miri, M. Tavakkoli and L. Saso. 2011. Antioxidant therapy: current status and future prospects. Curr Med Chem 18: 3871-3888.

Fisher, G.J. and J.J. Voorhees. 1998. Molecular mechanisms of photoaging and its prevention by retinoic acid: ultraviolet irradiation induces MAP kinase signal transduction cascades that induce Ap-1-regulated matrix metalloproteinases that degrade human skin *in vivo*. J Investig Dermatol Symp Proc 3: 61-68.

Fisher, G.J., S.C. Datta, H.S. Talwar, Z.Q. Wang, J. Varani, S. Kang, et al. 1996. Molecular basis of sun-induced premature skin ageing and retinoid antagonism. Nature 379: 335-339.

Fisher, G.J., Z.Q. Wang, S.C. Datta, J. Varani, S. Kang and J.J. Voorhees. 1997. Pathophysiology of premature skin aging induced by ultraviolet light. N Engl J Med 337: 1419-1428.

Fisher, G., S. Datta, Z. Wang, X. Li, T. Quan, J. Chung, et al. 2000a. c-Jun dependent inhibition of cutaneous procollagen transcription following ultraviolet irradiation is reversed by all-*trans* retinoid acid. J Clin Invest 106: 661-668.

Fisher, G.J., S. Datta, Z. Wang, X.Y. Li, T. Quan, J.H. Chung, et al. 2000b. c-Jun-dependent inhibition of cutaneous procollagen transcription following ultraviolet irradiation is reversed by all-trans retinoic acid. J Clin Invest 106: 663-670.

Fisher, G.J., S. Kang, J. Varani, Z. Bata-Csorgo, Y. Wan, S. Datta, et al. 2002. Mechanisms of photoaging and chronological skin aging. Arch Dermatol 138: 1462-1470.

Fisher, G.J., T. Quan, T. Purohit, Y. Shao, M.K. Cho, T. He, et al. 2009. Collagen fragmentation promotes oxidative stress and elevates matrix metalloproteinase-1 in fibroblasts in aged human skin. Am J Pathol 174: 101-114.

Franceschi, C., M. Capri, D. Monti, S. Giunta, F. Olivieri, F. Sevini, et al. 2007. Inflammaging and anti-inflammaging: a systemic perspective on aging and longevity emerged from studies in humans. Mech Ageing Dev 128: 92-105.

Ghaffari, A., R.T. Kilani and A. Ghahary. 2009. Keratinocyte-conditioned media regulate collagen expression in dermal fibroblasts. J Invest Dermatol 129: 340-347.

Giancotti, F.G. and E. Ruoslahti. 1999. Integrin signaling. Science 285: 1028-1032.

Gilchrest, B.A. and M. Yaar. 1992. Ageing and photoageing of the skin: observations at the cellular and molecular level. Br J Dermatol 127 Suppl 41: 25-30.

Grotendorst, G. 1997a. Connective tissue growth factor: a mediator of TGF-β action on fibroblasts. Cytokine Growth Factor Rev 8: 171-179.

Grotendorst, G.R. 1997b. Connective tissue growth factor: a mediator of TGF-beta action on fibroblasts. Cytokine Growth Factor Rev 8: 171-179.

Grotendorst, G.R., H. Okochi and N. Hayashi. 1996. A novel transforming growth factor beta response element controls the expression of the connective tissue growth factor gene. Cell Growth Differ 7: 469-480.

Grzeszkiewicz, T.M., D.J. Kirschling, N. Chen and L.F. Lau. 2001. CYR61 stimulates human skin fibroblast migration through Integrin alpha vbeta 5 and enhances mitogenesis through integrin alpha vbeta 3, independent of its carboxyl-terminal domain. J Biol Chem 276: 21943-21950.

Gupta, S., M. Clarkson, J. Duggan and H. Brady. 2000a. Connective tissue growth factor: Potential role in glomerulosclerosis and tubulointerstitial fibrosis. Kidney Intl 58: 1389-1399.

Gupta, S., M.R. Clarkson, J. Duggan and H.R. Brady. 2000b. Connective tissue growth factor: potential role in glomerulosclerosis and tubulointerstitial fibrosis. Kidney Int 58: 1389-1399.

Hall, M.C., D.A. Young, J.G. Waters, A.D. Rowan, A. Chantry, D.R. Edwards, et al. 2003. The comparative role of activator protein 1 and Smad factors in the regulation of Timp-1 and MMP-1 gene expression by transforming growth factor-beta 1. J Biol Chem 278: 10304-10313.

Han, J.S., E. Macarak, J. Rosenbloom, K.C. Chung and B. Chaqour. 2003. Regulation of Cyr61/CCN1 gene expression through RhoA GTPase and p38MAPK signaling pathways. Eur J Biochem 270: 3408-3421.

Harman, D. 1981. The aging process. Proc Natl Acad Sci USA 78: 7124-7128.

Harman, D. 1992. Free radical theory of aging. Mutat Res 275: 257-266.

Harrison, C.A., F. Gossiel, A.J. Bullock, T. Sun, A. Blumsohn and S. Mac Neil. 2006. Investigation of keratinocyte regulation of collagen I synthesis by dermal fibroblasts in a simple *in vitro* model. Br J Dermatol 154: 401-410.

Herrmann, G., M. Wlaschek, T.S. Lange, K. Prenzel, G. Goerz and K. Scharffetter-Kochanek. 1993. UVA irradiation stimulates the synthesis of various matrix-metalloproteinases (MMPs) in cultured human fibroblasts. Exp Dermatol 2: 92-97.

Holmes, A., S. Sa, X. Shiwen, C. Black, D. Abraham and A. Leask. 2001. CTGF and Smads: Maintenance of scleroderma phenotype is independent of Smad signalling. J Biol Chem 276: 10594-10601.

Honda, A., R. Abe, T. Makino, O. Norisugi, Y. Fujita, H. Watanabe, et al. 2008. Interleukin-1beta and macrophage migration inhibitory factor (MIF) in dermal fibroblasts mediate UVA-induced matrix metalloproteinase-1 expression. J Dermatol Sci 49: 63-72.

Ichihashi, M., M. Ueda, A. Budiyanto, T. Bito, M. Oka, M. Fukunaga, et al. 2003. UV-induced skin damage. Toxicology 189: 21-39.

Jay, P., J. Berge-Lefranc, C. Mejean, S. Taviaux and P. Berta 1997. The human growth factor-inducible immediate early gene, CYR61, maps to chromosome 1p. Oncogene 14: 1753-1757.

Jin, H. and J. Varner 2004. Integrins: roles in cancer development and as treatment targets. Br J Cancer 90: 561-565.

Jun, J.I. and L.F. Lau. 2010. The matricellular protein CCN1 induces fibroblast senescence and restricts fibrosis in cutaneous wound healing. Nat Cell Biol 12: 676-685.

Juric, V., C.C. Chen and L.F. Lau. 2012. TNFalpha-induced apoptosis enabled by CCN1/CYR61: pathways of reactive oxygen species generation and cytochrome c release. PLoS One 7: e31303.

Kafi, R., H.S. Kwak, W.E. Schumacher, S. Cho, V.N. Hanft, T.A. Hamilton, et al. 2007. Improvement of naturally aged skin with vitamin A (retinol). Arch Dermatol 143: 606-612.

Kang, S., J.H. Chung, J.H. Lee, G.J. Fisher, Y.S. Wan, E.A. Duell, et al. 2003. Topical N-acetyl cysteine and genistein prevent ultraviolet-light-induced signaling that leads to photoaging in human skin *in vivo*. J Invest Dermatol 120: 835-841.

Kang, S., S. Cho, J.H. Chung, C. Hammerberg, G.J. Fisher and J.J. Voorhees. 2005. Inflammation and extracellular matrix degradation mediated by activated transcription factors nuclear factor-kappaB and activator protein-1 in inflammatory acne lesions *in vivo*. Am J Pathol 166: 1691-1699.

Kireeva, M.L., B.V. Latinkic, T.V. Kolesnikova, C.C. Chen, G.P. Yang, A.S. Abler, et al. 1997. Cyr61 and Fisp12 are both ECM-associated signaling molecules: activities, metabolism and localization during development. Exp Cell Res 233: 63-77.

Kireeva, M.L., S.C. Lam and L.F. Lau. 1998. Adhesion of human umbilical vein endothelial cells to the immediate-early gene product Cyr61 is mediated through integrin alphavbeta3. J Biol Chem 273: 3090-3096.

Kondo, S. 2000. The roles of cytokines in photoaging. J Dermatol Sci 23 Suppl 1: S30-36.

Kondo, S. and D.N. Sauder. 1995. Keratinocyte-derived cytokines and UVB-induced immunosuppression. J Dermatol 22: 888-893.

Kondo, S., D.N. Sauder, T. Kono, K.A. Galley and R.C. McKenzie. 1994. Differential modulation of interleukin-1 alpha (IL-1 alpha) and interleukin-1 beta (IL-1 beta) in human epidermal keratinocytes by UVB. Exp Dermatol 3: 29-39.

Kouba, D.J., K.Y. Chung, T. Nishiyama, L. Vindevoghel, A. Kon, J.F. Klement, et al. 1999. Nuclear factor-kappa B mediates TNF-alpha inhibitory effect on alpha 2 (I) collagen (COL1A2) gene transcription in human dermal fibroblasts. J Immunol 162: 4226-4234.

Kripke, M.L. 1984. Immunological unresponsiveness induced by ultraviolet radiation. Immunol Rev 80: 87-102.

Krutmann, J. 2000. Ultraviolet A radiation-induced biological effects in human skin: relevance for photoaging and photodermatosis. J Dermatol Sci 23 Suppl 1: S22-26.

Kular, L., J. Pakradouni, P. Kitabgi, M. Laurent and C. Martinerie. 2011. The CCN family: a new class of inflammation modulators? Biochimie 93: 377-388.

Kunz, M., S. Moeller, D. Koczan, P. Lorenz, R.H. Wenger, M.O. Glocker, et al. 2003. Mechanisms of hypoxic gene regulation of angiogenesis factor Cyr61 in melanoma cells. J Biol Chem 278: 45651-45660.

Lau, L.F. 2011. CCN1/CYR61: the very model of a modern matricellular protein. Cell Mol Life Sci 68: 3149-3163.

Lau, L.F. and S.C. Lam. 1999. The CCN family of angiogenic regulators: the integrin connection. Exp Cell Res 248: 44-57.

Leask, A. and D.J. Abraham. 2006. All in the CCN family: essential matricellular signaling modulators emerge from the bunker. J Cell Sci 119: 4803-4810.

Leask, A., A. Holmes, C. Black and D. Abraham. 2003. Connective tissue growth factor gene regualtion. Requirements for its induction by transforming growth factor-beta 2 in fibroblasts. J Biol Chem 278: 13008-13015.

Lee, H.Y., J.W. Chung, S.W. Youn, J.Y. Kim, K.W. Park, B.K. Koo, et al. 2007. Forkhead transcription factor FOXO3a is a negative regulator of angiogenic immediate early gene CYR61, leading to inhibition of vascular smooth muscle cell proliferation and neointimal hyperplasia. Circ Res 100: 372-380.

Leivonen, S., L. Hakkinen, D. Lui and V. Kahari. 2001. Smad3 and extracellular signal-regulated kinase 1/2 coordinately mediate transforming growth factor-β-induced expression of connective tissue growth factor in human fibroblasts. J Invest Dermatol 124: 1162-1169.

Leu, S.J., S.C. Lam and L.F. Lau. 2002. Pro-angiogenic activities of CYR61 (CCN1) mediated through integrins alphavbeta3 and alpha6beta1 in human umbilical vein endothelial cells. J Biol Chem 277: 46248-46255.

Maggio, M., J.M. Guralnik, D.L. Longo and L. Ferrucci. 2006. Interleukin-6 in aging and chronic disease: a magnificent pathway. J Gerontol A Biol Sci Med Sci 61: 575-584.

Martin, R., C. Pierrard, F. Lejeune, P. Hilaire, L. Breton and F. Bernerd. 2008. Photoprotective effect of a water-soluble extract of Rosmarinus officinalis L. against UV-induced matrix metalloproteinase-1 in human dermal fibroblasts and reconstructed skin. Eur J Dermatol 18: 128-135.

Matrisian, L. 1994. Matrix metalloproteinase gene expression. Ann N Y Acad Sci 732: 42-50.

Mauviel, A. 1993. Cytokine regulation of metalloproteinase gene expression. J Cell Biochem 53: 288-295.

Menendez, J.A., I. Mehmi, D.W. Griggs and R. Lupu. 2003. The angiogenic factor CYR61 in breast cancer: molecular pathology and therapeutic perspectives. Endocr Relat Cancer 10: 141-152.

Mo, F.-E., A. Muntean, C.-C. Chen, D. Stolz, S. Watkins and L. Lau. 2002. CYR61 (CCN1) is essential for placental development and vascular integrity. Mol Cell Biol 22: 8709-8720.

Narayanan, D.L., R.N. Saladi and J.L. Fox. 2010. Ultraviolet radiation and skin cancer. Int J Dermatol 49: 978-986.

Nowinski, D., P. Hoijer, T. Engstrand, K. Rubin, B. Gerdin and M. Ivarsson. 2002. Keratinocytes inhibit expression of connective tissue growth factor in fibroblasts *in vitro* by an interleukin-1alpha-dependent mechanism. J Invest Dermatol 119: 449-455.

O'Brien, T., G. Yang, L.C. Sanders and L. Lau. 1990. Expression of cyr61, a growth factor-inducible immediate-early gene. Mol Cell Biol 10: 3569-3577.

Pashkow, F.J. 2011. Oxidative stress and inflammation in heart disease: do antioxidants have a role in treatment and/or prevention? Int J Inflam 2011: 514623.

Perbal, B. 2004. CCN proteins: multifunctional signalling regulators. Lancet 363: 62-64.

Perbal, B., D.R. Brigstock and L.F. Lau. 2003. Report on the second international workshop on the CCN family of genes. Mol Pathol 56: 80-85.

Perumal, S., O. Antipova and J.P. Orgel. 2008. Collagen fibril architecture, domain organization and triple-helical conformation govern its proteolysis. Proc Natl Acad Sci USA 105: 2824-2829.

Qin, Z., G.J. Fisher and T. Quan. 2013. Cysteine-rich protein 61 (CCN1) domain-specific stimulation of matrix metalloproteinase-1 expression through alphaVbeta3 integrin in human skin fibroblasts. J Biol Chem 288: 12386-12394.

Qin, Z., T. Okubo, J.J. Voorhees, G.J. Fisher and T. Quan. 2014a. Elevated cysteine-rich protein 61 (CCN1) promotes skin aging via upregulation of IL-1beta in chronically sun-exposed human skin. Age (Dordr) 36: 353-364.

Qin, Z., T. Okubo, J.J. Voorhees, G.J. Fisher and T. Quan. 2014b. Elevated cysteine-rich protein 61 (CCN1) promotes skin aging via upregulation of IL-1beta in chronically sun-exposed human skin. Age (Dordr) 36: 353-364.

Qin, Z., P. Robichaud, T. He, G.J. Fisher, J.J. Voorhees and T. Quan. 2014c. Oxidant exposure induces cysteine-rich protein 61 (CCN1) via c-Jun/AP-1 to reduce collagen expression in human dermal fibroblasts. PloS one 9: e115402.

Quan, T. 2013. Skin connective tissue aging and dermal fibroblasts. Dermal Fibroblasts: Histological Perspectives, Characterization and Role in Disease: 31-55.

Quan, T. and G.J. Fisher. 2015. Role of Age-Associated Alterations of the Dermal Extracellular Matrix Microenvironment in Human Skin Aging: A Mini-Review. Gerontology 61: 427-34.

Quan, T., T. He, J. Voorhees and G. Fisher. 2001a. Ultraviolet irradiation blocks cellular responses to transforming growth factor-β by down-regulating its type-II receptor and inducing Smad7. J Biol Chem 276: 26349-26356.

Quan, T., T. He, J.J. Voorhees and G.J. Fisher. 2001b. Ultraviolet irradiation blocks cellular responses to transforming growth factor-β by down-regulating its type-II receptor and inducing Smad7. J Biol Chem 276: 26349-26356.

Quan, T., T. He, S. Kang, J.J. Voorhees and G.J. Fisher. 2002. Connective tissue growth factor: expression in human skin *in vivo* and inhibition by ultraviolet irradiation. J Invest Dermatol 118: 402-408.

Quan, T., T. He, S. Kang, J.J. Voorhees and G.J. Fisher. 2004. Solar ultraviolet irradiation reduces collagen in photoaged human skin by blocking transforming growth factor-beta type II receptor/Smad signaling. Am J Pathol 165: 741-751.

Quan, T., T. He, Y. Shao, L. Lin, S. Kang, J.J. Voorhees, et al. 2006. Elevated cysteine-rich 61 mediates aberrant collagen homeostasis in chronologically aged and photoaged human skin. Am J Pathol 169: 482-490.

Quan, T., S. Shin, Z. Qin and G.J. Fisher 2009. Expression of CCN family of genes in human skin *in vivo* and alterations by solar-simulated ultraviolet irradiation. J Cell Commun Signal 3: 19-23.

Quan, T., Z. Qin, Y. Xu, T. He, S. Kang, J.J. Voorhees, et al. 2010a. Ultraviolet irradiation induces CYR61/CCN1, a mediator of collagen homeostasis, through activation of transcription factor AP-1 in human skin fibroblasts. J Invest Dermatol 130: 1697-1706.

Quan, T., Z. Qin, Y. Xu, T. He, S. Kang, J.J. Voorhees, et al. 2010b. Ultraviolet irradiation induces CYR61/CCN1, a mediator of collagen homeostasis, through activation of transcription factor AP-1 in human skin fibroblasts. J Invest Dermatol 130: 1697-1706.

Quan, T., Y. Shao, T. He, J.J. Voorhees and G.J. Fisher. 2010c. Reduced expression of connective tissue growth factor (CTGF/CCN2) mediates collagen loss in chronologically aged human skin. J Invest Dermatol 130: 415-424.

Quan, T., S. Shin, Z. Qin and G.J. Fisher. 2010d. Gene expression of CCN family members in young and aged human skin *in vivo*. CCN Proteins in Health and Disease: An Overview of the Fifth International Workshop on the CCN Family of Genes: 133-140.

Quan, T., Z. Qin, P. Robichaud, J.J. Voorhees and G.J. Fisher. 2011a. CCN1 contributes to skin connective tissue aging by inducing age-associated secretory phenotype in human skin dermal fibroblasts. J Cell Commun Signal 5: 201-207.

Quan, T., Z. Qin, P. Robichaud, J.J. Voorhees and G.J. Fisher. 2011b. CCN1 contributes to skin connective tissue aging by inducing Age-Associated Secretory Phenotype in human skin dermal fibroblasts. Journal of Cell Communication and Signaling 5: 201-207.

Quan, T., Z. Qin, J.J. Voorhees and G.J. Fisher. 2012a. Cysteine-rich protein 61 (CCN1) mediates replicative senescence-associated aberrant collagen homeostasis in human skin fibroblasts. J Cell Biochem 113: 3011-3018.

Quan, T., Z. Qin, J.J. Voorhees and G.J. Fisher. 2012b. Cysteine-rich protein 61 (CCN1) mediates replicative senescence-associated aberrant collagen homeostasis in human skin fibroblasts. J Cell Biochem 113: 3011-3018.

Quan, T., E. Little, H. Quan, Z. Qin, J.J. Voorhees and G.J. Fisher. 2013. Elevated matrix metalloproteinases and collagen fragmentation in photodamaged human skin: impact of altered extracellular matrix microenvironment on dermal fibroblast function. J Invest Dermatol 133: 1362-1366.

Rippe, R.A., L.W. Schrum, B. Stefanovic, J.A. Solis-Herruzo and D.A. Brenner. 1999. NF-kappaB inhibits expression of the alpha1 (I) collagen gene. DNA Cell Biol 18: 751-761.

Rittie, L., B. Perbal, J.J., Jr. Castellot, J.S. Orringer, J.J. Voorhees and G.J. Fisher. 2011. Spatial-temporal modulation of CCN proteins during wound healing in human skin *in vivo*. J Cell Commun Signal 5: 69-80.

Scharffetter-Kochanek, K., P. Brenneisen, J. Wenk, G. Herrmann, W. Ma, L. Kuhr, et al. 2000. Photoaging of the skin from phenotype to mechanisms. Exp Gerontol 35: 307-316.

Shi-Wen, X., A. Leask and D. Abraham. 2008. Regulation and function of connective tissue growth factor/CCN2 in tissue repair, scarring and fibrosis. Cytokine Growth Factor Rev 19: 133-144.

Uitto, J. and E.F. Bernstein. 1998. Molecular mechanisms of cutaneous aging: connective tissue alterations in the dermis. J Investig Dermatol Symp Proc 3: 41-44.

Underhill, G.H., G. Peter, C.S. Chen and S.N. Bhatia. 2012. Bioengineering methods for analysis of cells *in vitro*. Annu Rev Cell Dev Biol 28: 385-410.

Urbanski, A., T. Schwarz, P. Neuner, J. Krutmann, R. Kirnbauer, A. Kock, et al. 1990. Ultraviolet light induces increased circulating interleukin-6 in humans. J Invest Dermatol 94: 808-811.

Varani, J., R.L. Warner, M. Gharaee-Kermani, S.H. Phan, S. Kang, J.H. Chung, et al. 2000. Vitamin A antagonizes decreased cell growth and elevated collagen-degrading matrix metalloproteinases and stimulates collagen accumulation in naturally aged human skin. J Invest Dermatol 114: 480-486.

Varga, J., J. Rosenbloom and S.A. Jimenez. 1987. Transforming growth factor beta (TGF beta) causes a persistent increase in steady-state amounts of type I and type III collagen and fibronectin mRNAs in normal human dermal fibroblasts. Biochem J 247: 597-604.

Verrecchia, F., M. Pessah, A. Atfi and A. Mauviel. 2000. Tumor necrosis factor-α inhibits transforming growth factor-β/Smad signaling in human dermal fibroblasts via AP-1 activation. J Biol Chem 275: 30226-30231.

Vicentini, F.T., T. He, Y. Shao, M.J. Fonseca, W.A., Jr. Verri, G.J. Fisher, et al. 2011. Quercetin inhibits UV irradiation-induced inflammatory cytokine production in primary human keratinocytes by suppressing NF-kappaB pathway. J Dermatol Sci 61: 162-168.

White, L.A., T.I. Mitchell and C.E. Brinckerhoff. 2000. Transforming growth factor beta inhibitory element in the rabbit matrix metalloproteinase-1 (collagenase-1) gene functions as a repressor of constitutive transcription. Biochim Biophys Acta 1490: 259-268.

Wlaschek, M., I. Tantcheva-Poor, L. Naderi, W. Ma, L.A. Schneider, Z. Razi-Wolf, et al. 2001. Solar UV irradiation and dermal photoaging. J Photochem Photobiol B 63: 41-51.

Yaar, M. and B.A. Gilchrest. 2007. Photoageing: mechanism, prevention and therapy. Br J Dermatol 157: 874-887.

6

CHAPTER

Fibroblasts as Drivers of Healing and Cancer Progression: From *In vitro* Experiments to Clinics

Eliška Krejčí,[1,a] *Barbora Dvořánková,*[1,b] *Pavol Szabo,*[1,c] *Ondřej Naňka,*[1,d] *Hynek Strnad,*[2,e] *Ondřej Kodet,*[3,f] *Lukáš Lacina,*[3,g] *Michal Kolář*[2,h] *and Karel Smetana, jr*[1,i]

❏ Introduction

Tissues and organs are composed of cells as building stones. Biased by previous education in classical descriptive histology, we tend to see tissues as fairly stable structures. We admit certain dynamics and rapid changes during the lifetime especially through growth period of childhood and also in lesser extent during normal ageing. The reality is far more different. All the seeming tissue stability is resulting from a very complex orchestration of various, frequently counteracting, events. All the cells located in distinct types of tissues and organs, including skin, are participating on those

[1] Charles University, 1st Faculty of Medicine, Institute of Anatomy, U Nemocnice 3, 128 00 Prague 2, Czech Republic.
[2] Institute of Molecular Genetics, Academy of Sciences vvi., Vídeňská 1083, 142 20 Prague, Czech Republic.
[3] Charles University, 1st Faculty of Medicine, Institute of Anatomy and Department of Dermatovenerology, U Nemocnice 2 and 3, 128 00 Prague 2, Czech Republic.
[a] E-mail: eliska.krejci@lf1.cuni.cz
[b] E-mail: barbora.dvorankova@lf1.cuni.cz
[c] E-mail: pavol.szabo@lf1.cuni.cz
[d] E-mail: ondrej.nanka@lf1.cuni.cz
[e] E-mail: strnad@img.cas.cz
[f] E-mail: ondrej.kodet@lf1.cuni.cz
[g] E-mail: lukas.lacina@lf1.cuni.cz
[h] E-mail: kolarmi@img.cas.cz
* Corresponding author: karel.smetana@lf1.cuni.cz

events by mutual crosstalk mediated by numerous molecular messengers. This extensive conversation is conveyed by growth factors and molecules of extracellular matrix and reflects the actual position of an individual in wide ontogeny from prenatal stages of life till decease. Precise deciphering of this message can be complicated as individual components frequently reveal great context dependency. The crosstalk integrates internal impulses from the body and exogenous stimuli from the macroenvironment, including the interactions with e.g. microorganisms. Harmony of these signals and the optimal cellular response is necessary for the maintenance of proper homeostasis of the whole organism.

The progress of research in normal-tissue/cancer stem cells has resulted in a remarkable accumulation of scientific data on the influence of the microenvironment on cellular function. This chapter summarizes data on the intercellular interactions in human skin and other squamous epithelia and focuses predominantly on the role of fibroblasts in the course of wound healing and cancer formation.

❑ Functional Anatomy of Human Skin and its Appendages

Human skin is formed by epidermis, dermis with adjacent subcutaneous fat and skin appendageal organs. Epidermis is a multi-layered squamous epithelium. Given its structure and mechanical resistance, it protects our body against mechanical stress, excessive loss of water and invasion of pathogenic microorganisms. It is composed predominantly of specialized epithelial cells called keratinocytes. Keratinocytes of the basal epidermal layer are attached by hemidesmosomes to the basement membrane separating epidermis from dermis, the connective tissue component of skin. These basal keratinocytes are able to proliferate, but they enter mitosis only under specific tightly regulated physiological conditions. Keratinocytes of suprabasal layers are interconnected by desmosomes and they are keratinizing in direction to surface layers of epithelium. Fully keratinized cells of stratum corneum are continuously shed from the skin surface. Next to keratinocytes, the stratified epithelium contains also a minor populations of other cell types, such as intraepithelial leukocytes and professional antigen-presenting Langerhans cells, which protect the skin against invasion of microorganisms. Pigment cells, melanocytes, are located in the basal epithelial layer, where they protect the pool of proliferating keratinocytes against UV-light damage by pigment production and distribution. Mechanoreceptor Merkel cells are also located in basal layer. While keratinocytes are of ectodermal origin, the intraepidermal leukocytes and Langerhans cells originate from bone marrow and melanocytes and Merkel cells from neural crest (Szeder et al. 2003). These cells or their particular precursors colonize the epidermis, which represents a convenient microenvironment for their correct function.

Dermis is the connective tissue component of human skin. It is composed from numerous fibroblasts producing extracellular matrix molecules such as collagen and fibronectin. Dermis is rich in blood capillaries required for nutrition and oxygen supply for avascular epithelium. Oxygen, nutrients and metabolites diffuse to epidermis through the basement membrane. Leukocytes, predominantly tissue macrophages, are also present in dermis. Dermoepidermal junction is folded into rete ridges, this arrangement further reinforce contact and cohesivity of both layers. Dermis continues deeply to the subcutaneous connective tissue rich in adipocytes participating in the thermoprotection of body.

The hair, nails and sebaceous and sweat glands represent the main skin appendages. With respect to the topic of the chapter, we only discuss hair follicle. It is an invagination of epidermis composed from two layers, inner and outer root sheaths. Both epithelial layers are responsible for growth of hair from a widened region called the hair bulb. Hair bulb is tightly adjacent to dermal papilla containing loops of blood capillaries providing nutrition for the growing hair. Hair follicle represents the site of the attachment of smooth muscle (arrector pili muscle). The sebaceous gland opens to the hair follicle, where the secreted product covers surface of the hair. The part of outer root sheath between the arrector pili muscle insertion and opening of sebaceous gland is more voluminous and is called the bulge. It is important for the control of hair growth cycle and also represents a home site of stem cell populations (Bannister 1995).

❏ Stem Cells in Human Epidermis

Adult tissue stem cells are responsible for self-renewal of tissues and participate also in tissue repair. Stem cells usually undergo asymmetric mitosis. In such scenario the first daughter cell maintains the stem-cell properties and the second undergoes several mitoses and gives rise to population of so called transit amplifying cells. This progeny is the beginning of the differentiation cascade. At least three different populations of stem cells are located in human epidermis. Stem cells resident in the basal layer are more progenitor than the truly stem cells. The hair follicle epidermal stem cells are present in the bulge of hair follicle. They are multipotent with the potential to form keratinocytes and cells of sebaceous glands (Alonso and Fuchs 2003; Watt et al. 2006; Blanpain and Fuchs 2006). The differentiation potential of neural crest-originated stem cells present in the bulge of hair follicle is wide. *In vitro*, they have potency similar to neural crest cells, i.e., to create lineages ranging from chondrocytes to neurons (Sieber-Blum et al. 2004).

❏ Development of Human Epidermis and Hair Follicle

Epidermis develops from the embryonic surface ectoderm. This epithelial monolayer quickly changes to two-layered and subsequently further to multi-layered epithelium. Factors such as TGF-α, keratinocyte growth factor and endogenous lectin galectin-7 stimulate the growth of keratinocytes and formation of the epithelial multi-layer (Saussez and Kiss 2006; Visscher and Narendran 2014). Fibroblasts of prospective dermis influence the type of neighboring epidermis. For example, plantar fibroblasts are able to induce in co-culture the expression of palmar/plantar specific keratins in keratinocytes from other body sites (Yamaguchi et al. 1999). Development of hair follicles is quite similar to the development of other epithelial organs, like teeth and mammary glands. The epithelium thickens and forms a so called placode, which is growing as an epithelial bud against mesenchyme. It is surrounded by mesenchymal cells, which condense to form future dermal papilla. Intensive crosstalk between mesenchymal and epithelial cells regulating this morphogenetic process is mediated by many factors, namely BMP-4, members of fibroblasts growth factors family, Wnt family and Hedgehog family (Sonic hedgehog) is involved in this process (Mikkola and Millar 2006; Biggs and Mikkola 2014). In birds, it has been observed that the fine specificity of appendage is determined by the type of mesenchyme: mesenchyme from the body induces formation of feathers while the mesenchyme of the foot promotes formation of skin scales as verified by ectopic grafting of mesenchyme in chick embryos (Rawles 1963). These data demonstrate that the crosstalk between mesenchyme and epithelium is important for morphogenesis of cutaneous appendages and that the fibroblasts have a determinative role.

❑ Wound Healing

Damage to the skin compromises the barrier against the invasion of pathogenic microorganisms to the body. In case of extensive body surface injury, e.g., severe burns, the infection is complicated also by loss of water and minerals. The patient is subsequently endangered by the development of septic and hypovolemic shock syndrome. There highlights an urgent need for early wound closure.

   Wound healing can be characterized as a sequence of several steps resulting in the definitive closure of the wound (Cohen et al. 1975). Provisionally, the defect is covered by blood clot that later turns into a scab. The wound bed is readily colonized by the inflammatory cells responsible for removal of tissue debris and enhancement of an active barrier against pathogens. The dermal defect must be filled by granulation tissue, a soft connective tissue rich in fibroblasts producing extracellular matrix (molecules such as collagen, fibronectin and galectin-1) and plethora of growth factors, inflammatory cells as well as sprouting capillaries. Some fibroblasts undergo here transformation to myofibroblasts responsible for wound contraction (Kwon et al. 2006). This process is connected with activation of epidermal stem cells and mainly transit amplifying cells. The newly formed keratinocytes migrate from the hair follicles to superficial wounds or from the wound periphery to large and deep wounds (Brakebusch 2005). Remodeling of the defect follows after the final reepithelization is the last and also the longest step of the wound healing. Prolonged healing is usually connected with higher level of inflammation and incidence of myofibroblasts that could lead to formation of hypertrophic/keloid scars (van Beurden et al. 2005; Hinz 2007). Notably, adult skin usually repairs with occurrence of scars in contrast to prenatal scarless healing (Satish and Kathju 2010).

❑ Myofibroblasts in Wound Healing

In granulation tissue, the process of fibroblasts to myofibroblasts transition is under the paracrine control of other cell types including keratinocytes. The control is mediated predominantly by TGF-β1 and –3 (Lanning et al. 2000). These cytokines seem to be crucial for formation of the myofibroblasts. In addition to these factors galectin-1 (Gal-1), an endogenous lectin, is able to induce formation of myofibroblasts from the dermal fibroblasts. This Gal-1 activity is TGF-β1 independent, but synergistic (Dvořánková et al. 2011). Fibroblasts (and myofibroblasts) activated by TGF-β1 and/or by galectin-1 extensively produce fibrous ECM rich in fibronectin, tenascin and, as positive feedback loop, also Gal-1 (Fig. 1) (Dvořánková et al. 2011; Mifková et al. 2014). This ECM landscape influences also the phenotype of normal adherent keratinocytes *in vitro*. The cells turn small and express keratins typical for lowly differentiated keratinocytes. Gal-1 application to the experimental wound in rat model improved wound healing (Dvořánková et al. 2011). Gal-1 biological activity is dependent on lectin mechanism as depicted by inactivity of Gal-1 mutated in carbohydrate-recognition domain in the same experiment (Dvořánková et al. 2011). Immunocytochemical analysis of the granulation tissue confirmed presence of Gal-1 in experimental skin wound in rat and swine (Klíma et al. 2009; Gál et al. 2011). The role of Gal-1 in the process of wound healing is not specific for skin wound as similar observation was also reported during the healing of trachea in rat (Grendel et al. 2012). Gal-1 is also able to stimulate tissue fibrosis (Lim et al. 2014). When the wounded individuals are stimulated by estrogens, the role of fibroblasts/ myofibroblasts in granulation tissue seems to be sex-dependent. While transition of fibroblasts to myofibroblasts is stimulated by the agonists of oestrogen-α receptor, the production of extracellular matrix is supported by estrogen-β receptor agonists (Novotný et al. 2011). Some plant extracts used in herbalism and ethno medicine are also able to stimulate myofibroblast formation (Kováč et al. 2015).

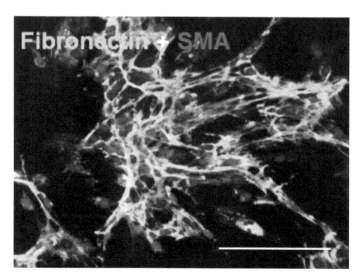

FIG. 1 *Human dermal fibroblasts treated by TGF-β1 produce extracellular matrix rich in fibronectin (green signal). Some cells are transformed to myofibroblasts exhibiting α-smooth muscle actin (SMA, red signal). Bar denotes 100 µm.*

Prolonged presence of myofibroblast in the wound leads to the formation of hypertrophic/keloid scars, which might be of clinical significance. In this line, the inactivation of TGF-β1 by inhibitors of DPP-IV has some therapeutic relevance (Seifert and Mrowietz 2009). Similarly, basic fibroblast growth factor (bFGF) is able to induce the apoptosis in myofibroblasts and reduce the tissue fibrosis (Akasaka et al. 2007). A synthetic low molecular weight polyamine BPA-C8 seems to have a similar effect (Nedeva et al. 2013). The polyamine reduces transition of fibroblasts to myofibroblasts (Mifková et al. 2014) and inhibits production of extracellular matrix molecules as fibronectin and tenascin. Moreover, it acts only on the cells that are in the process of transition to myofibroblasts. Pre-existing cells with α-smooth muscle actin (SMA), such as smooth muscle cells from the aorta, are not affected.

❏ Healing in Neonates

As mentioned above, the prenatal healing is virtually scarless. Neonates of up to age of one week heal rapidly with minimal scarring in comparison to older children and also adults (Borský et al. 2012). The observation is also supported by very rare anecdotic reports of regeneration of third digital phalanx in early postnatal mammals including humans (Han et al. 2008). Many pieces of evidence indicate that the virtually scarless healing is also related to reduced inflammatory response in fetuses (Liechty et al. 2000; Bukovsky et al. 2009; Kathju et al. 2012). High level of anti-inflammatory interleukin IL-10 seems to have a significant role (King et al. 2014). Reduced production of Gal-1 has been observed in neonatal fibroblasts in comparison to adult cells (Ho et al. 2014).

Fibroblasts prepared from early neonates, older children and adults exhibited *in vitro* similar morphology. However, the human neonatal dermal fibroblasts are rich in nestin, marker of immature cells (Krejčí et al. 2015). The number of nestin-positive cells decreases with ageing and only exceptional fibroblasts are positive in 5-years-old children. Production of extracellular matrix is also somewhat reduced in neonatal fibroblasts when compared to fibroblasts isolated from the skin of 9-months old baby. In other report neonatal fibroblasts isolated from the lip expressed pluripotency markers Oct-4 and Nanog when they were cultured according to protocol for neural crest-originated stem cells including chicken embryonic extract (Krejčí et al. 2015). Fibroblasts harvested from neonatal boys produced significantly lower quantity of pro-inflammatory cytokine IL-6 and chemokine IL-8 than those prepared from older boys (Bermudez et al. 2011). This observation clearly suggests that the fibroblasts actively participate in establishment of the pro-inflammatory tissue milieu. This is not so strong in fetuses and neonates. Neonatal and fetal fibroblasts also extensively produce matrix proteases that facilitate remodelation phase of wound healing and minimize the resulting scar (Cullen et al. 1997).

Although this chapter focuses predominantly on fibroblasts, we must inevitably comment also on neonatal keratinocytes as they form the indispensable partner for the cellular crosstalk. Porcine prenatal and human neonatal epidermis contains a population of remarkably small keratinocytes (Klíma et al. 2007; Krejčí et al. 2015). They fulfil criteria for epithelial-derived pop-up keratinocytes with stem cell-like properties (Marcelo et al. 2012). These cells are, in negligible proportion, present in adult human epidermis, where they are resistant to loss-of-anchorage dependent cell death, the anoikis (Dvořánková et al. 2005). *In vitro,* these small keratinocytes are positive not only for obligatory keratins but also for a mesenchymal marker vimentin (Krejčí et al. 2015). This observation can explain their ability to form colonies where vimentin is a necessary factor (Castro-Muñozledo et al. 2015).

❑ Clinical Aspects on Epithelial-mesenchymal Interaction in Wound Therapy

As mentioned above, the epithelial-mesenchymal interactions play a major role in wound healing. Already 40 years ago, Rheinwald and Green (1975) published a protocol for growth of human keratinocytes in a large-scale culture, using mouse fibroblasts with restricted proliferation activity as feeder cells. This technology is suitable for clinical purposes to cover extensive burns or trophic skin defects with quite encouraging results (Dvořánková et al. 1998, 2003). Unfortunately, this original method is associated with biosafety concerns due to use of animal serum and feeder cells of non-human origin. Thus, novel cultivation protocols and new generation of bioactive cultivation lattices enabling growth of keratinocytes in feeder-cell and animal-serum-free conditions were prepared. Despite this remarkable progress, the most efficient cultivation of keratinocytes still utilizes fibroblasts (Labský et al. 2003; Vacík et al. 2008; De Corte et al. 2012).

❑ Skin Cancer

In last decades, increasing incidence of tumors including the malignancies originating from epidermal cells, keratinocytes and melanocytes, is continuously reported. Epidemiological studies have shown association between the cancer incidence and increased life expectancy in developed countries. Ageing is accompanied by disturbances of cellular mechanisms that protect the genome against accumulation of acquired mutations, the major agents of cancer development (Smetana et al. 2013a). The growth of tumors is usually assumed to be autonomous and not respecting the physiological needs of organism. Similarly to normal organs, the tumors represent a complex tissue. Normal organ growth is influenced by other systems of the organism (Egblad et al. 2010). The idea, that the tumor can be also influenced by specific microenvironment was first proposed by Stephen Paget in the second half of nineteenth century who published on the "seed and soil" hypothesis. Hereby he tried to explain the stereotypical sites for metastases of certain types of tumors (reviewed and commented in Weinberg 2007). In agreement to philosophy adopted in our chapter, Harold Dvorak (1986) published an article, in which he demonstrated the remarkable similarity between morphological appearance of tumor with its stroma and wound healing, in which the granulation tissue plays such an important role.

❑ Cancer Stem Cells and Microenvironment

In most solid tumors, including the tumors originating from squamous epithelium, stem cell-like cells or tumor progenitor cells initiate the disease (Boehnke et al. 2012). The cancer stem cell origin can be explained by two putative mechanisms: the first possibility is based on the acquisition of a set of critical mutations in normal tissue stem cells. The second explanation assumes that mutated cells, other than stem cells, re-acquire properties of stem cells (Sell 2010). Nevertheless, the cancer stem cells have finally properties similar to normal stem cells. They proliferate slowly which makes their targeting by chemo- or actinotherapy difficult, as they are vulnerable to those therapies in S-phase of cell cycle only. Cancer stem cells are also equipped by active transport mechanisms capable of various xenobiotics elimination. These properties of cancer stem cells result in severe clinical complications of cancer therapy as multidrug resistance and/or minimal residual disease (Motlík et al. 2007).

The cancer frequently originates in exhibiting certain morphological abnormalities. Occurrence of cutaneous cancer in chronically photodamaged skin or around long lasting ulceration might be easily expected and it is a paradigm for dermatologists. On the other hand structural abnormalities can be clinically invisible, but they can be easily detected by histology or by molecular biology. For example, histologically normal squamous epithelium of oral cavity of smoking cancer patients who also abuse ethanol exhibits highly aberrant expression of galectin-9 and also aberrant keratin expression pattern, even in long distance from the tumor (Fík et al. 2013). This observation correlates well with clinically relevant hypothesis of field cancerization (Califano et al. 1996). Such aberrant tissue represents supportive environment for cancer stem cells. Similarly to normal tissue stem cells, even the cancer stem cells vitally require supportive microenvironment (Plzák et al. 2010), otherwise their unique features are inevitably lost. This microenvironment enabling and probably also actively participating in the expansive growth of cancer cells is traditionally called the tumor stroma. Tumour stroma is in various aspects similar to the granulation tissue in wounds and includes these cell types: fibroblasts producing extracellular matrix, infiltrating immune cells and endothelia. Similarly to wound healing, there is also an extensive mutual crosstalk between the tumor stroma and the tumor cells. The stroma is not just a passive permissive environment, but it is significantly influencing biological properties of cancer cells which might be reflected in e.g. readiness to metastasation. Indeed, cancer-associated fibroblasts (CAF) present in tumor stroma have been widely characterized as stimulators of cancer growth and metastasation as has been demonstrated for example in breast (Karnoub et al. 2007), prostate (Cunha et al. 2003) and lung (El-Nikhely et al. 2012) cancer. On the other hand, the inhibitory effect of CAF on cancer growth has also been reported for example in pancreas (Özdemir et al. 2014; Rhim et al. 2014). The stroma is, conversely, dependent on signalization from the cancer cells (Polyak et al. 2009).

The fibroblasts located in the tumor stroma, similarly to the granulation-tissue-located myofibroblasts, frequently but not necessarily express SMA (Smetana et al. 2013b). Their origin is still unclear. Experimental as well as clinical data demonstrate a wide range of cell types able to give rise to CAF. Those cell types include local fibroblasts, monocytes, myoepithelial cells, endothelium, pericytes, smooth muscle cells, hepatic/pancreatic stellate cells, adipocytes, mesenchymal stem cells and cancer epithelial cells themselves (De Wever et al. 2008). Formation of myofibroblasts from local fibroblasts is not surprising, as commented earlier in the paragraph on wound healing and also on adnexal organogenesis. Similarly, the role of mesenchymal stem cells has been demonstrated and their role in squamous cell carcinoma of the head and neck has been established (De Boeck et al. 2010). Formation of CAF by epithelial-mesenchymal transition from tumor epithelium is widely discussed, however this topic remains controversial. Experimental study of Petersen et al. (2003) demonstrated that cancer cells can participate in the formation of stromal elements similar to CAF. Our own data are depicting this phenomenon *in vitro* as well (Lacina et al. 2007b), however, there is recently no exact evidence of this mechanism of CAF formation or estimation of its relevance at clinical level (Marsh et al. 2013). Further, our recent data obtained on mice xenografted with human cancer cells, illustrate that CAF originate from the cells of host and not from the grafted cancer cells (Dvořánková et al. 2015).

❑ Cancer Originating from Squamous Epithelium

In skin cancer and cancer originating from squamous epithelium of upper aerodigestive tract, the role of CAF is well established. In basal cell carcinoma, the stromal reaction reflects the local aggressiveness of tumor growth, which can be employed for decision on therapeutic strategy (Bertheim et al. 2004). The expression profile of stromal fibroblasts from basal cell carcinoma significantly differs from normal dermal fibroblasts with 640 differentially expressed genes detected *in situ* (Micke et al. 2007). Fibroblasts isolated from the basal cell carcinoma produce similarly to CAF *in situ* extracellular matrix rich in galectin-1. They influence differentiation pattern of normal human keratinocytes to resemble the cells of basal cell carcinoma and stimulate nuclear expression of nucleostemin in the keratinocytes (Lacina et al. 2007a). The CAF are also able to influence cancer unrelated co-cultured immortalized fibroblasts to acquire the differentiation plasticity similar to mesenchymal stem cells. This observation highlights complexity in regulation and maintenance of tumor microenvironment. The role of growth factors such as IGF-2, FGF-7, leptin, nerve growth factor and TGF-β has been established to participate in the activity of CAF (Szabo et al. 2011).

Fibroblasts isolated from the head and neck squamous cell carcinoma differ in activity of almost 600 genes from normal mucosal fibroblasts and they are able to influence the phenotype of normal keratinocytes and induce epithelial-mesenchymal transition (Lacina et al. 2007b; Strnad et al. 2010). On the other hand, when normal fibroblasts are cultured with cancer and/or normal keratinocytes, they significantly change expression of proteins related to cytoskeleton rearrangement. Moreover, they express proinflammatory cytokines and chemokines (IL-6, IL-8, CXCL-1) that are present also in human tumor biopsies. However, their production is transient and lasts shorter than in case of CAF co-cultured with keratinocytes (Szabo et al. 2013). Of note, many of those bioactive molecules are part of so called senescence associated secretory phenotype. This should not be misinterpreted as a straight forward proof of replicative senescence, but on the contrary should be seen as functional signature of fibroblasts interacting with epithelial cells. The prolonged dynamics of this interaction is probably important driving force in cancer progression. These substances are able to influence the phenotype of cultured keratinocytes, more intensely when administered simultaneously (Kolář et al. 2012). Similarly to wound healing and basal cell carcinoma formation, squamous cell carcinoma formation is associated with high occurrence of Gal-1 in tumor stroma (Valach et al. 2012). Its presence is reflected by high incidence of SMA-positive CAF in the stroma and high activity of genes, which indicate rapid tumor progression, in cancer cells. Gal-1-stimulated dermal fibroblasts and CAF positively influence growth of endothelial cells and can be important for tumor vascularization (Peржelová et al. 2014).

❑ Malignant Melanoma

Malignant melanoma, highly aggressive cutaneous tumor, is derived from melanocytes, a minor epidermal cell population. Melanoma is also significantly influenced by its microenvironment similar to more frequent keratinocytic tumors. Surprisingly, when melanoma cells are injected to the embryo, they lose their malignant behavior and migrate in pathways typical for embryonic neural crest cells, the precursors of normal melanocytes (Kulesa et al. 2006). In various models of microenviroment, fibroblasts, embryonic extract and human embryonic stem cells conditioned medium have a distinct influence on the phenotype of melanoma cells too (Kodet et al. 2013). Keratinocytes also influence their migratory activity (Sogabe et al. 2006). On the other hand, the melanoma cells are able to influence properties of fibroblasts (Li et al. 2009) and model the landscape of neighboring keratinocytes by induction of pseudohyperplastic changes in the epidermis overlaying nodular melanoma. An *in vitro* model explains the observation *in situ*, as melanoma cells and neural crest-originated stem cells influence the differentiation pattern of co-cultured keratinocytes by production of FGF-2, CXCL-1, IL-8 and VEGF-A (Kodet et al. 2015).

❑ Conclusion

The remarkable similarity between skin development, wound healing and cancer was demonstrated by multiple models with emphasis on intercellular crosstalk. Fibroblasts play here a significant role of structural and regulatory hubs (Fig. 2). In skin wound, the fibroblasts participate during the course of healing. Their function here has obvious effective timeframe and any deviation from this timeframe can lead to various consecutive pathologies. In cancer, a series of genetic errors starts up the cancerous programme, but the role of microenvironments with remarkable contribution of stromal fibroblast should not be overseen. They support the growth and metastasation of cancer cells. Mechanistically, similar and widely overlapping repertoire of cytokines can be seen in senescence, in wound healing and cancer. Better understanding to the role of fibroblasts and their temporal and spatial regulation in the above described situations may be useful for the development of new therapeutic strategies for management of signs of skin ageing, acute and chronic wounds and also for cancer therapy.

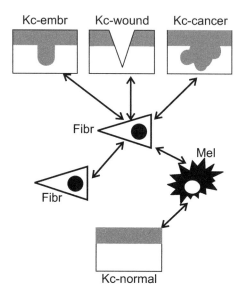

FIG. 2   *Extensive intercellular crosstalks between fibroblasts (Fibr) and keratinocytes in course of skin development (Kc-embr), keratinocytes in course of skin healing (Kc-wound), malignant keratinocytes (Kc-cancer), other fibroblasts (Fibr) and melanoma cells (Mel) have been demonstrated. Melanoma cells interact mutually also with normal keratinocytes.*

❑ Acknowledgements

Part of the results presented in this study was obtained with financial support of the Grant Agency of the Czech Republic (projects no. 304/12/1333 and 13-20293S), of the Charles University in Prague (projects PRVOUK-27 and UNCE 204013), Grant Agency of the Ministry of Health (project no. NT-13488-4), Agency for Medical Research of the Czech Republic (project no. 15-28933A) and EC project BIOCEV (Biotechnology and Biomedicine Centre of the Academy of Sciences and Charles University in Vestec -CZ.1.05/1.1.00/02.0109 from the European Regional Development Fund). Authors are grateful to Professor Jiri Stork for critical reading of the manuscript.

❏ References

Akasaka, Y., I. Ono, A. Tominaga, Y. Ishikawa, K. Ito, T. Suzuki, et al. 2007. Basic fibroblast growth factor in an artificial dermis promotes apoptosis and inhibits expression of α–smooth muscle actin, leading to reduction of wound contraction. Wound Rep Reg 15: 378-389.

Alonso, L. and E. Fuchs. 2003. Stem cells of the skin epithelium. Proc Natl Acad Sci USA 100 (Suppl 1): 11830-11835.

Bannister, L.H. 1995. Integumental system. pp 375-424. *In*: Williams, P.L. [ed.]. Gray´s Anatomy. Churchill Livingstone, New York, NY, USA.

Bermudez, D.M., D.A. Canning and K.W. Liechty. 2011. Age and pro inflammatory cytokine production: Wound-healing implications for scar-formation and the timing of genital surgery in boys. J Pediatric Urol 7: 324e331.

Bertheim, U., P.A. Hoferb, A. Engström-Laurentc and S. Hellström. 2004. The stromal reaction in basal cell carcinomas. A prerequisite for tumour progression and treatment strategy. Br Ass Plast Surg 57: 429-439.

Biggs, L.C. and M.L. Mikkola. 2014. Early inductive events in ectodermal appendage morphogenesis. Semin Cell Dev Biol 25-26: 11-21.

Blanpain, C. and E. Fuchs. 2006. Epidermal stem cells of the skin. Annu Rev Cell Dev Biol 22: 339-73.

Boehnke K., B. Falkowska-Hanseny, H.-J. Stark and P. Boukamp. 2012. Stem cells of the human epidermis and their niche: composition and function in epidermal regeneration and carcinogenesis. Carcinogenesis 33: 1247-1258.

Borský, J., J. Velemínská, M. Jurovčík, J. Kozák, D. Hechtová, M. Tvrdek, et al. 2012. Successful early neonatal repair of cleft lip within first 8 days of life. Int J Ped Otorhinolaryngology 76: 1616-1626.

Brakebusch, C. 2005. Keratinocyte migration in wound healing. pp 275-298. *In*: Wedlich, D. [ed.]. Cell Migration in Development and Disease. Wiley-WCH, Weinheim, Germany.

Bukovsky, A., M.R. Caudle, R.J. Carson, F. Gaytán, M. Huleihel, A. Kruse, et al. 2009. Immune physiology in tissue regeneration and aging, tumor growth and regenerative medicine. Aging 1: 157-181.

Califano, J., P. van der Riet, W. Westra, H. Nawroz, G. Clayman, S. Piantadosi, et al. 1996. Genetic progression model for head and neck cancer: implications for field cancerization. Cancer Res 56: 2488-2492.

Castro-Muñozledo, F., C. Velez-DelValle, M. Marsch-Moreno, M. Hernández-Quintero and W. Kuri-Harcuch. 2015. Vimentin is necessary for colony growth of human diploid keratinocytes. Histochem Cell Biol 143: 45-57.

Cohen, B.H., L.A. Lewis and S.S. Resnik. 1975. Wound healing: a brief review. Int J Dermatol 14: 722-726.

Cullen, B., D. Silcock, L.J. Brown, A. Gosiewska and J.C. Geesin. 1997. The differential regulation and secretion of proteinases from fetal and neonatal fibroblasts by growth factors. Int J Biochem Cell Biol 29: 241-50.

Cunha, G.R., S.W. Haywards, Y.Z. Wang and W.A. Ricke. 2003. Role of the stromal microenvironment in cancerogenesis of the prostate. Int J Cancer 107: 1-10.

De Boeck, A., K. Narine, W. De Neve, M. Mareel, M. Bracke and O. De Wever. 2010. Resident and bone marrow-derived mesenchymal stem cells in head and neck squamous cell carcinoma. Oral Oncol 46: 336-342.

De Corte, P., G. Verween, G. Verbeken, T. Rose, S. Jennes, A. De Coninck, et al. 2012. Feeder layer- and animal product-free culture of neonatal foreskin keratinocytes: improved performance, usability, quality and safety. Cell Tissue Bank 13: 175-89.

De Wever, O., P. Demetter, M. Mareel and M. Bracke. 2008. Stromal myofibroblasts are drivers of invasive cancer growth. Int J Cancer 123: 2229-2238.

Dvorak, H.F. 1986. Tumors: wounds that do not heal. Similarities between tumor stroma generation and wound healing. N Engl J Med 315: 1650-1659.

Dvořánková, B., K. Smetana Jr, R. Königová, H. Singerová, J. Vacík, M. Jelínková, et al. 1998. Cultivation and grafting of human keratinocytes on a poly (hydroxyethyl methacrylate) support to the wound bed: a clinical study. Biomaterials 19: 141-146.

Dvořánková, B., Z. Holíková, J. Vacík, R. Königová, Z. Kapounková, J. Michálek, et al. 2003. Reconstruction of epidermis by grafting of keratinocytes cultured on polymer support-clinical study. Int J Dermatol 42: 219-23.

Dvořánková, B., P. Szabo, L. Lacina, P. Gal, J. Uhrová, T. Zima, et al. 2011. Human galectins induce conversion of dermal fibroblasts into myofibroblasts and production of extracellular matrix: potential application in tissue engineering and wound repair. Cells Tissues Organs 194: 469-480.

Dvořánková, B., K. Smetana Jr., B. Říhová, J. Kučera, R. Mateu and P. Szabo. 2015. Cancer-associated fibroblasts are not formed from cancer cells by epithelial-to-mesenchymal transition in nu/nu mice. Histochem Cell Biol 143: 463-469.

Dvořánková, B., K. Smetana Jr., M. Chovanec, L. Lacina, J. Štork, Z. Plzáková, et al. 2005. Transient expression of keratin K19 is induced in originally negative interfollicular epidermal cells by adhesion of suspended cells. Int J Mol Med 16: 525-531.

Egblad, M., E.S. Nakasone and Z. Werb. 2010. Tumors as organs: complex tissues that interface with the entire organism. Dev Cell 18: 884-901.

El-Nikhely, N., L. Larzabal, W. Seeger, A. Calvo and R. Savai. 2012. Tumor-stromal interactions in lung cancer: novel candidate targets for therapeutic intervention. Expert Opin Investig Drugs 21: 1107-1122.

Fík, Z., J. Valach, M. Chovanec, J. Mazánek, R. Kodet, O. Kodet, et al. 2013. Loss of adhesion/growth-regulatory galectin-9 from squamous cell epithelium in head and neck carcinomas. J Oral Pathol Med 42: 166-173.

Gál, P., T. Vasilenko, M. Kostelníková, J. Jakubčo, I. Kováč, F. Sabol, et al. 2011. Open wound healing *in vivo*: monitoring, binding and presence of adhesion/growth-regulatory galectins in rat skin during the course of complete re-epithelialization. Acta Histochem Cytochem 44: 191-199.

Grendel, T., J. Sokolský, A. Vaščáková, V. Hudák, M. Chovanec, F. Sabol, et al. 2012. Early stages of trachea healing process: (immuno/lectin) histochemical monitoring of selected markers and adhesion/growth-regulatory endogenous lectins. Folia Biol 58: 135-143.

Han, M., X. Yang, J. Lee, C.A. Allan and K. Muneoka. 2008. Development and regeneration of the neonatal digit tip in mice. Dev Biol 315: 125-135.

Hinz, B. 2007. Formation and function of the myofibroblast during tissue repair. J Invest Dermatol 127: 526-537.

Ho, S., H. Marçal and L.J. Foster. 2014. Towards scarless wound healing: a comparison of protein expression between human, adult and foetal fibroblasts. Biomed Res Int 2014: 676493.

Karnoub, A.E., A.B. Dash, A.P. Vo, A. Sullivan, M.W. Brooks, G.W. Bell, et al. 2007. Mesenchymal stem cells within tumour stroma promote breast cancer metastasis. Nature 449: 557-565.

Kathju, S., P.H. Gallo and L. Satish. 2012. Scarless integumentary wound healing in the mammalian fetus: molecular basis and therapeutic implications. Birth Defects Res C Embryo Today 96: 223-236.

King, A., S. Balaji, L.D. Le, T.M. Crombleholme and S.G. Keswani. 2014. Regenerative wound healing: the role of interleukin-10. Adv Wound Care 3: 315-323.

Klíma, J., J. Motlík, H.-J. Gabius and K. Smetana Jr. 2007. Phenotypic characterization of porcine interfollicular keratinocytes separated by elutriation: a technical note. Folia Biol 53: 33-36.

Klíma, J., L. Lacina, B. Dvořánková, D. Herrmann, J.W. Carnwath, H. Niemann, et al. 2009. Differential regulation of galectin expression/reactivity during wound healing in porcine skin and in cultures of epidermal cells with functional impact on migration. Physiol Res 58: 873-884.

Kodet, O., B. Dvořánková, E. Krejčí, P. Szabo, P. Dvořák, J. Štork, et al. 2013. Cultivation-dependent plasticity of melanoma phenotype. Tumor Biol 34: 3345-3355.

Kodet, O., L. Lacina, E. Krejčí, B. Dvořánková, M. Grim, J. Štork, et al. 2015. Melanoma cells influence the differentiation pattern of human epidermal keratinocytes. Molecular Cancer 14: 1.

Kolář, M., P. Szabo, B. Dvořánková, L. Lacina, H.-J. Gabius, H. Strnad, et al. 2012. Upregulation of IL-6, IL-8 and CXCL-1 production in dermal fibroblasts by normal/malignant epithelial cells *in vitro*, immunohistochemical and transcriptomic analyses. Biol Cell 104: 738-751.

Kováč, I., J. Ďurkáč, M. Hollý, K. Jakubčová, V. Peržeľová, P. Mučaji, et al. 2015. *Plantagolanceolata L.* water extract induces transition of fibroblasts into myofibroblasts and increases tensile strength of healing skin wounds. J Pharm Pharmacol 67: 117-125.

Krejčí, E., O. Kodet, P. Szabo, J. Borský, K. Smetana Jr., M. Grim, et al. 2015. *In vitro* differences of neonatal and later postnatal keratinocytes and dermal fibroblasts. Physiol Res 64: 561-569.

Kulesa, P.M., J.C. Kasemeier-Kulesa, J.M. Teddy, N.V. Margaryan, E.A. Seftor, R.E. Seftor, et al. 2006. Reprogramming metastatic melanoma cells to assume a neural crest cell-like phenotype in an embryonic microenvironment. Proc Natl Acad Sci USA 103: 3752-3757.

Kwon, Y.-B., H.-W. Kim, D.-H. Roh, S.-Y. Yoon, R.-M. Baek, J.-Y. Kim, et al. 2006. Topical application of epidermal growth factor accelerates wound healing by myofibroblast proliferation and collagen synthesis in rat. J Vet Sci 7: 105-109.

Labský, J., B. Dvořánková, K. Smetana Jr., Z. Holíková, L. Broz and H.-J. Gabius. 2003. Mannosides as crucial part of bioactive supports for cultivation of human epidermal keratinocytes without feeder cells. Biomaterials 24: 863-872.

Lacina, L., K. Smetana Jr, B. Dvořánková, R. Pytlík, L. Kideryová, L. Kučerová, et al. 2007a. Stromal fibroblasts from basal cell carcinoma affect phenotype of normal keratinocytes. Brit J Dermatol 156: 819-829.

Lacina, L., B. Dvořánková, K. Smetana Jr, M. Chovanec, J. Plzák, R. Tachezy, et al. 2007b. Marker profiling of normal keratinocytes identifies the stroma from squamous cell carcinoma of the oral cavity as a modulatory microenvironment in co-culture. Int J Radiat Biol 83: 837-848.

Lanning, D.A., R.F. Digelmann, D.R. Yager, M.L. Wallace, C.E. Bagwell and J.H. Hayens. 2000. Myofibroblast induction with transforming growth factor-β1 and -β3 in cutaneous fetal excisional wounds. J Ped Surg 35: 183-188.

Li, L., B. Dragulev, P. Zigrino, C. Mauch and J.W. Fox. 2009. The invasive potential of human melanoma cell lines correlates with their ability to alter fibroblast gene expression in vitro and the stromal microenvironment in vivo. Int J Cancer 125: 1796-804.

Liechty, K.W., N.S. Adzick and T.M. Crombleholme. 2000. Diminished interleukin 6 (IL-6) production during scarless human fetal wound repair. Cytokine 12: 671-676.

Lim, M.J., J. Ahn, J.Y. Yi, M.H. Kim, A.R. Son, S.L. Lee, et al. 2014. Induction of galectin-1 by TGF-β1 accelerates fibrosis through enhancing nuclear retention of Smad2. Exp Cell Res 326: 125-135.

Marcelo, C.L., A. Peramo, A. Ambati and S.E. Feinberg. 2012. Characterization of a unique technique for culturing primary adult human epithelial progenitor/"stem cells." BMC Dermatol 12: 8.

Marsh, T., K. Pietras and S.S. McAllister. 2013. Fibroblasts as architects of cancer pathogenesis. Biochim Biophys Acta 1832: 1070-1078.

Micke, P., K. Kappert, M. Ohshima, C. Sundquist, S. Scheidl, P. Lindahl, et al. 2007. *In situ* identification of genes regulated specifically in fibroblasts of human basal cell carcinoma. J Invest Dermatol 127: 1516-1523.

Mifková, A., O. Kodet, P. Szabo, J. Kučera, B. Dvořánková, S. André, et al. 2014. Synthetic polyamine BPA-C8 inhibits TGF-β1-mediated conversion of human dermal fibroblast to myofibroblasts and establishment of galectin-1-rich extracellular matrix in vitro. Chem Bio Chem 15: 1465-1470.

Mikkola, M.L. and S.E. Millar. 2006. The mammary bud as a skin appendage: unique and shared aspects of development. J Mammary Gland Biol Neoplasia 11: 187-203.

Motlík, J., J. Klíma, B. Dvořánková and K. Smetana Jr. 2007. Porcine epidermal stem cells as a biomedical model for wound healing and normal/malignant epithelial cell propagation. Theriogenology 67: 105-111.

Nedeva, I., G. Koripelly, D. Caballero, L. Chièze, B. Guichard, B. Romain, et al. 2013. Synthetic polyamines promote rapid lamellipodial growth by regulating actin dynamics. Nat Commun 4: 2165.

Novotný, M., T. Vasilenko, L. Varinská, K. Smetana Jr., P. Szabo, M. Šarišský, et al. 2011. ER-α agonist induces conversion of fibroblasts into myofibroblasts, while ER-β agonist increases ECM production and wound tensile strength of healing skin wounds in ovarectomised rats. Exp Dermatol 20: 703-708.

Özdemir, B.C., T. Pentcheva-Hoang, J.L. Carstens, X. Zheng, C.C. Wu, T.R. Simpson, et al. 2014. Depletion of carcinoma-associated fibroblasts and fibrosis induces immunosuppression and accelerates pancreas cancer with reduced survival. Cancer Cell 25: 719-734.

Peržélová, V., L. Varinská, B. Dvořanková, P. Szabo, P. Spurný, J. Valach, et al. 2014. Extracellular matrix of galectin-1-exposed dermal and tumor-associated fibroblasts favors growth of human umbilical vein endothelial cells *in vitro*: A short report. Anticancer Res 34: 3991-3996.

Petersen, O.W., H.L. Nielsen, T. Gudjonsson, R. Villadsen, F. Rank, E. Niebuhr et al. 2003. Epithelial to mesenchymal transition in human breast cancer can provide a nonmalignant stroma. Am J Pathol 162: 391-402.

Plzák, J., L. Lacina, M. Chovanec, B. Dvoránková, P. Szabo, Z. Cada, et al. 2010. Epithelial-stromal interaction in squamous cell epithelium-derived tumors: an important new player in the control of tumor biological properties. Anticancer Res 30: 455-462.

Polyak, K., I. Haviv and I.G. Campbell. 2009. Co-evolution of tumor cells and their microenvironment. Trends Genet 25: 30-38.

Rawles, M.E. 1963. Tissue interactions in scale and feather development as studied in dermal-epidermal recombinations. J Embryol Exp Morphol 11: 765-789.

Rheinwald, J.G. and H. Green. 1975. Serial cultivation of strains of human epidermal keratinocytes: the formation of keratinizing colonies from single cells. Cell 6: 331-343.

Rhim, A.D., P.E. Oberstein, D.H. Thomas, E.T. Mirek, C.F. Palermo, S.A. Sastra, et al. 2014. Stromal elements act to restrain, rather than support, pancreatic ductal adenocarcinoma. Cancer Cell 25: 735-747.

Satish, L. and S. Kathju. 2010. Cellular and molecular characteristics of scarless versus fibrotic wound healing. Dermatol. Res. Pract. 2010: Article ID 790234.

Saussez, S. and R. Kiss. 2006. Galectin-7. Cell Mol Life Sci 63: 686-697.

Seifert, O. and U. Mrowietz. 2009. Keloid scarring: bench and bedside. Arch Dermatol Res 301: 259-272.

Sell, S. 2010. On the stem cell origin of cancer. Am J Pathol 176: 2584-2594.

Sieber-Blum, M., M. Grim, Y.F. Hu and V. Szeder. 2004. Pluripotent neural crest stem cells in the adult hair follicle. Dev Dyn 231: 258-269.

Smetana, K. Jr., B. Dvoránková and L. Lacina. 2013a. Phylogeny, regeneration, ageing and cancer: role of microenvironment and possibility of its therapeutic manipulation. Folia Biol 59: 207-216.

Smetana, K. Jr., B. Dvoránková, P. Szabo, H. Strnad and M. Kolár. 2013b. Role of stromal fibroblasts in cancer originated from squamous epithelia. pp 83-84. *In*: Bai, X. [ed.]. Dermal Fibroblasts: Histological Perspectives, Characterization and Role in Disease. Nova Sciences Publishers, New York, NY, USA.

Sogabe, Y., M. Abe, Y. Yokoyama, O. Ishikawa. 2006. Basic fibroblast growth factor stimulates human keratinocyte motility by Rac activation. Wound Repair Regen 14: 457-462.

Strnad, H., L. Lacina, M. Kolár, Z. Cada, C. Vlcek, B. Dvoránková, et al. 2010. Head and neck squamous cancer fibroblasts produce growth factors influencing phenotype of normal human keratinocytes. Histochem. Cell Biol 133: 201-211.

Szabo, P., M. Kolár, B. Dvoránková, L. Lacina, J. Stork, C. Vlcek, et al. 2011. Mouse 3T3 fibroblasts under the influence of fibroblasts isolated from stroma of human basal cell carcinoma acquire properties of multipotent stem cells. Biol Cell 103: 233-248.

Szabo, P., J. Valach, K. Smetana Jr., B. Dvoránková. 2013. Comparative analysis of IL-8 and CXCL-1 production by normal and cancer stromal fibroblasts. Folia Biol 59: 134-137.

Szeder, V., M. Grim, Z. Halata and M. Sieber-Blum. 2003. Neural crest origin of mammalian Merkel cells. Dev Biol 253: 258-263.

Vacík, J., B. Dvořánková, J. Michálek, M. Přádný, E. Krumbholcová, T. Fenclová, et al. 2008. Cultivation of human keratinocytes without feeder cells on polymer carriers containing ethoxyethyl methacrylate: in vitro study. J Mater Sci Mater Med 19: 883-888.

Valach, J., Z. Fík, H. Strnad, M. Chovanec, J. Plzák, Z. Čada, et al. 2012. Smooth muscle actin expressing stromal fibroblasts in head and neck squamous cell carcinoma: increased expression of galectin-1 and induction of poor prognosis factors. Int J Cancer 131: 2499-2508.

van Beurden, H.E., J.W. Von den Hoff, R. Torensma, J.C. Maltha and A.M. Kuijpers-Jagtman. 2005. Myofibroblasts in palatal wound healing: Prospects for the reduction of wound contraction after cleft palate repair. J Dent Res 84: 871-880.

Visscher, M. and V. Narendran. 2014. The ontogeny of skin. Adv Wound Care 3: 291-303.

Watt, F.M., C.L. Celso and V. Silva-Vargas. 2006. Epidermal stem cells: an update. Current Opinion Genet Develop 16: 518-524.

Weinberg, R.A. 2007. The Biology of Cancer. Garland Science, New York, NY, USA.

Yamaguchi, Y., S. Itami, M. Tarutani, K. Hosokawa, H. Miura and K. Yoshikaw. 1999. Regulation of keratin 9 in nonpalmoplantar keratinocytes by palmoplantar fibroblasts through epithelial-mesenchymal interactions. J Invest Dermatol 112: 483-488.

Mitochondrial DNA Common Deletion in Human Skin Connective Tissue Aging

Chunji Quan

❑ Introduction

Human skin is the largest and heaviest organ of the human body. Skin provides a protective barrier from environmental stressors, such as heat, solar ultraviolet (UV) irradiation, infection, injury and water loss. Human skin undergoes a natural aging process with the passage of time. However, unlike other organs, human skin is constantly exposed environment insults, such as solar UV irradiation that leads to accelerate aging process (Berneburg et al. 2000; Fisher et al. 1996). Based on its causes, skin aging is classified into two types: natural aging and photoaging (Chung 2003; Yaar et al. 2002). Natural aging refers to those changes observed in all individuals resulting from the passage of time, whereas photoaging refers to those changes attributable to habitual sun exposure. Both of these processes are cumulative, therefore photoaging is superimposed on intrinsic aging.

Histological studies have revealed that the major alterations in aged skin are localized to the collage-rich connective tissue and are manifested as a thin and damaged dermis (Fisher et al. 2008; Fisher et al. 1997). These features are derived directly from deleterious alterations in collagen, the most abundant structural protein in skin. Impairment of the dermal collagenous ECM microenvironment directly relate to the development of age-related skin pathologies by causing increased fragility, impaired vasculature support, poor wound healing and a tissue microenvironment that promotes epithelial cancer (Bissell and Hines 2011; Bissell et al. 2005; Kudravi and Reed 2000).

Department of Pathology, Affiliated Hospital of Yanbian University, Yanji 133000, Jilin Province, China.
E-mail: chunjiquan@163.com

In cellular levels, alterations of the collagenous ECM microenvironment significantly disrupt cell-extracellular matrix (ECM) interaction and thus impair cellular function.

As dermal fibroblasts are largely responsible for collagen homeostasis, impaired dermal fibroblast function is a major contributing factor in human skin connective tissue aging (Quan 2013; Quan and Fisher 2015; Quan et al. 2010). Impaired dermal fibroblast function is largely resulted from loss of cell shape and size, due to disruption of cell-ECM interaction (Fisher et al. 2008; Qin et al. 2014; Varani et al. 2004). In young healthy skin, dermal fibroblasts attach to intact collagen fibrils and achieve normal cell spreading/shape and maintain typical elongated spindle-like morphology. However, in aged dermis the collagen fibrils are fragmented, which impairs fibroblast-collagen interactions and thus become shorter with a rounded and collapsed morphology. While cell spreading is known to regulate many cellular functions (Butcher et al. 2009; Iskratsch et al. 2014; Janmey et al. 2013; Mammoto and Ingber 2009), the molecular basis of their impact on dermal fibroblast function and on skin connective tissue aging are not well understood.

Mitochondrial DNA (mtDNA) mutations and deletions have been has been proposed to be involved in many human diseases (Cha et al. 2015; Chan 2006; Enns 2003; Wallace 1992) including aging process (Berneburg et al. 2004; Birch-Machin et al. 1998; Lee and Wei 2012; Sastre et al. 2003; Yang et al. 1994). A 4977 base pair deletion of mtDNA, the so-called common deletion mtDNA, is one of the most frequently observed mtDNA mutations (Cortopassi and Arnheim 1990; Wallace 1992) and have been reported to be prevalent in human skin aging (Berneburg et al. 2000; Berneburg et al. 2004; Lu et al. 1999; Yang et al. 1994). The levels of mtDNA common deletions in epidermal keratinocytes would result in little time to accumulate due to the high turnover of keratinocytes. Therefore, mtDNA common deletions in epidermal keratinocytes may be not accurately reflect the actual mtDNA common deletions in skin. Although an increased frequency of mtDNA mutations has been reported in naturally and photoaged aged human skin (Berneburg et al. 2000; Berneburg et al. 2004; Birch-Machin et al. 1998; Yang et al. 1994), the frequency of mtDNA common deletion in the dermal compartment in naturally and photoaged skin has not been well documented until recently. Dermal fibroblasts have a very low proliferative rate and thus mtDNA common deletion might be accumulated in the cell.

❑ Accumulation of mtDNA Common Deletion in Naturally-aged and Photoaged Human Skin Dermis *In vivo*

Recently, Quan et al. reported that the average level of mtDNA common deletion in aged dermis is 5-fold greater compared to young skin dermis

(Quan et al. 2015). Similarly, the levels of mtDNA common deletion is much higher in sun-exposed photodamaged skin dermis (forearm) than in sun-protected skin dermis (underarm). The average level of mtDNA common deletion in photodamaged skin dermis is 7-fold larger compared to sun-protected skin dermis. These results demonstrate the accumulation of mtDNA common deletion in the dermis of both naturally aged and photoaged human skin *in vivo*. It should be noted that increased mtDNA common deletion in the dermis has significant implication for skin connective tissue aging, as described below.

❑ Reduced Cell Spreading Induces mtDNA Common Deletion Associated with Increased Reactive Oxygen Species (ROS) in Human Skin Dermal Fibroblasts

Human skin is largely composed of collagen-rich ECM, which provides structural and functional support for skin. The collagen-rich ECM is synthesized, organized and maintained by dermal fibroblasts. During aging process, collagenous ECM proteins undergo progressive loss and fragmentation, leading to thin and damaged dermis (connective tissue aging). Dermal fibroblasts in young human dermis intimately interact with intact collagen fibrils and thus maintain normal cell shape and size. In contrast, fibroblasts in aged human dermis have a collapsed and small largely due to fragmented collagen fibrils are unable to support normal cell morphology (Fisher et al. 2008; Qin et al. 2014; Varani et al. 2004). Reduced fibroblast spreading/size has significant consequences in human skin connective tissue aging; up-regulates matrix metalloproteinase-1 (MMP-1) (Fisher et al. 2009), which contributes to damaged skin and down-regulates collagen production (Quan and Fisher 2015; Quan et al. 2010; Quan et al. 2013), which contributes to thinning of the skin. To explore the connection between age-related reduced fibroblast shape/size and mtDNA common deletion, Quan et al. modulated the shape and size of the dermal fibroblasts by disrupting the actin cytoskeleton with latrunculin-A (Lat-A), which rapidly blocks actin polymerization (Gieni and Hendzel 2008). Interestingly, reduced cell spreading results in significant elevation of mtDNA common deletion (Quan et al. 2015). The levels of mtDNA common deletions are increased more than 3-fold by interruption of cell shape/size. These data suggest that reduced cell spreading/size leads to elevated mtDNA common deletion in human dermal fibroblasts. Cellular damage from reactive oxygen species (ROS) likely plays an important role in mtDNA deletions as well as in the aging process (Ishikawa et al. 2008; Murphy and Smith 2007; Sastre et al. 2003). Interestingly, interruption of dermal fibroblasts shape/size displays increased mitochondria ROS, suggesting that cell-shape/size-dependent increase of mtDNA common deletion is accompanied by elevated mitochondrial ROS levels. A strong co-localization of Mitotracker, a marker of mitochondria and RedoxSensor, a maker of ROS, indicating that the mitochondria are the primary source of cell-shape/size-dependent increase of ROS.

❑ Antioxidant Treatment Protects Against Cell-shape-dependent mtDNA Common Deletion in Human Dermal Fibroblasts

Furthermore, treatment of fibroblasts with N-acetyl-cysteine (NAC), an antioxidant and metabolic precursor of glutathione (De Vries and De Flora 1993), markedly diminishes the elevation of endogenous ROS levels and thus prevents cell-shape/size-dependent mtDNA common deletion. These results indicate that the deleterious effects of endogenous oxidative exposure are responsible, at least in part, for cell-shape/size-dependent mtDNA common deletion. Antioxidant treatments to either retard the aging process or to treat age-related disorders are subjects of heightened interest. NAC is safe for human use and NAC easily penetrates human skin and effectively mitigates ROS-driven responses to acute UV irradiation in human skin *in vivo* (Kang et al. 2003). Antioxidant NAC may be able to retard skin connective tissue aging through reduction of mtDNA common deletion. Slowing the accumulation of mtDNA common deletion would likely result in less functional decline in dermal fibroblasts over time. It is tempting to speculate that the combination of an antioxidant and an agent that promotes features of cell spreading/ size would promote normal dermal fibroblast function and rejuvenate aged human skin. Additionally, it is also of interest to test whether mitochondrial-targeted antioxidants, such as MitoQ and SkQ1, effectively protect against mtDNA common deletion induced by reduced cell shape and size. Together, mtDNA common deletion is significantly increased in both naturally aged and photoaged human skin dermis *in vivo* and that reduced fibroblasts spreading/size causes mtDNA common deletion through increased endogenous ROS.

Accumulating evidence suggests that mtDNA mutations/deletions can lead to ROS generation, while at the same time oxidative stress can also induce mtDNA mutations/deletions (Cortopassi et al. 1992; Ishikawa et al. 2008; Lee et al. 1994; Linnane et al. 1989; Terzioglu and Larsson 2007; Wei and Lee 2002). Cell spreading/size-dependent mtDNA common deletion is mediated by elevated ROS. These data suggest that the possibility of a positive feedback loop between ROS and mtDNA common deletion in response to reduced cell spreading/size. The mechanism by which impaired cell spreading/ size leads to increased endogenous ROS levels remains to be determined. Cell spreading/size impacts a multitude of cellular processes including signal transduction, gene expression and metabolism (Butcher et al. 2009; Iskratsch et al. 2014; Janmey et al. 2013; Mammoto and Ingber 2009). Recent evidence suggests that cytoskeletal tension plays a key role in translation of mechanical information into cell function (Ingber 2006; Silver et al. 2003;

Wang et al. 1993). In general, intracellular redox homeostasis is maintained by enzymatic antioxidant defenses such as superoxide dismutase (SOD), glutathione peroxidase (GPx) and catalase (CAT). SODs are responsible for the dismutation of superoxide radicals, generated by NAD(P) H oxidases, to hydrogen peroxide. CAT converts hydrogen peroxide into water and oxygen. Impairment or imbalance of the enzymatic antioxidant defenses could contribute to elevated ROS generation in response to impaired cell shape/size. An imbalance of antioxidant enzyme levels may contribute to elevated ROS levels in dermal fibroblasts in response to impaired cell shape/size. Currently, knowledge regarding the relationship among impaired cell shape/size, ROS and mtDNA common deletion is in a nascent state. Further studies are needed to understand the mechanisms that couple impaired cell shape/size to oxidative stress and mtDNA common deletion in human dermal fibroblasts, their role in skin connective tissue aging and possible therapeutic implications. In addition, future work should focus on types of mtDNA deletions/mutations other than common deletion, which may be considerably more prevalent.

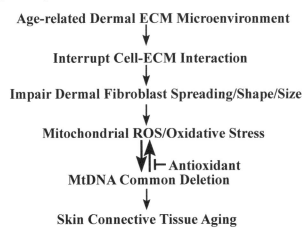

FIG. 1 *Proposed model for age-related reduction of dermal fibroblast spreading/shape/size induces mtDNA common deletion through ROS/oxidative stress (see **Conclusion and Outlook** for details).*

❑ Conclusion and Outlook

Aged related impairment of dermal collagenous ECM microenvironment directly interrupts cell-ECM interaction, which leads to disruption of dermal fibroblast spreading/shape/size (Figure 1). Impairment of dermal fibroblast spreading/shape/size brings about numerous alterations including increased mitochondrial ROS/oxidative stress, which promotes mtDNA common deletion. Increased mtDNA common deletion could further induce

ROS/oxidative stress through a positive feedback mechanism, forming a critical mechanism of human skin aging. This mechanism extends current understanding of the oxidative theory of aging by recognizing that age-related impairment of dermal fibroblast spreading/shape/size induces mtDNA common deletion through mitochondrial ROS/oxidative stress.

Accumulating evidence suggests that aging is associated with increased frequency of mitochondrial DNA mutations/deletions and increased production of ROS (Cortopassi et al. 1992; Ishikawa et al. 2008; Lee et al. 1994; Linnane et al. 1989; Terzioglu and Larsson 2007; Wei and Lee 2002). However, such observations have been made primarily in tissues with high rates of oxidative metabolism such as brain and muscle. ROS is intimately associated with accumulation of mtDNA common deletion in the dermis of both naturally and photoaged human skin *in vivo*. These data are consistent with previous report that oxidant levels are indeed increased in dermal fibroblasts in aged skin *in vivo* (Fisher et al. 2009). The magnitude of mtDNA common deletion seems to be 10-fold higher in photoaged skin compared to naturally aged skin, which is consistent with the general concept that more severe dermal connective tissue damage occurs in photoaged skin than in naturally aged skin (Quan et al. 2015). The work from Quan et al. (Quan et al. 2015) provides new insight into the connection between age-related impaired cell shape/size and the mtDNA common deletion/ROS axis, implicating the involvement of mtDNA common deletion in the pathophysiology of human skin connective tissue aging. These data extend current understanding of the mitochondrial theory of aging by identifying the connection among mtDNA common deletion and age-related reduction of cell shape/size and ROS. Slowing the accumulation of mtDNA common in aged skin, such as antioxidant, would be benefit to prevent functional decline in dermal fibroblasts over time. Furthermore, the combination of an antioxidant and an agent that improve cell spreading/shape/size would be an interesting strategy in promoting normal dermal fibroblast function and rejuvenating aged human skin.

❑ Acknowledgments

This study is supported by the National Institutes of Health (Bethesda, MD) Grants: ES014697 and ES014697 30S1 to Taihao Quan, AG019364. The author would like to thank Drs Taihao Quan, Moon Kyun Cho, Daniel Perry their help and support.

❑ References

Berneburg, M., H. Plettenberg and J. Krutmann. 2000. Photoaging of human skin. Photodermatol Photoimmunol Photomed 16: 239-244.

Berneburg, M., H. Plettenberg, K. Medve-Konig, A. Pfahlberg, H. Gers-Barlag, O. Gefeller, et al. 2004. Induction of the photoaging-associated mitochondrial common deletion *in vivo* in normal human skin. J Invest Dermatol 122: 1277-1283.

Birch-Machin, M.A., M. Tindall, R. Turner, F. Haldane and J.L. Rees. 1998. Mitochondrial DNA deletions in human skin reflect photo-rather than chronologic aging. J Invest Dermatol 110: 149-152.

Bissell, M.J. and W.C. Hines. 2011. Why don't we get more cancer? A proposed role of the microenvironment in restraining cancer progression. Nat Med 17: 320-329.

Bissell, M.J., P.A. Kenny and D.C. Radisky. 2005. Microenvironmental regulators of tissue structure and function also regulate tumor induction and progression: the role of extracellular matrix and its degrading enzymes. Cold Spring Harb Symp Quant Biol 70: 343-356.

Butcher, D.T., T. Alliston and V.M. Weaver. 2009. A tense situation: forcing tumour progression. Nat Rev Cancer 9: 108-122.

Cha, M.Y., D.K. Kim and I. Mook-Jung. 2015. The role of mitochondrial DNA mutation on neurodegenerative diseases. Exp Mol Med 47: e150.

Chan, D.C. 2006. Mitochondria: dynamic organelles in disease, aging and development. Cell 125: 1241-1252.

Chung, J.H. 2003. Photoaging in Asians. Photodermatol photoimmunol photomed 19: 109-121.

Cortopassi, G., D. Shibata, N.-W. Soong and N. Arnheim. 1992. A pattern of accumulation of a somatic deletion of mitochondrial DNA in aging human tissues. Proc Nat Acad Sci USA 89: 7370-7374.

Cortopassi, G.A. and N. Arnheim. 1990. Detection of a specific mitochondrial DNA deletion in tissues of older humans. Nucleic Acids Res 18: 6927-6933.

De Vries, N. and S. De Flora. 1993. N-acetyl-l-cysteine. J Cellular Biochem Suppl 17F: 270-277.

Enns, G.M. 2003. The contribution of mitochondria to common disorders. Mol Genet Metab 80: 11-26.

Fisher, G.J., S.C. Datta, H.S. Talwar, Z.Q. Wang, J. Varani, S. Kang, et al. 1996. Molecular basis of sun-induced premature skin ageing and retinoid antagonism. Nature 379: 335-339.

Fisher, G.J., Z.Q. Wang, S.C. Datta, J. Varani, S. Kang and J.J. Voorhees. 1997. Pathophysiology of premature skin aging induced by ultraviolet light. N Engl J Med 337: 1419-1428.

Fisher, G.J., J. Varani and J.J. Voorhees. 2008. Looking older: fibroblast collapse and therapeutic implications. Arch Dermatol 144: 666-672.

Fisher, G.J., T. Quan, T. Purohit, Y. Shao, K.C. Moon, T. He, et al. 2009. Collagen fragmentation promotes oxidative stress and elevates matrix metalloproteinase-1 in fibroblasts in aged human skin. American Journal of Pathology 174: 101-114.

Gieni, R.S. and M.J. Hendzel. 2008. Mechanotransduction from the ECM to the genome: are the pieces now in place? J Cell Biochem 104: 1964-1987.

Ingber, D.E. 2006. Cellular mechanotransduction: putting all the pieces together again. FASEB J 20: 811-827.

Ishikawa, K., K. Takenaga, M. Akimoto, N. Koshikawa, A. Yamaguchi, H. Imanishi, et al. 2008. ROS-generating mitochondrial DNA mutations can regulate tumor cell metastasis. Science 320: 661-664.

Iskratsch, T., H. Wolfenson and M.P. Sheetz. 2014. Appreciating force and shape-the rise of mechanotransduction in cell biology. Nat Rev Mol Cell Biol 15: 825-833.

Janmey, P.A., R.G. Wells, R.K. Assoian and C.A. McCulloch. 2013. From tissue mechanics to transcription factors. Differentiation 86: 112-120.

Kang, S., J.H. Chung, J.H. Lee, G.J. Fisher, Y.S. Wan, E.A. Duell, et al. 2003. Topical N-acetyl cysteine and genistein prevent ultraviolet-light-induced signaling that leads to photoaging in human skin *in vivo*. J Invest Dermatol 120: 835-841.

Kudravi, S.A. and M.J. Reed. 2000. Aging, cancer and wound healing. *In vivo* 14: 83-92.

Lee, H.C. and Y.H. Wei. 2012. Mitochondria and aging. Adv Exp Med Biol 942: 311-327.

Lee, H.-C., C.-Y. Pang, H.-S. Hsu and Y.-H. Wei. 1994. Differential accumulations of 4,977bp deletion in mitochondrial DNA of various tissues in human ageing. Biochima Biophysica Acta 1226: 37-43.

Linnane, A., S. Marzuki, T. Ozawa and M. Tanaka. 1989. Mitochondrial DNA mutations as an important contributor to ageing and degenerative diseases. Lancet: 1(8639)642-645.

Lu, C.Y., H.C. Lee, H.J. Fahn and Y.H. Wei. 1999. Oxidative damage elicited by imbalance of free radical scavenging enzymes is associated with large-scale mtDNA deletions in aging human skin. Mutat Res 423: 11-21.

Mammoto, A. and D.E. Ingber. 2009. Cytoskeletal control of growth and cell fate switching. Curr Opin Cell Biol 21: 864-870.

Murphy, M.P. and R.A. Smith. 2007. Targeting antioxidants to mitochondria by conjugation to lipophilic cations. Annual Rev Pharmacol Toxicol 47: 629-656.

Qin, Z., J.J. Voorhees, G.J. Fisher and T. Quan. 2014. Age-associated reduction of cellular spreading/mechanical force up-regulates matrix metalloproteinase-1 expression and collagen fibril fragmentation via c-Jun/AP-1 in human dermal fibroblasts. Aging Cell 13: 1028-1037.

Quan, C., M.K. Cho, D. Perry and T. Quan. 2015. Age-associated reduction of cell spreading induces mitochondrial DNA common deletion by oxidative stress in human skin dermal fibroblasts: implication for human skin connective tissue aging. J Biomed Sci 22: 62.

Quan, T. 2013. Skin connective tissue aging and dermal fibroblasts. Dermal Fibroblasts: Histological Perspectives, Characterization and Role in Disease: 31-55.

Quan, T. and G.J. Fisher. 2015. Role of Age-Associated Alterations of the Dermal Extracellular Matrix Microenvironment in Human Skin Aging: A Mini-Review. Gerontology. 61: 427-34.

Quan, T., Y. Shao, T. He, J.J. Voorhees and G.J. Fisher. 2010. Reduced expression of connective tissue growth factor (CTGF/CCN2) mediates collagen loss in chronologically aged human skin. J Invest Dermatol 130: 415-424.

Quan, T., F. Wang, Y. Shao, L. Rittié, W. Xia, J.S. Orringer, et al. 2013. Enhancing structural support of the dermal microenvironment activates fibroblasts, endothelial cells and keratinocytes in aged human skin *in vivo*. Journal of Investigative Dermatology 133: 658-667.

Sastre, J., F.V. Pallardo and J. Vina. 2003. The role of mitochondrial oxidative stress in aging. Free Radic Biol Med 35: 1-8.

Silver, F.H., L.M. Siperko and G.P. Seehra. 2003. Mechanobiology of force transduction in dermal tissue. Skin Res Technol 9: 3-23.

Terzioglu, M. and N.G. Larsson. 2007. Mitochondrial dysfunction in mammalian ageing. Novartis Found Symp 287: 197-208; discussion 208-113.

Varani, J., L. Schuger, M.K. Dame, C. Leonard, S.E. Fligiel, S. Kang, et al. 2004. Reduced fibroblast interaction with intact collagen as a mechanism for depressed collagen synthesis in photodamaged skin. J Invest Dermatol 122: 1471-1479.

Wallace, D.C. 1992. Mitochondrial genetics: a paradigm for aging and degenerative diseases? Science 256: 628-632.

Wang, N., J.P. Butler and D.E. Ingber. 1993. Mechanotransduction across the cell surface and through the cytoskeleton. Science 260: 1124-1127.

Wei, Y.-H. and H.-C. Lee. 2002. Oxidative stress, mitochondrial DNA mutation and impairment of antioxidant enzymes in aging. Exp Biol Med 227: 671-682.

Yaar, M., M.S. Eller and B.A. Gilchrest. 2002. Fifty years of skin aging. J Investig Dermatol Symp Proc 7: 51-58.

Yang, J.H., H.C. Lee, K.J. Lin and Y.H. Wei. 1994. A specific 4977-bp deletion of mitochondrial DNA in human ageing skin. Arch Dermatol Res 286: 386-390.

8

Nanodermatology: Nanoscale Therapeutics for Topical Application

Angelo Landriscina, BA,[1,a] *Jamie Rosen, BA*[1,b] and
Adam J. Friedman, MD[2,3,*]

❑ Introduction

Topical drug delivery is the cornerstone of dermatologic therapy. Application of drugs to the skin provides several benefits including localization of treatment, avoidance of first-pass metabolism, minimization of toxicity and ease of use (Nolan and Feldman 2009). However, topical therapies are limited in the treatment of many dermatologic disease processes. Many drugs are not easily solubilized in water- or oil-based topical formulations—a factor that limits the development of topical versions of many drugs. One of the primary functions of the skin is that of a barrier and as such, many drugs that can be solubilized are not able to easily access their molecular targets, or may be degraded en route. Drugs that are able to overcome these difficulties may be nonspecifically distributed within tissues, leading to minimal efficacy and adverse outcomes. Furthermore, efficacy is often impacted by patient compliance, a factor that is strongly influenced by the ease of use and cosmetic elegance of a particular topical formulation. These difficulties result in longer treatment times, increased healthcare costs and rigorous dosing schedules.

[1] Department of Medicine (Division of Dermatology), Albert Einstein College of Medicine, Bronx, New York.
[2] Department of Dermatology, George Washington School of Medicine and Health Sciences, Washington, DC.
[3] Department of Physiology and Biophysics, Albert Einstein College of Medicine, Bronx, New York.
[a] E-mail: angelo.landriscina@med.einstein.yu.edu
[b] E-mail: jamie.rosen@mssm.edu
[*] Corresponding author: Ajfriedman@mfa.gwu.edu

The aforementioned obstacles have led to the development of innovative vehicles for topical drug delivery. One approach to the development of these vehicles is nanotechnology- the use of molecules at the nanoscale (1-100 nm). Nanomaterials allow for the use of potent drugs with targeted delivery and minimal side effects (Han et al. 2011). These nanoplatforms have been investigated for use as wound healing adjuvants, antimicrobial therapies, anti-inflammatory therapeutics, antineoplastic agents and cosmetics. This chapter aims to provide an overview of nanotechnology and the use of nanotechnology in dermatologic disorders (nanodermatology).

❑ Characteristics of Nanomaterials

Interestingly, nanomaterials have been used by humans for thousands of years. Cosmetic applications of nanomaterials date back to the Greco-Roman period, when a recipe of slaked lime, litharge and water was used to color hair black, a phenomenon attributed to the synthesis of PbS quantum dots within the hair shaft (Walter et al. 2006). Through this historical lens, we can see that the introduction of nanomaterials into the body is not revolutionary. In fact, many of the drugs currently used measure on the nanoscale and nanoscaled molecules abound in the natural biological environment—including inside the human body.

However, the use of nanomaterials in topical therapeutic agents is a relatively new phenomenon allowing for the exploitation of unique characteristics of matter at the nanoscale. Decreasing the size of matter increases the surface area-to-volume ratio. As many of these molecules are only a few atoms thick, the result is the localization of most atoms in the molecule to the surface—a factor associated with many unique nanoscale properties (Roduner 2006; Kim et al. 2010). Atoms at the surface are highly reactive, possessing fewer neighboring atoms with which to bond. This property allows for the electrostatic attachment of a variety of compounds on the molecular surface (Huh and Kwon 2011). For example, positively charged chitosan has been conjugated to a variety of nanoparticles for both enhanced absorption and antimicrobial activity (Martinez et al. 2010; Barhate et al. 2014). Additionally, the size of nanomaterials alone provides an added penetration benefit, with the size of nanomaterials able to be tailored to particular routes or levels of penetration through the skin, hair and nails. They can be targeted for specific molecular structures, allowing for minimization of side effects (Zhou et al. 2013). Nanomaterials also allow for encapsulation of drugs—enabling sustained release and the use of previously insoluble substances (Krausz et al. 2015). Taken together, these characteristics allow these flexible platforms to produce tailored treatments for a variety of dermatologic disorders.

Nanomaterials for Dermatology

Nanoplatforms

Nanoplatforms take on several physical forms, each with their own advantages and unique applications, with nanosize as a commonality. Prominent classes of nanomaterials are outlined below:

Nanoemulsions

An emulsion is a traditional topical vehicle that employs oil and water in varying amounts, unified by an emulsifier such as a surfactant or detergent. When emulsions are topically applied, the aqueous portion evaporates, leaving behind active ingredients and an occlusive lipophilic film. This mechanism is the basis for traditional topical delivery, with different ratios of oil and water tailored for texture, transparency, occlusion and cosmesis (ointment, cream, lotion etc). Nanoemulsions exploit these same principles. However, the droplets found in nanoemulsions range on the nanoscale (<100 nm) (Tadros et al. 2004). The size of these droplets influences opacity of the emulsion, providing a transparent product when the droplets measure below 70 nm. The stratum corneum is an excellent barrier to lipophilic substances due to the abundance of intra and extracellular lipids—making penetration of lipophilic substances difficult. Nanoemulsions help to overcome this barrier by delivering hydrophobic substances at small sizes (Sonneville-Aubrun et al. 2004).

Nanoliposomes

Liposomes are spherical vesicles consisting of a bilayer of amphilic phospholipids. This bilayer is analogous to biological cell membranes and confers the ability to encapsulate both hydrophilic and hydrophobic substances (Gupta et al. 2010). As drug carriers, liposomes increase drug stability, promote uptake of drugs to target tissues and augment therapeutic efficacy (Manosroi et al. 2003; Gupta et al. 2010). While liposomes confer all of these advantages, studies have shown that their topical use is limited due to aggregation within the stratum corneum, indicating limited penetration of the epidermal barrier (Kirjavainen et al. 1996). This difficulty is overcome by synthesis of nanosized liposomes. Nanoliposomes provide additional benefits such as the ability to release drugs at a desired pH or temperature, or customization with surface ligands to influence phagocytosis by specific cell types (Draelos 2013). Use of these vehicles is challenged by their instability—nanoliposomes are easily lysed by pressure or vibration, can form aggregates beyond the nano range and easily leave their evenly distributed state in emulsions (Draelos 2013).

Nanoparticles

While nanoliposomes represent an easily synthesized nanoparticle, the use of polymer science techniques has resulted in the formulation of stabile nanoparticles for topical use. There are a variety of nanoparticles including nanoparticles based on solid lipids and polymeric nanoparticles. Solid lipid nanoparticles (SLN), nanostructured lipid carriers (NLC) and lipid drug conjugated particles (LDC) are carrier nanoparticles that are based on a solid lipid matrix and therefore inherently solid at body temperature (Wilczewska et al. 2012). The physical stability of lipid nanoparticles is an advantageous characteristic, though they have fairly low loading capacity. Polymeric nanoparticles employ the formation of a polymeric skeleton in which drugs are encapsulated and released through gaps or "pores" in the skeleton. Nanoparticle platforms synthesized in this way are easily customizable with multiple polymer choices as well as the addition of reagents to control pore size and surface characteristics. Polymers utilized for nanoparticle synthesis include silicates, chitosan, gelatin and proteins such as albumin (Wilczewska et al. 2012).

Nanopigments

Nanopigments are nanosized aggregates of metals and metallic compounds used to impart color. Metals such as silver, gold, titanium and zinc are often used. Colors reflected by these compounds differ with differening nanoscale size, allowing for a myriad of color options. Some nanopigments such as titanium dioxide (TiO2) and zinc oxide (ZnO) are naturally occurring minerals that have been used for years as physical sunscreens due to their ability to reflect and scatter ultraviolet (UV) light. Their cosmetic elegance has been improved by nanoscale sized and will be covered later in this chapter.

Quantum Dots

Quantum dots are the smallest of nanomaterials, measuring ≤ 10 nm. At this scale, they exhibit unique magnetic and electrical properties, with the ability to change direction of magnetism at room temperature. These properties lend to uses in imaging and therapeutics, with the ability to concentrate quantum dots in areas exposed to magnetic fields. Quantum dots have also been designed which release multiple drugs in response to different strength magnetic pulses (Draelos 2013).

Nanodrug Delivery, Penetration and Absorption

The primary hurdle for topical drug delivery is the epidermal barrier, a feature predominantly conferred by the stratum corneum. The stratum corneum is the outermost layer of the epidermis, comprised of a lipid-rich extracellular space and corneocytes tightly bonded by corneodesmosomes. These elements together compose a formidable barrier to extracorporeal substances with a strong preference for lipophilic, nonpolar and small sized molecules. Despite this efficient barrier, substances are able to traverse the stratum corneum via three distinct routes (Fig. 1): transcellular (through corneocytes), intercellular (through the lipid-rich extracellular space) and transappengeal (via accessory structures such as the pilosebaceous unit). Furthermore, permeability of the stratum corneum can be altered via hydration and the use of permeabilizing agents like detergents (Mihranyan et al. 2012).

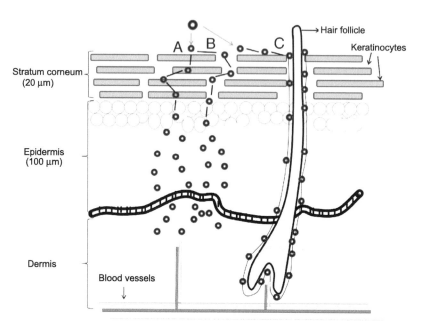

FIG. 1   Routes of entry for nanomaterials. *(A) intercellular, (B) transcellular and (C) transappengeal. Reprinted with permission from Valenuela et al. Nanoparticle delivery for transdermal HRT. Nanomedicine. 2012; 8(suppl 1): S83-9.*

Recent progress in nanotechnology has allowed for the development of drugs that are able to not only penetrate, but also collect within the epidermis. The efficiency of the barrier can be overcome by the creation of particles with favorable charge, size and structure. Transcellular penetration is especially difficult due to limitations of cellular absorption, with charge and lipophilicity of molecules being especially limiting. However, decreases in size result in exponential increases in permeability through this route, making materials at the smaller end of the nanoscale attractive (Potts and Guy 1992). Materials smaller than 36 nm are able to transit the intercellular route providing another option for cutaneous penetration (Baroli 2010). Nevertheless, a significant amount of drug may penetrate via the transappendageal route. Follicular openings represent 0.1% of the cutaneous surface and have a wide distribution, with hair-bearing skin showing greater penetration of traditional topicals (Tenjarla et al. 1999; Contri et al. 2011). The follicular opening is an orifice 200 nm in diameter, though it has been shown that particles much larger in size are able to penetrate and collect within the pilosebaceous unit, with size being inversely proportional to depth of penetration (Fig. 2) (Vogt et al. 2006; Patzelt et al. 2011). The follicular unit not only serves as a gateway for topically applied nanomaterials, but also as an important reservoir. It has been suggested that the follicular unit offers enhanced storage of nanoparticles, with a delay in the movement of particles from the follicular unit compared to their non-particle formulations (Lademann et al. 2007).

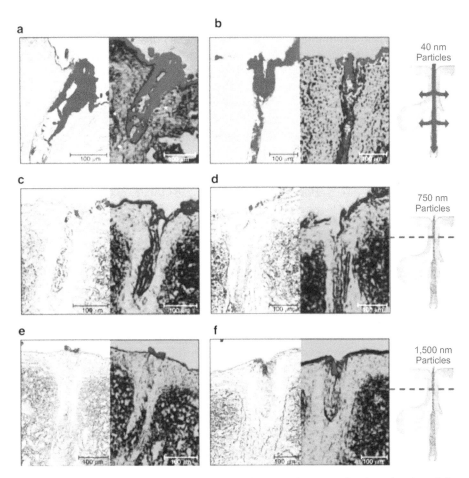

FIG. 2 **Follicular penetration of nanoparticles is inversely proportional to the size of the nanoparticle.** *(A and B) 40 nm nanoparticles are capable of penetrating deep into the hair follicle. However, 750 nm particles (C and D) and 1500 nm particles (E and F) collected within the infundibulum. Scale Bar = 100 um. Reprinted with permission from Vogt et al. 40 nm, but not 750 or 1,500 nm, Nanoparticles Enter Epidermal CD1a+ Cells after Transcutaneous Application on Human Skin. J Invest Dermatol 2006; 126: 1316-1322.*

The small size of nanoparticles raises concerns about systemic absorption of topical applications. There is currently a paucity of data about the penetration of nanoparticles beyond the stratum corneum. Once the nanoparticles penetrate the follicular orifice, follicular depletion can be achieved by penetration into the deeper layers of the epidermis or via exiting the hair follicle by sebum flow or hair growth. Studies have shown limited systemic absorption of TiO2 microparticles, in spite of enhanced penetration into the hair follicle, with *in vivo* data showing inability to cross the intact epidermal barrier (Lademann et al. 1998; Labouta and Schneider 2013). Nevertheless, it has been hypothesized that materials at an extremely small scale (1-10 nm) take on unique properties causing lipid modulation and therefore allow absorption (Huang et al. 2010). The delayed exiting of the majority of nanomaterials enhances contact time of the active ingredient, adding to the sustained release benefit of nanotherapeutics. This is a direct advantage over traditional topical therapeutics whose efficacy may be limited given the relatively short interaction with the epidermis due to rapid turnover of the stratum corneum. Current literature indicates the possibility of extended release with promising early toxicological data.

Toxicological Evaluation of Nanomaterials

Given the information above, it is easy to theorize that decreases in particulate size would enable deeper penetration of active ingredients into the skin, with the potential for systemic absorption. However, the literature does not support this notion. For example, there has been considerable concern about the use of ZnO and TiO2 nanoparticles (described in detail below) in consumer products, though *in vitro* and *in vivo* studies have shown that these materials do not penetrate beyond the stratum corneum (Mavon et al. 2006). Furthermore, toxicity of nanoparticles to mammalian cells is dependent on their cellular uptake; Keratinocytes, for example, are able to phagocytose small molecules such as nanomaterials, which may result in DNA damage due to accumulation of the materials within the nuclei (Görög et al. 1987). In fact, *in vitro* toxicological investigations have demonstrated a significant impact on cell survival with a variety of nanoparticle formulations (Yu et al. 2009; Samberg et al. 2010). However, a study by Krausz et al. found that curcumin-nanoparticles did not affect viability of keratinocytes *in vitro* (Krausz et al. 2015). Authors confirmed the biocompatibility of their nanoparticles *in vivo* using embryonic zebrafish (*Daniorerio)*, showing a lack of toxic responses following exposure. Taken together, these results suggest that current *in vitro* methods may not be sufficient for evaluating toxicity of nanomaterials—with *in vitro* studies not correlating with the limited *in vivo* data. Furthermore, there is lack of standardized methods to assess permeation and penetration of nanomaterials. The development of new methods of evaluation may help to elucidate toxicological data and alleviate concerns about systemic absorption.

Applications of Nanomaterials in Dermatology

The nanodermatological literature is rapidly growing with the development of new delivery systems leading to therapeutic advances for wound healing, cutaneous infection, inflammatory disorders, skin cancer and cosmetic concerns. Nanotechnology has allowed for the delivery of previously unusable substances, as well as the optimization of traditional therapies with enhanced penetration and limited toxicity.

Wound Healing

Wounds represent a major concern in healthcare, causing considerable morbidity, mortality and healthcare costs ($25 billion) each year (Sen et al. 2009). Wound healing can be understood in several phases, first starting with hemostasis in which platelet aggregation results in the formation of a fibrin clot and the aggregation of many growth factors and inflammatory cytokines (Broughton et al. 2006). These soluble signals result in the recruitment of several cell types including neutrophils, whose predominance defines the inflammatory phase of wound healing. During this stage neutrophils have important roles in the scavenging of damaged tissues structures and clearance of microbes. The balance of pro- and anti-inflammatory cytokines is crucial for the progression from the inflammatory to the proliferative phase of wound healing. The proliferative phase is dominated by macrophages, whose primary role is to clear cellular debris. Meanwhile, fibroblasts lay the groundwork of the extracellular matrix composed of type III collagen and an extensive network of capillaries develops. Eventually, type III collagen is replaced by the more permanent type I collagen in order to restore the normal dermal collagen composition. Remodeling of the wound can last from around 2 weeks to 2 years, with the residual tissue gaining around 80% of its original strength 1 year following injury (Levenson et al. 1965).

Wound healing is governed by the complex interplay of several cell types. Coordination of their many processes is carried out through the production of soluble molecular signals such as cytokines and growth factors. One such molecule is epidermal growth factor (EGF), whose influence spans from keratinocyte migration to granulation tissue deposition (Hardwicke et al. 2008). While exogenous EGF administration has been shown beneficial in wound healing, its use has been limited by rapid degradation, dilution and leakage from the wound bed. To overcome these difficulties, one group has developed a recombinant human EGF (rhEGF) nanoparticle, capable of accelerating wound healing in a diabetic mouse model compared to conventional rhEGF (Chu et al. 2010). Furthermore, rhEGF nanoparticle treatment resulted in more positive histologic features including more rapid re-epithelialization, angiogenesis and fibroblast migration, suggesting its benefit in the proliferative and remodeling stages of wound healing (Fig. 3).

Tissue regeneration is also dependent on the removal of damaged extracellular structures and regeneration of a functional extracellular matrix. Nanomaterials have been developed to aid this process by providing a 3 dimensional "scaffold" which serves to assist in the reconstruction of a functional tissue architecture. One such nanomaterial described by Khil et al. is a polyurethane nanofibrous membrane synthesized by electrospinning (Khil et al. 2003). This membrane was found to accelerate dermal organization and re-epithelization compared to untreated wounds in a guinea pig model. This membrane also provided added benefits as a dressing, minimizing water loss, increasing oxygenation and promoting drainage of exudate.

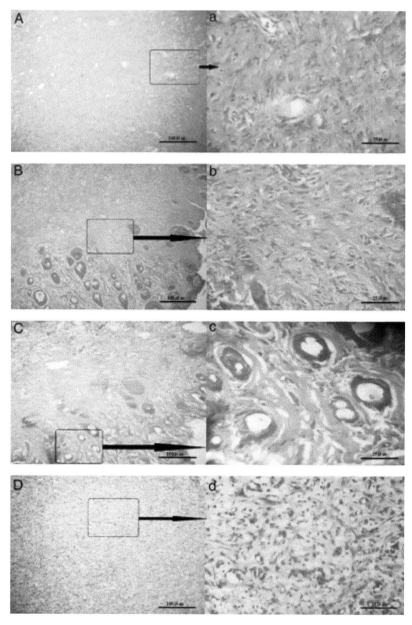

FIG. 3   rhEGF nanoparticles accelerate wound healing in a diabetic mouse model with positive histologic features after 14 days of treatment as compared to controls: *PBS-control (A, a), rhEGF nanoparticles (B, b), rhEGF stock solution (C, c) and empty nanoparticles (D, d) at 100 nm (left) and 400 nm (right). Reprinted with permission from Chu et al. Nanotechnology promotes the full-thickness diabetic wound healing effect of recombinant human epidermal growth factor in diabetic rats. Wound Repair Regen. 2010; 18(5): 499-505.*

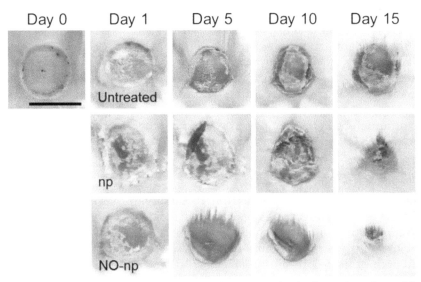

FIG. 4   NO-np accelerates wound healing in BALB/c mice in the setting of *Candida albicans* infected burn wounds. *Reprinted under the Creative Commons Attribution Non Commerical License from Macherla et al. Nitric Oxide Releasing Nanoparticles for Treatment of Candida Albicans Burn Infections. Front Microbiol 2012; 3: 193.*

As mentioned above, nanotechnology has allowed for the use of beneficial, but unstable substances. One such substance is nitric oxide (NO), a biologically ubiquitous, short-lived, diatomic gas with a myriad of roles in virtually all organ systems. NO's primary mechanism in the body is nitrosation—the addition of an NO group to thiol or sulfhydryl residues. Wound healing efficacy has been shown with the use of nanomaterials harnessing the power of nitrosation both by the production of NO and donation by molecules such as n-acetylcysteine. Our group has developed and characterized a sol gel-based platform for the creation of a nanoparticulate system capable of sustained release of nitric oxide over time (NO-np) (Friedman et al. 2008). This platform was used to accelerate healing of both burn and excision wounds in a murine model in a variety of settings including both bacterial and fungal infections (Fig. 4) (Han et al. 2009; Mihu et al. 2010; Blecher et al. 2012; Han et al. 2012; Macherla et al. 2012). Another study showed that NO-np exert their effect partially through a positive influence on leukocyte and fibroblast migration, transforming growth factor β (a promoter of angiogenesis) and collagen deposition, indicating a role for NO-np treatment throughout the wound healing process (Han et al. 2012). Similar results have been seen in a study which investigated the burn healing efficacy of nanoencapsulated n-acetylcysteine-s-nitrosothiol (NAC-SNO-np), a potent NO donor. NAC-SNO-np was shown not only to accelerate wound healing but also to attenuate neutrophil infiltration while augmenting macrophage migration, indicating a swift progression from the inflammatory to proliferative stage of wound healing (Landriscina et al. 2015).

While inflammation is an integral part of wound healing, excesses of inflammation can result in the diffusion of inflammatory cytokines and proteases into the tissue surrounding the wound and subsequent wound expansion/delayed wound healing. The inflammatory stage can be partially kept in check by lowering microbial burden. Much research has focused on the antimicrobial efficacy of a variety of nanotherapeutics. These therapies are covered in detail in the next section.

Skin and Soft Tissue Infections

Interest in nanotechnology for antimicrobial therapy has increased in recent years, as resistant infections have grown in incidence both in the nosocomial and community settings. Nanotechnology is an especially attractive antimicrobial strategy, since the multi-mechanistic activity of many nanoparticles is hypothesized to prevent resistance (Huh and Kwon 2011). Furthermore, the small size of nanomaterials compared to microbes which range in size from the higher end of the nanoscale to the micron scale maximizes interaction between microbes and drug. These advantages along with those mentioned above allow for the creation of tailored antimicrobial therapies with enhanced efficacy and low resistance potential.

The most straightforward approach for harnessing nanotechnology to combat resistance is encapsulating already widely-used drugs in order to enhance their efficacy. Such strategies have been used in order to harness drugs such as ampicillin, (Tonegawa et al. 2015) cephaolsporins, (Abeylath 2007) macrolides (Valizadeh et al. 2012) and amphotericin B (Sanchez et al. 2014). For example, Tonegawa et al. showed increased antibacterial activity of ampicillin nanoparticles versus traditional ampicillin against methicillin-resistant *Staphylococcus aureus* (MRSA), a highly-resistant bacterium with β-lactamase activity (Tonegawa et al. 2015). Furthermore, the investigators found unique cell wall changes in bacteria treated with the nanoparticle preparation, leading to the hypothesis that the nanoencapsulated drug was able to more easily penetrate the cell wall. Nanoencapsulation has also allowed for new applications of known drugs. Our group has optimized a nanopreparation of amphotericin B, a potent, nephrotoxic antifungal only available for parenteral administration. These amphotericin B nanoparticles have been shown efficacious against *Candida spp.* when applied topically in a murine burn infection model (Sanchez et al. 2014). These and many other studies indicate the increased efficacy and new modes of use for these well known antimicrobial agents.

The potential for encapsulation has also led to the use of molecules with intrinsic antimicrobial activity that were previously unusable. Curcumin (diferuloylmethane), a crystalline compound derived from the plant *Curcuma longa*, is the molecule that gives the East Asian spice turmeric its bright yellow color. Its medicinal properties have been referenced in alternative medicine for centuries, but have not yet allowed it to emerge as a component of the mainstream therapeutic repertoire. Given its limited oral bioavailability, poor solubility in water, instability at high pH and unsightly yellow color, its utility is limited, in spite of evidence showing antimicrobial, antioxidant and antineoplastic activity (Aggarwal et al. 2007). Nanoencapsulation has overcome these pitfalls allowing for sustained release and efficacy against MRSA and *Pseudomonas aeruginosa in vitro* and MRSA *in vivo* (Fig. 5) (Krausz et al. 2015).

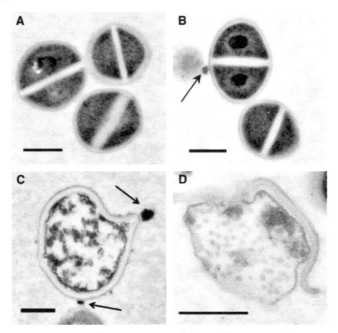

FIG. 5   **Curc-np disrupts MRSA cellular architecture.** *High power transmission electron microscopy reveals curc-np's interaction with MRSA. (A) Untreated MRSA reveals intact cellular architecture and uniform cytoplasmic density. (B) MRSA incubated with control-np, without any changes in cellular architecture after 24 hours. (C and D) Cells incubated with curc-np and MRSA demonstrated distortion and edema of architecture and eventually lysis and extrusion of contents after 6 and 24 hours respectively. Scale bars = 500 nm. Reprinted with permission from Krausz et al. Curcumin-encapsulated nanoparticles as innovative antimicrobial and wound healing agent. Nanomedicine 2015; 11(1): 195-206.*

Nanotherapies utilizing nanoscaled versions of other natural agents such as the polysaccharide chitosan have shown improved antimicrobial efficacy against a variety of gram positive and gram negative bacteria and fungi—likely owing to higher surface charge and increased interaction with microbial elements (Qi et al. 2004; Hernández-Lauzardo et al. 2008). Similar results have been seen with the use of nanosized metals. Interestingly, antibacterial effect of silver nanoparticles has been found inversely proportional to particle size, with smaller silver nanoparticles demonstrating higher antimicrobial efficacy (Ruparelia et al. 2008).

Inflammatory Disease

Unchecked and inappropriate inflammation is the primary pathological feature of several of the most common dermatologic disorders including atopic dermatitis, contact dermatitis and psoriasis. Current treatments rely heavily on modulation of inflammation in order to provide relief from these disease processes. Many patients begin treatment with topical therapies due to their tolerability and low risk for side effects. However, the therapeutic potential of topical agents is often limited, causing many patients to fail treatment with traditional therapies. Nanotherapeutics are being investigated in order to provide more efficacious topical applications.

Corticosteroids are a mainstay of topical immunomodulatory therapy and are used widely for both treatment and prevention in the setting of conditions such as psoriasis and atopic dermatitis (Schlupp et al. 2011). While use of topical corticosteroids is generally safe, side effects including cutaneous atrophy due to fibroblast inhibition and collagen cross-linking do occur. Investigators have begun to turn to nanotechnology in order to provide a topical glucocorticoid formulation with predictable concentration and penetration characteristics. For example, solid lipid nanoparticle glucocorticoid formulations have been found to localize to the epidermis *in vitro*, which may prevent atrophy (Santos Maia et al. 2002). Several other studies have shown that these formulations may penetrate into the dermis (Maia et al. 2000; Schlupp et al. 2011) This may be offset by the added benefit of sustained release, allowing for controlled drug concentration within tissues (Schlupp et al. 2011). Further study is needed to fully elucidate the benefits and side effect profiles of these nanotherapies.

Allergic contact dermatitis is another common inflammatory cutaneous process, with a significant portion of the population exhibiting allergies to metals such as nickel. In order to offset the allergenicity of nickel exposure, Vemula et al. described a nanoparticulate system harnessing calcium carbonate/phosphate in order to bind nickel and prevent penetration into the skin (Vemula et al. 2011). Investigators hypothesize that the high surface area and charge density of the particles allows for greater interaction with nickel ions. Results of assays employing pig skin showed that coating with the nanoparticle preparation prevented cutaneous permeation of nickel. *In vivo* studies using a mouse model that was sensitized to nickel showed improved dermatitis scores with the nanoparticle treatment versus untreated controls, indicating reduced exposure to nickel ions (Fig. 6) (Vemula et al. 2011).

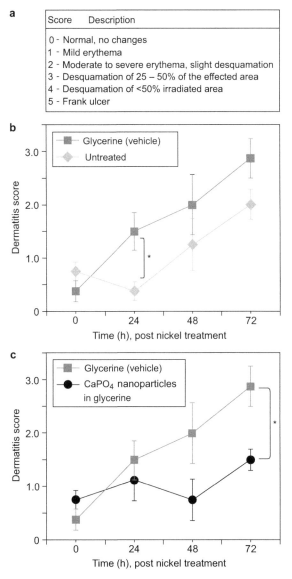

FIG. 6 Mice treated with CaPO4 nanoparticles demonstrated improved dermatitis scores as compared to controls. *(A) Dermatitis was evaluated by blinded observers based on the following scale. Animals sensitized to nickel were randomized into 3 groups: untreated, glycerine (vehicle) or CaPO4 nanoparticles (B) Temporal dermatitis scores between vehicle and untreated control (*P<0.05) and (C) temporal dermatitis scores between vehicle and CaPO4 nanoparticles (*P<0.05). Reprinted with permission from Vemula et al. Nanoparticles reduce nickel allergy by capturing metal ions. Nature 2011; 6: 291-295.*

Acne vulgaris represents the most common dermatologic disorder, with a multifactorial etiology. While the debate continues, new research has suggested that all types of acne have an inflammatory component (Qin et al. 2014). One of the key initiators of this inflammatory response is the bacterium *Propionibacterium acnes*, an anaerobic, gram-positive bacillus that comprises part of the normal skin flora. *P. acnes* orchestrates a multifactorial, extra- and intra-cellular response through activation of toll-like receptor 2 (TLR2) and the inflammasome, an intracytoplasmic complex that induces the secretion of pro-inflammatory cytokines (Kim et al. 2002; Kistowska et al. 2014; Qin et al. 2014). The use of nanomaterials has been shown efficacious against *P. acnes* and its immunologic sequelae. Friedman et al. found that chitosan-alginate nanoparticles had anti-inflammatory properties, attenuating IL-6 and IL-12 secretion in human keratinocytes and monocytes, respectively, which were exposed to *P. acnes* (Friedman et al. 2013). Investigators posited that former results showing chitosan's ability to attenuate NF-κβ signaling indicate the anti-inflammatory activity of the nanoparticles may be due to inhibition of toll-like receptor signaling.

Cutaneous Neoplasms

According to the American Cancer Society, skin cancer is one of the leading causes of morbidity and mortality worldwide, with projections of 9,940 deaths from melanoma and 3,400 deaths from other types of skin cancer by the end of 2015 (American Cancer Society 2015). Chemotherapy continues to be the hallmark of cancer treatment, though it is indiscriminately cytotoxic to both neoplastic and normal cells. Furthermore, since cancer is a biological disease with unregulated cell replication, cancer cells are extremely quick to develop mechanisms for drug resistance. The rapidity with which tumors grow is reflected in their structure. Tumor architecture is inherently leaky; tumors stimulate the growth of new blood vessels, but because of the rapid growth associated, the vessels tend to be irregular and extremely permeable. Nanotechnology is able to exploit this weakness as a result of their observed ability to selectively accumulate in tumor tissue from the enhanced penetration and retention (EPR) effect (Chen et al. 2013). Nanomaterials that measure less than 100 nm are capable of passing through the relatively large gaps in tumor blood vessels. Interestingly, the pores in normal blood vessels range from 2-6 nm and therefore nanotherapeutics are unable to significantly penetrate healthy tissue, thus limiting their toxicity (Grossman and McNeil 2012). This phenomenon has been demonstrated in several studies. For example, abraxane, an albumin bound nanoparticle formulation of the drug paclitaxel, was found to have increased anti-tumor activity while limiting the common taxane-associated toxicities such as myelosupression, peripheral neuropathy, nausea and vomiting as compared to the non-nano form of the drug (Miele et al. 2009).

Applications of nanotechnology to skin cancer seek to engineer nanoparticles that are capable of imaging and selectively targeting melanoma cells. For example, the use of interleukin (IL)-2, a glycoprotein which causes enhanced tumor immunogenicity and tumor regression in the setting of metastatic melanoma, is limited as a therapeutic by its relatively short half-life in serum (Dummer et al. 2008). A recent study by Yao et al. found that a nanopolymer IL-2 delivery system was capable of suppressing tumor growth and prolonging survival of mice bearing melanoma grafts (Yao et al. 2011). Nanomedicine has also shown promise in the selective delivery of small-interfering RNA (siRNA) specifically to silence the expression of cancer related genes or regulate the pathways involved in the development of malignant melanoma (Chen et al. 2010a/b; Davis et al. 2010). Studies have found that liposome-polycation-hyaluronic acid nanoparticles modified with a tumor-targeting human monoclonal antibody are able to effectively deliver siRNA and microRNA to lung metastases of murine melanoma (Chen et al. 2010a/b). Authors found that the nanoparticles suppressed the growth of the metastatic nodules in the lung by downregulating target genes including c-myc, MDM2 and vascular endothelial growth factor (VEGF) (Chen et al. 2010a/b). Nanotherapeutics maintain several advantages over conventional monoclonal antibodies or small molecules as they are able to penetrate the targeted site with high specificity and affinity and low toxicity. Nanoparticle-based materials, such as diagnostic probes, are also of great interest in the oncology world given their ability to selectively target tumors while limiting toxicity and exhibiting favorable clearance profiles. The use of radiolabeled silica nanoparticles has recently been approved for human clinical trials for tumor targeting, differential tumor burden, nodal mapping and lymphatic drainage patterns—representing an advantage of this platform for staging metastatic melanoma within the clinical setting (Benezra et al. 2011).

Nanotherapeutics tailored for cancer treatment hold the potential to overcome several limitations of conventional chemotherapeutics. The emergence of multi-drug resistant cutaneous neoplasms has limited the use of traditional chemotherapies. Even the revolutionary melanoma treatment that targeted oncogenic mutations in v-raf murine sarcoma viral oncogene homolog B1 (BRAF) has met severe setbacks due to the development of resistance (Sullivan and Flaherty 2013). Nanotechnology is one such avenue to overcome or reduce the development of drug resistance. It has been proposed that nanoparticles are able to circumvent resistance mechanisms by bypassing recognition of the drug efflux transporter P-glycoprotein, one of the major mediators of drug resistance and therefore accumulate within tumor cores (Chen et al. 2010a/b; Shapira et al. 2011). Taken together, the existing research on the use of tailored nanotherapeutics for targeting melanoma represents an advance in the treatment of melanoma and non-melanoma skin cancer. Nanotechnology has generated a remarkable number of advancements in cancer therapy with important roles in diagnostics, prognostics and management.

Cosmetics

Regardless of the data presented above, cosmetics companies are the largest stakeholders in nanotechnology. In fact, a cosmetics company is the sixth largest patent holder for nano-based technologies and each of the top 10 cosmetics companies currently have nano-related products on the market (Raj et al. 2012). Increasingly, nanomaterials are being exploited in the development of advanced cosmetic products for skin, hair and nails to harness the unique properties of matter on the nanoscale and improve on previous technologies.

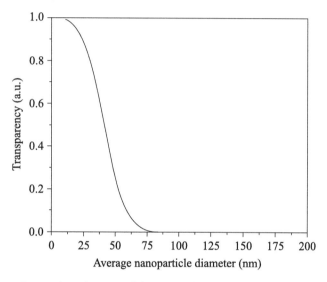

FIG. 7   Size of nanoparticle preparation predicts transparency. *The smaller the nanoparticle, the more transparent the preparation. 10 nm TiO2 nanoparticles are almost completely transparent, while 85 nm nanoparticles are opaque. Reprinted with permission from Barnard. One-to-one comparison of sunscreen efficacy, aesthetics and potential nanotoxicity. Nat Nanotech 2010; 5: 271-274.*

The largest area of interest for the utilization of nanomaterials in consumer products has been in the area of sunscreen. As discussed above, melanoma is a major source of morbidity and mortality and the use of sunscreen is a primary prevention tactic for this and other cutaneous neoplasms, as well as photoaging and a host of other cosmetic concerns. TiO2 and ZnO are inorganic, physical UV filters that have been used in commercial sunscreens for decades to protect against UVA and UVB radiation. The use of these UV filters has been limited by a lack of cosmetic elegance—both of these UV filters are coarse white powders that reflect light in the visible spectrum, resulting in products that leave an opaque white layer on the skin. This lack of transparency leads many consumers to choose other sunscreen products that may not be as effective (Dransfield 2000).

Nanotechnology has allowed for the production of new ZnO and TiO2 sunscreens that overcome this difficulty, with nanopreparations enhancing optical transparency and therefore cosmetic elegance (Fig. 7). Studies have found that nanopreparations using particles between 40 and 60 nm exhibit favorable transparency without compromising UV protection (Wiechers and Musee 2010). While there has been some concern among consumers about the toxicity of these preparations, it has been shown that penetration through the stratum corneum does not occur (Filipe et al. 2009).

The use of nanomaterials in makeup has also garnered considerable interest. Makeup is widely used in order to even skin tone, color correct imperfections such as erythema and hyperpigmentation and augment cosmetic appeal with products like eye shadow and lipstick. Several patents describe the use of metallic nanomaterials for color cosmetics (Cassin and Simonnet 2006; Alfano et al. 2007; Ha et al. 2007). For instance, Alfano et al. proposed a two-color system for color correction using nanopreparations of various metals, exploiting their specific optical properties at different nanoscale sizes (Alfano et al. 2007). This system uses one metal to achieve a base color, with a second silver nanopreparation in order to provide undertones that neutralize unwanted hues. While these technologies are promising, toxicity studies should be carried out prior to introduction to the commercial space.

One of the primary cosmetic concerns of consumers is signs of aging. To address these concerns, countless products have been introduced to the consumer and clinical space, with injectable botulinum toxin becoming a staple of the latter. While administration of botulinum toxin is successful at removing fine lines, there are a plethora complications that may arise including dipolopia, dysphagia and temporal artery pseudoaneurysm (Sorensen and Urman 2015). Nanotechnology has allowed for the creation of a topical preparation of botulinum toxin that can avoid these potentially serious side effects (Chajchir et al. 2008). This topical preparation allows for transepidermal flux of the toxin into the dermis and has shown a significant improvement of wrinkling of the lateral canthal lines when compared to placebo (Atamoros 2009). Additional benefits include the potential for at home use and fewer office visits which may help to decrease incurred costs. Furthermore this may represent a potential treatment for hyperhydrosis, with topical application of this drug reducing sweating by 80-90% following 5 applications (Modi 2010).

❑ Conclusion

The above studies demonstrate the potential for the improvement of topical drug delivery using nanotechnology. Nanotherapies have allowed for improved efficacy, minimized toxicity and enhanced cosmetic elegance for a variety of applications. Furthermore, the ability to stabilize previously unusable compounds and control tissue concentration via timed release is attractive for a multitude of pathological processes. While the above data is promising, there remains a paucity of human clinical trials, which limit the current translatability to the bedside. Future studies should focus on clinical efficacy as well as toxicity in order to ensure translatability.

❑ References

Abeylath, T.W.S.C. 2007. Glyconanobiotics: novel carbohydrated nanoparticle polymers.

Aggarwal, B.B., C. Sundaram, N. Malani and H. Ichikawa. 2007. Curcumin: the Indian solid gold. The molecular targets and therapeutic uses of curcumin in health and disease, Springer 1-75.

Alfano, R., X. Ni and M. Zevallos. 2007. Changing skin-color perception using quantum and optical principles in cosmetic preparations, Google Patents.

American Cancer Society. Cancer Facts and Figures 2015. American Cancer Society.

Atamoros, F. 2009. Botulinum toxin type A for the treatment of moderate to severe lateral canthal lines: prelimary safety and efficacy results of a blinded, randomized, placebo controlled trial. The American Academy of Dermatology's 2009 Summer Academy. Boston, Massachusetts.

Barhate, G., M. Gautam, S. Gairola, S. Jadhav and V. Pokharkar. 2014. Enhanced mucosal immune responses against tetanus toxoid using novel delivery system comprised of chitosan-functionalized gold nanoparticles and botanical adjuvant: characterization, immunogenicity and stability assessment. J Pharm Sci 103(11): 3448-3456.

Barnard, A.S. 2010. One-to-one comparison of sunscreen efficacy, aesthetics and potential nanotoxicity. Nat Nanotech 5(4): 217-4.

Baroli, B. 2010. Penetration of nanoparticles and nanomaterials in the skin: fiction or reality? J Pharm Sci 99(1): 21-50.

Benezra, M., O. Penate-Medina, P.B. Zanzonico, D. Schaer, H. Ow, A. Burns, et al. 2011. Multimodal silica nanoparticles are effective cancer-targeted probes in a model of human melanoma. J Clin Invest 121(7): 2768.

Blecher, K., L.R. Martinez, C. Tuckman-Vernon, P. Nacharaju, D. Schairer, J. Chouake, et al. 2012. Nitric oxide-releasing nanoparticles accelerate wound healing in NOD-SCID mice. Nanomed Nanotech Biol Med 8(8): 1364-1371.

Broughton, G., J.E. Janis and C.E. Attinger. 2006. The basic science of wound healing. Plast Reconstr Surg 117(7 Suppl): 12S-34S.

Cassin, G. and J.T. Simonnet. 2006. Cosmetic compositions comprising photoluminescent nanoparticles and at least one rare-earth metal, Google Patents.

Chajchir, I., P. Modi and A. Chajchir. 2008. Novel topical BoNTA (CosmeTox, toxin type A) cream used to treat hyperfunctional wrinkles of the face, mouth and neck. Aesthet Plast Surg 32(5): 715-722.

Chen, J., R. Shao, X.D. Zhang and C. Chen. 2013. Applications of nanotechnology for melanoma treatment, diagnosis and theranostics. Int J Nanomedicine 8: 2677-2688.

Chen, Y., S.R. Bathula, J. Li and L. Huang. 2010a. Multifunctional nanoparticles delivering small interfering RNA and doxorubicin overcome drug resistance in cancer. J Biol Chem 285(29): 22639-22650.

Chen, Y., X. Zhu, X. Zhang, B. Liu and L. Huang. 2010b. Nanoparticles modified with tumor-targeting scFv deliver siRNA and miRNA for cancer therapy. Mol Ther 18(9): 1650-1656.

Chu, Y., D. Yu, P. Wang, J. Xu, D. Li and M. Ding. 2010. Nanotechnology promotes the full-thickness diabetic wound healing effect of recombinant human epidermal growth factor in diabetic rats. Wound Repair Regen 18(5): 499-505.

Contri, R.V., L.A. Fiel, A. Pohlmann, S. Guterres and R. Beck. 2011. Nanocosmetics and nanomedicines: new approaches for skin care. Transport of Substances and Nanoparticles across the Skin and In Vitro Models to Evaluate Skin Permeation and/or Penetration, Springer: 3-35.

Davis, M.E., J.E. Zuckerman, C.H.J. Choi, D. Seligson, A. Tolcher, et al. 2010. Evidence of RNAi in humans from systemically administered siRNA via targeted nanoparticles. Nature 464(7291): 1067-1070.

Draelos, Z. 2013. Enhancement of topical delivery with nanocarriers. pp 87-93. *In*: Nasir, A., A. Friedman and S. Wang [eds.]. Nanotechnology in Dermatology. Springer, New York.

Dransfield, G.P. 2000. Inorganic sunscreens. Radiation Protection Dosimetry 91(1-3): 271-273.

Dummer, R., C. Rochlitz, T. Velu, B. Acres, J.-M. Limacher, P. Bleuzen, et al. 2008. Intralesional adenovirus-mediated interleukin-2 gene transfer for advanced solid cancers and melanoma. Mol Ther 16(5): 985-994.

Filipe, P., J.N. Silva, R. Silva, J.L. Cirne de Castro, M. Marques Gomes, et al. 2009. Stratum corneum is an effective barrier to TiO2 and ZnO nanoparticle percutaneous absorption. Skin Pharmacol Physiol 22(5): 266-275.

Friedman, A.J., G. Han, M.S. Navati, M. Chacko, L. Gunther, A. Alfieri, et al. 2008. Sustained release nitric oxide releasing nanoparticles: characterization of a novel delivery platform based on nitrite containing hydrogel/glass composites. Nitric Oxide 19(1): 12-20.

Friedman, A.J., J. Phan, D.O. Schairer, J. Champer, M. Qin, A. Pirouz, et al. 2013. Antimicrobial and anti-inflammatory activity of chitosan-alginate nanoparticles: a targeted therapy for cutaneous pathogens. J Invest Dermatol 133(5): 1231-1239.

Görög, P., J.D. Pearson and V.V. Kakkar. 1987. Generation of reactive oxygen metabolites by phagocytosing endothelial cells. Atherosclerosis 72(1): 19-27.

Grossman, J.H. and S.E. McNeil. 2012. Nanotechnology in cancer medicine. Physics Today 65(8): 38.

Gupta, M., A.K. Goyal, S.R. Paliwal, R. Paliwal, N. Mishra, B. Vaidya, et al. 2010. Development and characterization of effective topical liposomal system for localized treatment of cutaneous candidiasis. J Liposome Res 20(4): 341-350.

Ha, T.H., J.Y. Jeong, B.H. Jung, J.K. Kim and Y.T. Lim. 2007. Cosmetic pigment composition containing gold or silver nano-particles, Google Patents.

Han, G., L.R. Martinez, M.R. Mihu, A.J. Friedman, J.M. Friedman and J.D. Nosanchuk. 2009. Nitric oxide releasing nanoparticles are therapeutic for Staphylococcus aureus abscesses in a murine model of infection. PLoS One 4(11): e7804.

Han, G., A.J. Friedman and J.M. Friedman. 2011. Nitric oxide releasing nanoparticle synthesis and characterization. pp. 187-195. In: McCarthy, H.O. and J.A. Coulter [eds.]. Nitric Oxide: Methods in Molecular Biology. Springer, New York, NY, USA.

Han, G., L.N. Nguyen, C. Macherla, Y. Chi, J.M. Friedman, J.D. Nosanchuk, et al. 2012. Nitric oxide–releasing nanoparticles accelerate wound healing by promoting fibroblast migration and collagen deposition. American J Path 180(4): 1465-1473.

Hardwicke, J., D. Schmaljohann, D. Boyce and D. Thomas. 2008. Epidermal growth factor therapy and wound healing--past, present and future perspectives. Surgeon 6(3): 172-177.

Hernández-Lauzardo, A.N., S. Bautista-Baños, M.G. Velázquez-del Valle, M.G. Méndez-Montealvo, M.M. Sánchez-Rivera and L.A. Bello-Pérez. 2008. Antifungal effects of chitosan with different molecular weights on in vitro development of Rhizopus stolonifer (Ehrenb.:Fr.) Vuill. Carbohydrate Polymers 73(4): 541-547.

Huang, Y., F. Yu, Y.-S. Park, J. Wang, M.-C. Shin, H.S. Chung, et al. 2010. Co-administration of protein drugs with gold nanoparticles to enable percutaneous delivery. Biomaterials 31(34): 9086-9091.

Huh, A.J. and Y.J. Kwon. 2011. "Nanoantibiotics": a new paradigm for treating infectious diseases using nanomaterials in the antibiotics resistant era. J Control Release 156(2): 128-145.

Khil, M.-S., D.-I. Cha, H.-Y. Kim, I.-S. Kim and N. Bhattarai. 2003. Electrospun nanofibrous polyurethane membrane as wound dressing. J Biomed Mater Res B Appl Biomater 67B(2): 675-679.

Kim, B.Y., J.T. Rutka and W.C. Chan. 2010. Nanomedicine. N Engl J Med 363(25): 2434-2443.

Kim, J., M.T. Ochoa, S.R. Krutzik, O. Takeuchi, S. Uematsu, A.J. Legaspi, et al. 2002. Activation of toll-like receptor 2 in acne triggers inflammatory cytokine responses. J Immunol 169(3): 1535-1541.

Kirjavainen, M., A. Urtti, I. Jääskeläinen, T. Marjukka Suhonen, P. Paronen, R. Valjakka-Koskela, et al. 1996. Interaction of liposomes with human skin in vitro — The influence of lipid composition and structure. Biochimica et Biophysica Acta. (BBA) - Lipids and Lipid Metabolism 1304(3): 179-189.

Kistowska, M., S. Gehrke, D. Jankovic, K. Kerl, A. Fettelschoss, L. Feldmeyer, et al. 2014. IL-1beta drives inflammatory responses to propionibacterium acnes in vitro and in vivo. J Invest Dermatol 134(3): 677-685.

Krausz, A.E., B.L. Adler, V. Cabral, M. Navati, J. Doerner, R. Charafeddine, et al. 2015. Curcumin-encapsulated nanoparticles as innovative antimicrobial and wound healing agent. Nanomedicine 11(1): 195-206.

Labouta, H.I. and M. Schneider. 2013. Interaction of inorganic nanoparticles with the skin barrier: current status and critical review. Nanomed Nanotech Biol Med 9(1): 39-54.

Lademann, J., H.-J. Weigmann, C. Rickmeyer, H. Barthelmes, H. Schaefer, et al. 1998. Penetration of titanium dioxide microparticles in a sunscreen formulation into the horny layer and the follicular orifice. Skin Pharmacol Appl Skin Physiol 12(5): 247-256.

Lademann, J., H. Richter, A. Teichmann, N. Otberg, U. Blume-Peytavi, J. Luengo, et al. 2007. Nanoparticles–an efficient carrier for drug delivery into the hair follicles. Eur J Pharm Biopharm 66(2): 159-164.

Landriscina, A., T. Musaev, J. Rosen, A. Ray, P. Nacharaju, J.D. Nosanchuk, et al. 2015. N-acetylcysteine S-nitrosothiol nanoparticles prevent wound expansion and accelerate wound closure in a murine burn model. J Drugs Dermatol 14(7): 726-32.

Levenson, S.M., E.F. Geever, L.V. Crowley, J.F. Oates, C.W. Berard and H. Rosen. 1965. Healing of rat skin wounds. Ann Surg 161(2): 293-308.

Macherla, C., D.A. Sanchez, M.S. Ahmadi, E.M. Vellozzi, A.J. Friedman, J.D. Nosanchuk, et al. 2012. Nitric oxide releasing nanoparticles for treatment of Candida albicans burn infections. Front Microbiol 3: 193.

Maia, C.S., W. Mehnert and M. Schäfer-Korting. 2000. Solid lipid nanoparticles as drug carriers for topical glucocorticoids. Int Journal Pharm 196(2): 165-167.

Manosroi, A., P. Wongtrakul, J. Manosroi, H. Sakai, F. Sugawara, M. Yuasa, et al. 2003. Characterization of vesicles prepared with various non-ionic surfactants mixed with cholesterol. Colloids Surf, B. 30(1–2): 129-138.

Martinez, L.R., M.R. Mihu, M. Tar, R.J. Cordero, G. Han, A.J. Friedman, et al. 2010. Demonstration of antibiofilm and antifungal efficacy of chitosan against candidal biofilms, using an in vivo central venous catheter model. J Infect Dis 201(9): 1436-1440.

Mavon, A., C. Miquel, O. Lejeune, B. Payre and P. Moretto. 2006. In vitro percutaneous absorption and in vivo stratum corneum distribution of an organic and a mineral sunscreen. Skin Pharmacol Physiol (1): 10-20.

Miele, E., G.P. Spinelli, E. Miele, F. Tomao and S. Tomao. 2009. Albumin-bound formulation of paclitaxel (Abraxane(®) ABI-007) in the treatment of breast cancer. Int J Nanomedicine 4: 99-105.

Mihranyan, A., N. Ferraz and M. Strømme. 2012. Current status and future prospects of nanotechnology in cosmetics. Prog Mater Sci 57(5): 875-910.

Mihu, M.R., U. Sandkovsky, G. Han, J.M. Friedman, J.D. Nosanchuk and L.R. Martinez. 2010. The use of nitric oxide releasing nanoparticles as a treatment against Acinetobacter baumannii in wound infections. Virulence 1(2): 62-67.

Modi, P. 2010. Technical overview of topical botulinum toxin. from http://www.transdermalcorp.com/.

Nolan, B.V. and S.R. Feldman. 2009. Dermatologic medication adherence. Dermatol Clin. 27(2): 113-120, v.

Patzelt, A., H. Richter, F. Knorr, U. Schäfer, C.-M. Lehr, L. Dähne, et al. 2011. Selective follicular targeting by modification of the particle sizes. J Control Release 150(1): 45-48.

Potts, R.O. and R.H. Guy. 1992. Predicting skin permeability. Pharm Res 9(5): 663-669.

Qi, L., Z. Xu, X. Jiang, C. Hu and X. Zou. 2004. Preparation and antibacterial activity of chitosan nanoparticles. Carbohydr Res 339(16): 2693-2700.

Qin, M., A. Pirouz, M.H. Kim, S.R. Krutzik, H.J. Garban and J. Kim. 2014. Propionibacterium acnes Induces IL-1beta secretion via the NLRP3 inflammasome in human monocytes. J Invest Dermatol 134(2): 381-388.

Raj, S., S. Jose, U.S. Sumod and M. Sabitha. 2012. Nanotechnology in cosmetics: Opportunities and challenges. J. Pharm. Bioall. Sci. 4(3): 186-193.

Roduner, E. 2006. Size matters: why nanomaterials are different. Chem Soc Rev 35(7): 583-592.

Ruparelia, J.P., A.K. Chatterjee, S.P. Duttagupta and S. Mukherji. 2008. Strain specificity in antimicrobial activity of silver and copper nanoparticles. Acta Biomaterialia 4(3): 707-716.

Samberg, M.E., S.J. Oldenburg and N.A. Monteiro-Riviere. 2010. Evaluation of silver nanoparticle toxicity in skin in vivo and keratinocytes in vitro. Environ Health Perspect 118(3): 407.

Sanchez, D.A., D. Schairer, C. Tuckman-Vernon, J. Chouake, A. Kutner, J. Makdisi, et al. 2014. Amphotericin B releasing nanoparticle topical treatment of Candida spp. in the setting of a burn wound. Nanomedicine 10(1): 269-277.

Santos Maia, C., W. Mehnert, M. Schaller, H.C. Korting, A. Gysler, A. Haberland, et al. 2002. Drug targeting by solid lipid nanoparticles for dermal use. J Drug Target 10(6): 489-495.

Schlupp, P., T. Blaschke, K.D. Kramer, H.D. Holtje, W. Mehnert and M. Schafer-Korting. 2011. Drug release and skin penetration from solid lipid nanoparticles and a base cream: a systematic approach from a comparison of three glucocorticoids. Skin Pharmacol Physiol 24(4): 199-209.

Sen, C.K., G.M. Gordillo, S. Roy, R. Kirsner, L. Lambert, T.K. Hunt, et al. 2009. Human skin wounds: a major and snowballing threat to public health and the economy. Wound repair and regeneration: official publication of the Wound Healing Society [and] the European Tissue Repair Society 17(6): 763-771.

Shapira, A., Y.D. Livney, H.J. Broxterman and Y.G. Assaraf. 2011. Nanomedicine for targeted cancer therapy: towards the overcoming of drug resistance. Drug Resist Updat 14(3): 150-163.

Sonneville-Aubrun, O., J.T. Simonnet and F.L. Alloret. 2004. Nanoemulsions: a new vehicle for skincare products. Adv Colloid Interface Sci 108-109: 145-149.

Sorensen, E. and C. Urman. 2015. Cosmetic complications: rare and serious events following botulinum toxin and soft tissue filler administration. J Drugs Dermatol 14(5): 486-491.

Sullivan, R.J. and K.T. Flaherty. 2013. Resistance to BRAF-targeted therapy in melanoma. Eur J Cancer 49(6): 1297-1304.

Tadros, T., P. Izquierdo, J. Esquena and C. Solans. 2004. Formation and stability of nano-emulsions. Adv Colloid Interface Sci 108-109: 303-318.

Tenjarla, S.N., R. Kasina, P. Puranajoti, M.S. Omar and W.T. Harris. 1999. Synthesis and evaluation of N-acetylprolinate esters—novel skin penetration enhancers. Int Journal Pharm 192(2): 147-158.

Tonegawa, J., K. Ohtuka, M. Nakano and S. Shirotake. 2015. Reinforcement of antibiotic activity by nanoencapsulation of ampicillin against β-lactamase producing and non-producing strains of methicillin-resistant Staphylococcus aureus. J of Pharm Pharmacol 9(7): 190-197.

Valenuela, P., J.A. Simon. 2012. Nanoparticle delivery for transdermal HRT. Nanomedicine 8(suppl1): S83-9.

Valizadeh, H., G. Mohammadi, R. Ehyaei, M. Milani, M. Azhdarzadeh, P. Zakeri-Milani, et al. 2012. Antibacterial activity of clarithromycin loaded PLGA nanoparticles. Pharmazie 67(1): 63-68.

Vemula, P.K., R.R. Anderson and J.M. Karp. 2011. Nanoparticles reduce nickel allergy by capturing metal ions. Nat Nanotechnol 6(5): 291-295.

Vogt, A., B. Combadiere, S. Hadam, K.M. Stieler, J. Lademann, H. Schaefer, et al. 2006. 40 nm, but not 750 or 1,500 nm, nanoparticles enter epidermal CD1a+ cells after transcutaneous application on human skin. J Invest Dermatol 126(6): 1316-1322.

Walter, P., E. Welcomme, P. Hallégot, N.J. Zaluzec, C. Deeb, J. Castaing, et al. 2006. Early use of PbS nanotechnology for an ancient hair dyeing formula. Nano Lett 6(10): 2215-2219.

Wiechers, J.W. and N. Musee. 2010. Engineered inorganic nanoparticles and cosmetics: facts, issues, knowledge gaps and challenges. J Biomed Nanotechnol 6(5): 408-431.

Wilczewska, A.Z., K. Niemirowicz, K.H. Markiewicz and H. Car. 2012. Nanoparticles as drug delivery systems. Pharmacol Rep 64(5): 1020-1037.

Yao, H., S.S. Ng, L.-F. Huo, B.K. Chow, Z. Shen, M. Yang, et al. 2011. Effective melanoma immunotherapy with interleukin-2 delivered by a novel polymeric nanoparticle. Mol Cancer Ther 10(6): 1082-1092.

Yu, K., C. Grabinski, A. Schrand, R. Murdock, W. Wang, B. Gu, et al. 2009. Toxicity of amorphous silica nanoparticles in mouse keratinocytes. J Nanopar Res 11(1): 15-24.

Zhou, W., Y. Wang, J. Jian and S. Song. 2013. Self-aggregated nanoparticles based on amphiphilic poly(lactic acid)-grafted-chitosan copolymer for ocular delivery of amphotericin B. Int J Nanomedicine 8: 3715-3728.

9
CHAPTER

Skin Conditions in Elderly

Aleksandar Godic, MD, PhD

❑ Introduction

As we are getting older, the population of elderly who live progressively longer is rapidly increasing and their chances of developing skin-related disorders increase (Chang et al. 2013). There are two types of skin aging (intrinsic and extrinsic), which are often overlapping. Intrinsic skin aging is genetically determined, it occurs in all individuals and includes changes due to normal maturity. On the other hand extrinsic aging is produced by extrinsic factors such as ultraviolet light exposure, smoking, diet, environmental pollutants and even sleep position. They cause a cumulative damage to the skin, which becomes clinically apparent as we age and are due to unbalance between oxidative stress and reparatory mechanisms (antioxidants). It is also worth to mention that decreased mobility, drug-induced disorders and many chronic diseases, which compromise vascular efficiency and decrease immune response, contribute (directly or indirectly) to increased risk for skin disorders in elderly (Chang et al. 2013).

Morphological changes in aging involve all tissues and cells in the skin. Some are related to intrinsic skin aging and others to extrinsic, e.g. photoaging due to sun exposure. Epidermal cells become pleomorphic (variability in cell size, shape and/or their nuclei) that can leads to nonspecific architectural abnormalities, precancerous lesions (actinic keratoses), or skin cancer. Epidermal atrophy (thinning of the epidermis) leads to skin transparency, increased transepidermal water loss (TEWL) and skin surface becomes dry and scaly. Skin becomes more fragile because of the flattening of the dermal-

Consultant Dermatologist Dermatology University Hospital Lewisham High Street London, SE13 6LH UK.
E-mail: aleksandar.godic@gmail.com

epidermal junction. There is also an increased incidence of benign skin tumors, e.g. seborrheic keratoses and stucco keratoses.

Number, function and density of melanocytes and Langerhans' cells in the skin (intradermal macrophages) decrease, which leads to pigmentary disorders and eczematous disorders. The dermis becomes relatively acellular, avascular and less dense and the loss of functional elastic tissue results in wrinkles and skin laxity. The nerves, microcirculation and sweat glands undergo a gradual decline, predisposing to decreased thermoregulation and sensitivity to burning. Nails become dystrophic, they grow slower, nail plates become thinner, their distal portions split (onycholysis) and their surface become rough (trachyonychia). The subcutaneous fat layer atrophies on the cheeks and distal extremities, but hypertrophies on the waist of men and thighs of women. Hair grow slower, they become thinned, brittle and sparse and the scalp is often inflamed (dandruff and seborrheic dermatitis) (Table 1) (Chang et al. 2013).

TABLE 1 Most common skin disorders in elderly.

Inflammatory Disorders	Vascular Disorders	Autoimmune Disorders	Infections	Skin Lesions and Sun Damage
– Xerosis	– Chronic venous insufficiency	– Bullous pemphigoid	– Herpes zoster	– Actinic keratosis
– Pruritus	– Pressure ulcers	– Mucous membrane pemphigoid		– Seborrheic keratosis
– Eczema	– Senile purpura	– Pemphigus vulgaris		– Stucco keratosis
– Seborrheic dermatitis		– Paraneoplastic pemphigus		– Chronic sun damage
– Stasis dermatitis (eczema)				

❑ Inflammatory Disorders

Xerosis

Dry skin (xerosis, asteatosis) is caused by exogenous and endogenous factors. It is mostly caused by low humidity (especially in winter), dry climate, excessive exposure to water and soap, if natural skin emollients are not replaced. Xerosis may be a sign of systemic illnesses (renal insufficiency, ichthyosis, atopic dermatitis, nutritional deficiencies, thyroid disease, neurological disorders, malignancies, human immunodeficiency virus infection), a consequence of treatment (radiation), or side effect of medications (anti-androgens, diuretics). It is often seen in elderly due to decreased intercellular lipids of the stratum corneum (SC), reduced water-binding capacity of the SC and increased transepidermal water loss (TEWL) (Rawlings and Harding 2004). It is often asymptomatic, but pruritus and stinging sensation may be present in more pronounced cases and in asteatotic eczema. It is characterized by dry, cracked and fissured skin with scaling. If more advanced, a criss-cross pattern of superficial cracks and fissures of the horny layer is seen and lesions appear as cracked porcelain. Subsequently, environmental allergens and pathogens can easily penetrate the skin, increasing the risk of allergic and irritant contact dermatitis, as well as infection. Patients with allergic and irritant contact dermatitis present with erythema, oozing, vesicles, excoriations and crusting and are more symptomatic. Xerosisfirst arises on the shins and may spread to the thighs, proximal extremities and trunk.

Topical moisturizers and steroids are the primary treatment of xerosis. It usually resolves within few days after application of topical corticosteroid ointment. Alternatively, topical calcineurin inhibitors mat also be used. Regular use of emollients, including petrolatum-, urea-, ceramide-, or lactic acid-containing preparations should be used in order to prevent relapses. Proper attention must be given to eliminate factors that aggravate dry skin, which include reduced frequency of bathing with lukewarm (not hot) water, minimal use of a nonirritant soap and avoidance of skin cleansers.

Pruritus

Pruritus (itching) is a sensation that elicits a desire to scratch. It is the most common skin-related symptom, which is associated with underlying skin conditions or may be a manifestation of systemic illnesses in 10% to 25% of affected individuals, which include hepatic, renal, thyroid disorders, lymphoma, myelopreoliferative disorders, human immunodeficiency virus infection, parasitic infections, diabetes mellitus, parathyroid disease, hypervitaminosis A, iron-deficiency anemia, neuropathy and neuropsychiatric disorders. In some patients, there are no visible skin lesions (psychogenic pruritus). Drug-induced pruritus should also be considered. Pruritic skin diseases are the most common dermatological problem in elderly and xerosis is the most common underlying dermatological condition. Characteristic features of pruritis are scratching and inflammation. Pruritus is thought to be induced by the histamine and is mediated exclusively by the peripheral nervous system. Scratching produces an immunology-based inflammatory response.

Initial treatment focuses on relief of pruritus and treatment strategy is to find the underlying cause. Unfortunately there is no specific antipruritic treatment and each individual patient requires specific management.

Elimination of provocative factors is necessary, which include wearing of soft clothing (cotton and silk), avoiding of excessive bathing and regular use of emollients, especially in elderly patients, who are prone to xerosis. It is important to educate patients on the itch-scratch cycle and measurements how to break it. A large variety of topical antipruritic preparations are available, including moisturizers, emollients, coal tars, corticosteroids, anaesthetics, dimethindene, doxepin, capsaicin, tacrolimus and pimecrolimus. Most systemic antipruritic drugs act centrally and have sedating effect. Ultraviolet (UV) light is also effective antipruritic treatment. Behavioral therapy is beneficial in patients with psychogenic pruritus (Chang et al. 2013).

Eczema

Eczema is a group of heterogeneous skin disorders. In each stage, patients may develop acute, subacute and chronic eczematous lesions, which are pruritic, often excoriated (due to scratching) or lichenified (due to rubbing) and may be secondary infected. Skin lesions in acute stage of eczema are oozing erythematous papules and patches with vesicles and crusts, which turn into red, scaly and cracked papules, patches and plaques in a chronic stage of a disease. Eczematous disorders include atopic, allergic contact, asteatotic, nummular, seborrheic, varicose and autoeczematization eczema. Several of these disorders are commonly seen in the elderly. Nummular eczema is characterized by pruritic, coin-shaped lesions that are most commonly found on the lower legs, upper extremities, dorsum of hands and the trunk. Adults with atopic eczema present with chronic, lichenified lesions, which involve flexural areas and commonly the dorsal aspect of hands, or the face, particularly the eyelids. In elderly there is commonly marked xerosis. Common complication of eczema is secondary infection because of impaired skin barrier and immune response in elderly. *Staphylococcus aureus* (and frequently *Streptococcus pyogenes*) commonly cause impetiginization of eczematous lesions. Patients with limited infected atopic eczema may be treated with topical fucidic acid (for no longer than two weeks to reduce the risk of drug resistance or skin sensitisation), or with mupirocin. In more extensive cases, flucloxacillin or erythromycin may be used; the latter in patients with penicillin allergy or resistance. Careful attention should be given to watch more severe infections such as methicillin-resistant *Staphylococcus aureus*. Treatment options of atopic eczema include topical steroids, pimecrolimus, tacrollimus, emollients, soap substitutes, phototherapy, or systemic immunosuppressants.

Seborrheic Dermatitis

Seborrheic dermatitis (SD) is the most common type of eczema and its prevalence is estimated at 5%. Several studies showed that it is strongly linked to *Pytirosporumovale* yeast (*Malassezia furfur*) and its direct causative role is today widely accepted (Shuster 1984; Faergemann 2000). It predominantly occurs in areas of the skin with active sebaceous glands, but patients with SD may have normal or excessive sebum production and *M. furfur* may or may not be increased in those areas. It presents as sharply demarcated pink-yellow, dull red or red brown scaly patches or thin plaques, which are symmetrically distributed. Predilection areas are areas rich in sebaceous glands (scalp, face, ears, presternal region) and, less often, intertriginous areas. On rare occasions, generalized or even erythrodermic forms can occur. Adult SD has a chronic relapsing course and exposure to sun, heat, febrile illnesses and overly aggressive topical therapy may precipitate flares and dissemination. It is commonly found in patients with Parkinson's disease, quadriplegia and emotional distress. Rebound flares of SD can be seen in patients treated with systemic corticosteroids when they are tapered off. Treatment includes topical azoles (e.g. ketoconazole), either as shampoos or creams (mainstay), or zinc pyrithione and tar shampoos as well as topical calcineurin inhibitors as a second-line treatment. In addition, low-potency topical corticosteroids and emollients may be used in symptomatic patients and/or disseminated SD.

❑ Vascular Disorders

Chronic Venous Insufficiency, Stasis Dermatitis and Varicose Eczema

Chronic venous insufficiency (CVI) is very common condition in elderly and its prevalence varies between 1% and 17% in men and 1% and 40% in women. The venous system of the lower extremities consists of superficial, deep and perforating veins, which are connected in a mesh-like structure. Valves in veins are responsible that the blood flow is directed from the superficial into the deep venous system and that there is no reflux (retrograde flow). Since veins are not as strong as arteries (the vessel walls are thinner and contain less tissue), the unidirectional blood flow is maintained by contraction of calf muscles, enabling proper venous return toward the heart. In the absence of competent valves and/or insufficient calf muscles contraction (e.g. in elderly who are not mobile), the increased venous pressure of the deep veins is transmitted to the superficial venous system and to the microcirculation within the skin (Bergan et al. 2006), which leads to venous hypertension (also called venous insufficiency). There are several factors which contribute to venous hypertension, like reflux through incompetent valves (primary or secondary due to deep venous thrombosis), venous outflow obstruction (e.g. due to obesity, pregnancy), or insufficient calf muscle contraction (e.g. obesity, leg immobility).

Patients with CVI complain of swelling of the legs, which is most prominent toward the end of the day after prolonged standing and is improved by leg elevation. Their legs may be painful and restless. In addition, they may have cramps and paraesthesias. In advanced stages of CVI, venous leg ulcers may appear, which are typically located above the medial malleolus and if untreated, are slowly getting larger and may be painful. Pedal pulses are usually palpable (which excludes peripheral artery disease). All patients with CVI have some teleangiectasias (in early stage of CVI) and varicose veins (in advanced stage of CVI). Associated features of CVI are pinpoint petechiae and hemosiderin deposition due to extravasation of erythrocytes, which is clinically visible as hyperpigmentation. If CVI lasts for a long time, stasis dermatitis with pruritus, erythema, scaling and weeping may develop, which is often misdiagnosed as cellulitis and treated with antibiotics. Stasis dermatitis and frequent usage of various topical preparations may cause allergic contact dermatitis. Atrophie blanche (white, stellate scars on the medial aspect of the ankles) may develop in up to 40% of patients with CVI. Patients with longstanding venous insufficiency may develop lipodermatosclerosis (sclerosing panniculitis), which begins on the lower medial aspect of the legs and may progress proximally. Clinically, it presents as red, warm, swollen legs (acute stage) and progress into a tender, painful and firm plaques, which may involve entire circumference of the lower legs and give appearance of "inverted champagne bottle" (chronic stage). One of the potential complications of CVI is "id" reaction or autosensitization dermatitis (eczema), which presents as itchy papulovesicular, often symmetrically distributed rash on the extremities. Duplex sonography of venous system in patients of CVI is useful for assessing reflux and obstruction.

In regard of treatment, support elastic stockings are the golden standard (if there is no associated peripheral artery disease), which enables unidirectional blood flow from the superficial into the deep venous system and from the ankles toward the thighs. Stasis dermatitis may be treated with low-potency steroids and emollients. Proper hygiene is crucial to prevent infections. Venous ulcers are treated with various wound dressings, according to the healing stage and concomitant infection.

Purpura

Purpura is visible hemorrhage into the skin or mucous membranes. It may be caused by decreased platelet count (thrombocytopenia), platelet abnormalities, vascular defects, trauma, or drug reactions. Elderly are especially susceptible to hemorrhage into the skin. Aging causes a gradual reduction in the number of blood vessels, loss of elastic fibers, dermal collagen and the subcutaneous fat. The atrophic skin offers reduced protection from external trauma and leads to senile purpura. It is also worth to mention that many elderly persons are taking medications that can cause thrombocytopenia, coagulopathies, or impaired collagen synthesys of vessel walls, leading to purpura. Drugs, which commonly cause thrombocytopenia are penicillins, quinine, quinidine, thiazide diuretics, methyldopa and heparin, in addition to corticosteroids, which may impair collagen synthesis leading to vessel fragility. Thrombocytopenic purpura (TP) presents as petechiae and/or ecchymoses. Petechiae are small, nonpalpable, nonblanchable, erythematous macules. Ecchymoses are larger (> 0.5 cm) hemorrhages into the skin.

Senile purpura is caused by burst blood vessels in the skin following negligible trauma to the extremities. It is very common in elderly persons. It is a benign condition characterized by recurrent formation of purple ecchymoses (bruises) on the extensor surfaces of forearms and affects both sexes equally. On examination patients present with well-defined, dark purple, irregularly-shape macules, which measure 1-4 cm in diameter and resolve spontaneously within three weeks following the trauma. The surrounding skin is usually atrophic, with signs of chronic sun damage (scales, hyperpigmentation and inelasticity). The lesions are most commonly distributed on the extensor surfaces of forearms and dorsal aspect of hand.

❑ Autoimmune Disorders

Bullous Pemphigoid

Bullous pemphigoid (BP) is the most common autoimmune blistering disease, which predominantly affects the elderly. It is a chronic disease characterized by exacerbations and remissions. Mortality rate among elderly is high and has been estimated between 10% and 40% during the first year, especially in those with multiple comorbidities and systemic treatments. It is caused by autoantibodies directed against BP antigen 180 (BP180, or type XVII collagen) and BP antigen 230 (BP230). The former is a transmembrane protein and the latter a cytoplasmic protein, which belongs to the plakin family (Giudice et al. 1992; Stanley et al. 1988). Both antigens are components of the hemidesmosomes, which attach an epithelial tissue to the surrounding stroma. When this attachment is disrupted due to an antibody-antigen complex, it leads to a subepidermal dysadhesions and bullae formation. BP can be triggered by trauma, burns, radiotherapy, UV irradiation (including phototherapy) and drugs; the latter is often observed in elderly.

BP is usually manifested in two phases: pre-bullous and bullous. Cutaneous manifestation and symptoms of pre-bullous phase are nonspecific and include mild to severe pruritus, excoriated eczematous papules, patches, urticarial lesions, which may persist for several months until the bullous phase became apparent. Cutaneous manifestations of bullous phase are characterized by vesicles or bullae, which may be arranged in annular or figurate pattern. Blisters can measure up to 4 cm, they contain clear fluid, may be present for several days and leave behind erosions after they rupture. They are symmetrically distributed and sites of involvement are flexural areas of the limbs and the lower back and abdomen. Occasionally, vegetating plaques may be observed in the intertriginous areas. Lesions heal with postinflammatory pigment alterations (hypo- or hyperpigmentations) and occasionally milia. Oral cavity is normally not affected, but lesions can be present in 10-30% of patients; other mucous membranes are rarely affected. Lesions are characteristically itchy and eosinophilia in peripheral blood may be noted in 50% of patients. In addition to classical BP presentation, there have been described several variants, which include dyshidrosiform (on palms and feet), vegetans (in the intertriginous areas), vesicular, nodular, papular, eczematous, erythrodermic and lichen planus pemphigoid.

Association with internal malignancies has been reported in elderly, but three case-control studies did not prove increase risk of malignancies in patients with BP (Marazza et al. 2009; Di Zenzo et al. 2007). In addition, BP has been rarely reported in patients with inflammatory bowel disease, rheumatoid arthritis, Hashimoto's thyroiditis, dermatomyositis, lupus erythematosus and autoimmune thrombocytopenia. In some patients with psoriasis and lichen planus, bullae may be localized to the lesions.

Treatment include superpotent topical corticosteroids, topical tacrolimus, oral corticosteroids, doxycycline or tetracycline, azathioprine, mycophenolatemofetil, methotrexate, to name some which are first and second line options.

❑ Skin Lesions

Actinic Keratosis

Actinic (or solar) keratosis (AK) is common lesion, commonly observed in individuals with lighter phototype, in those who have history of excessive sun exposure, which means that prevalence is increasing with aging due to a cumulative UV-induced damage of the skin (elderly). They can be found on sun-damaged skin of the head, neck, trunk and extremities. Lesions have been characterized as premalignant (precancerous), because atypical keratinocytes within the lesions are located in the epidermis and do not invade the dermis. The likelihood that they evolve into a skin cancer (squamous cell carcinoma) has been estimated to occur at a rate of 0.075-0.096% per lesion per year. They can also resolve spontaneously. They can be diagnosed by palpation (rough surface) rather than by a visual inspection.

They are initially thin, erythematous, slightly scaly clusters of papules and patches on sun exposed areas, which evolve into thicker small hyperkeratotic erythematous and well-defined plaques. There exist several variants of AKs: classic, hyperkeratotic, pigmented, lichenoid, bowenoid and actinic cheilitis if on the lips.

Treatment options include cryotherapy, curettage & cautery, shave excision, 5-fluorouracil cream, imiquimod, photodynamic therapy, diclofenac gel and ingenol mebutate gel.

Seborrheic Keratoses

Seborrheic keratosis (SK) is common benign skin lesion that is almost ubiquitous among older individuals. They occur on the face, neck, trunk (especially the upper back) and extremities, but not on the palms, feet and the mucous membranes. They can be usually diagnozed by clinical examination, but some lesions may mimic melanoma, so biopsy for histopatologic examination may be required, especially when there is a history of recent change. Typical morphological structures can be visible on dermoscopy, which is unfortunately not always helpful. They may occur frequently and earlier at sun-exposed areas (the head and the neck) in individuals residing in tropical climates. Their origin is rather neoplastic (clonal) than hyperplastic. In irritated SKs, apoptosis within areas of squamous differentiation has been found on histopathologic examination (Pesce and Scalora 2000).

Patients have usually more than one SK (although solitary SK is not impossible), which are more or less pigmented, sharply demarcated, flat or raised and have more or less prominent keratotic surface. They are usually light brown but may appear waxy yellow to brown–black in color. They typically evolve as a macule and may progress to become papular or verrucous. They can become large and evolve into plaques and may become inflamed. They are usually asymptomatic, although irritated SK may become tender, pruritic, erythematous and crusted.

They can be a marker of internal malignancies in particular of gastric or colonic adenocarcinoma, breast carcinoma and lymphoma (Leser–Trélat sign); if so, they appear abruptly and in increased number and/or size (Vielhauer et al. 2000; Heaphy et al. 2000; Grob et al. 1991).

Treatment options of symptomatic lesions include curettage, shave excision, cryotherapy, electrodesiccation and lasers (pulsed CO_2, erbium-YAG).

Stucco Keratosis

Stucco keratosis was first described by Koscard in 1958 in 24 affected men in an Australian study group of 240 geriatric patients. The name originates from "stuck-on" appearance. Lesions are benign and are characterized as grey-white papules, which are symmetrically distributed, mostly on the lower extremities and in elderly. Their number varies and they measure up to 4 mm. They are noted more frequently during winter months due to lower humidity and dry skin. They can easily be scraped off the skin surface by fingernails with minimal or no bleeding.

They do not need to be treated apart from cosmetic reason and common treatment options include curettage, cryotherapy and electrodessication.

❏ References

Bergan, J.J., G.W. Schmid-Schonbein, P.D. Smith, A.N. Nicolaides, M.R. Boisseau and B. Ekiof. 2006. Chronic venous disease. N Engl J Med 355: 488-498.

Chang, A.L., J.W. Wong, J.O. Endo and R.A. Norman. 2013. Geriatric dermatology review: Major changes in skin function in older patients and their contribution to common clinical challenges. J Am Med Dir Assoc 14: 724-30.

Di Zenzo G., G. Marazza and L. Borradori. 2007. Bullous pemphigoid: physiopathology, clinical features and management. Adv Dermatol 23: 257-288.

Faergemann, J. 2000. Management of seborrheic dermatitis and pityriasis versicolor. Am J Clin Dermatol 1: 75-80.

Giudice, G.J., D.J. Emery and L.A. Diaz. 1992. Cloning and primary structural analysis of the bullous pemphigoid autoantigen BP180. J Invest Dermatol 99: 243-250.

Grob, J.J., M.C. Rava, J. Gouvernet, P. Fuentes, L. Gamerre, J.C. Sarles, et al. 1991. The relation between seborrheic keratoses and malignant solid tumours. A case-control study. Acta Derm Venereol 71: 166-169.

Heaphy, M.R., J.L. Jr. Millns and A.L. Schroeter. 2000. The sign of Leser-Trélat in a case of adenocarcinoma of the lung. J Am Acad Dermatol 43: 386-390.

Marazza G., H.C. Pham, L. Schärer, P.P. Pedrazzetti, T. Hunziker, R.M. Trueb, et al. 2009. Incidence of bullous pemphigoid and pemphigus in Switzerland: a 2-year prospective study. Br J Dermatol 161: 861-868.

Pesce, C. and S. Scalora. 2000. Apoptosis in the areas of squamous differentiation of irritated seborrheic keratosis. J Cutan Pathol 27: 121-123.

Rawlings, A.V. and C.R. Harding. 2004. Moisturization and skin barrier function. Dermatol Ther 17: 43-48.

Shuster, S. 1984. The aetiology of dandruff and the mode of action of therapeutic agents. Br J Dermatol 111: 235-242.

Stanley, J.R., T. Tanaka, S. Mueller, V. Klaus-Kovtun and D. Roop. 1988. Isolation of complementary DNA for bullous pemphigoid antigen by use of patients' autoantibodies. J Clin Invest 82: 1864-1870.

Vielhauer, V., T. Herzinger and H.C. Korting. 2000. The sign of Leser-Trélat: a paraneoplastic cutaneous syndrome that facilitates early diagnosis of occult cancer. Eur J Med Res 5: 512-516.

10

CHAPTER

Regenerative Properties of Laser Light

Nicolette Nadene Houreld

❑ Introduction

Physical appearance is important to many individuals and can influence how individuals are perceived by others. Smooth, wrinkle free facial skin is correlated to supposed attractiveness, youthfulness and health, while facial wrinkles or rhytids have a negative impact on ones perceived appearance, image and self-esteem. Aesthetic procedures such as surgery, fillers and laser/light therapy have been utilized to achieve and obtain a more youthful appearance. Lasers have been used over the last 50 years for a variety of skin conditions and disorders, including skin rejuvenation. However it is only within the last two decades that lasers have been extensively used in dermatology. Currently there is a wide range of lasers and devices available for the regeneration and healing of skin conditions. Ablative lasers, which destroy the upper epidermis and simultaneously heat the dermis causing collagen to shrink, are typically used in skin resurfacing and rejuvenation. Non-ablative lasers, which stimulates collagen growth and tightens underlying skin and do not induce epidermal destruction, are also used. Fractional ablative lasers linked to ablative and non-ablative technologies, is associated with decreased risks. There is a dynamic balance between extracellular matrix (ECM) synthesis and destruction. The use of lasers in skin regeneration and rejuvenation decreases the appearance of fine lines and wrinkles and improves skin tone and complexion. There are however limitations to the treatment and the techniques and possible associated risks and results must be understood. The introduction of non-thermal, non-ablative low-level light therapy (LLLT), also known as photobiomodulation

Laser Research Centre Faculty of Health Sciences, University of Johannesburg PO Box 17011, Doornfontein, Johannesburg, 2028, South Africa.
E-mail: nhoureld@uj.ac.za

(PBM), has also shown positive results in decreasing the appearance of wrinkles and improving skin laxity. Understanding basic laser physics and principles will allow for the correct choice and use of devices and better results will be obtained. This chapter will look at the use of lasers for skin regeneration and healing and summarize relevant laser physics and laser tissue interaction.

❑ Basic Laser Physics

The term "laser" is an acronym for Light Amplification by Stimulated Emission of Radiation and is a source of non-ionizing electromagnetic radiation. In order to emit electromagnetic radiation, atoms of the active medium or gain medium, which resides within the optical cavity (optical resonator) of the laser, are excited by an external power source. These excited atoms are unstable and release the excess energy in the form of light/photons (electromagnetic radiation). Incident photons traveling along the laser cavity collide with other excited atoms, resulting in the rapid multiplication of photons all travelling in the same direction and of the same wavelength. This process is referred to as stimulated emission of radiation. At either end of the optical cavity are mirrors which reflect the photons, thus further increasing the intensity. Approximately 1-20 percent of the emitted photons are released from the optical cavity through a partially transparent mirror (output coupler), such that the light intensity inside the laser is higher than the output power (Tunér and Hode 2002) (Fig. 1). The active media may be a gas (e.g. CO_2 laser), liquid (dye lasers), solid (e.g. neodymium yttrium-aluminum-garnet, Nd:YAG, lasers), semiconductor (e.g. indium gallium arsenide, InGaAs, lasers) or plasma and is the determinant of not only the name of the laser, but also its wavelength. The light produced by the laser is bright (laser intensity as determined by the number of photons leaving the optical cavity), coherent (all the waves are synchronized and travel together), monochromatic (of a single colour) and collimated (has the same diameter throughout its entire length), (Fig. 2).

Wavelength is the distance from crest to crest of an electromagnetic wave and is measured in nanometres (nm). Light energy is expressed in joules (J) and its fluence or energy density in joules per square centimetre (J/cm^2). The output power of the laser is measured in watts (W) and the power density (light concentration) is the amount of optical energy incident upon a surface, divided by the area of the surface being irradiated and is measured in watts per centimetre square (W/cm^2), with the area being defined by the beam spot size (r^2) at the tissue surface. The energy which is delivered is constant but changing the spot size determines the surface area over which this energy is delivered (Stewart et al. 2013). Spreading laser light over a larger area leads to a directly proportional reduction in power density and fluence (Ohshiro 1991; Stewart et al. 2013). What this means is if the spot size is decreased all the photon energy will be delivered to a smaller area, thereby increasing the fluence and vice versa.

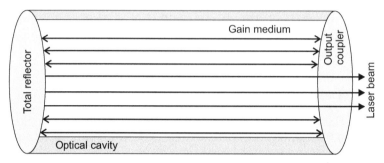

FIG. 1 *Electrons within the gain medium absorb energy from an electrical current and become excited and move to a higher orbital. As they return to their ground state, the electrons emit particles of light (photons). At either end of the optical cavity there are mirrors which bounce and reflect the photons, resulting in amplification of the energy. On one end of the optical cavity is an output coupler which is a partially transparent mirror and allows a certain percentage of the light to leave and produces the resultant laser beam.*

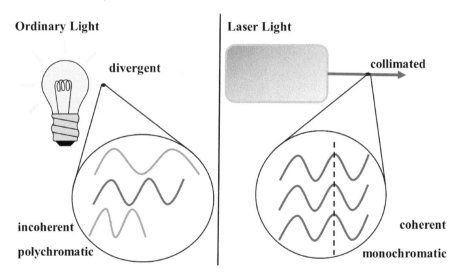

FIG. 2 *The properties of ordinary light as compared to laser light. Laser light is collimated (same diameter), coherent (all the waves are synchronized) and monochromatic (of a single wavelength), while ordinary light is divergent (emitted in many directions away from the source), incoherent (all the waves are out of phase with each other) and polychromatic (combination of many different wavelengths).*

Laser light can be administered as a continuous wave (CW), pulsed or quality switched (Q-switched). CW lasers emit continuously in time of relatively low power, while in pulsed lasers the beam is gated by mechanical shutters or electrically switched and the light is emitted in bursts of low energy with peak powers higher than CW (Acland and Barlow 2000). The pulse repetition rate is measured in Hertz (Hz) and can be adjusted and timed to allow cooling of the skin between pulses and thus reducing thermal damage (Acland and Barlow 2000). Q-switching is achieved by use of an electro-optical switch and produces extremely high peak power pulses in the nanosecond range (Fig. 3), (Stewart et al. 2013).

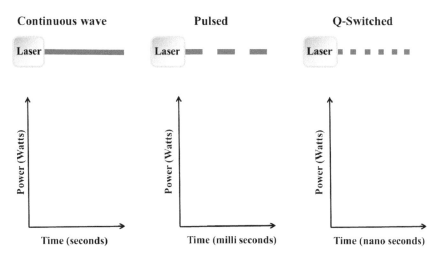

FIG. 3 *Modes of laser emission. Laser emission can be described as being continuous, pulsed, or quality switched (Q-switched).*

One also needs to understand the principle of selective photothermolysis, which is the thermal damage of target tissue without damaging the surrounding tissue. The photon energy is absorbed by a target chromophore such as melanin, water, oxyhaemoglobin, tattoo ink etc and sufficient heat is produced to damage the target chromophore. In order to achieve this the physical properties of the incident radiation (wavelength, fluence, pulse) must be manipulated and the absorption spectra of the target and surrounding tissue must be different. The tissue which is being irradiated must also be allowed to cool between pulses to allow for heat dissipation. The thermal relaxation time (TRT), which is chromophore specific, must also be taken into consideration. This is the time taken for the target chromophore to dissipate 50 percent of the thermal energy to the surrounding tissue and the laser pulse is selected to match the TRT of the chromophore of interest (Stewart et al. 2013; Acland and Barlow 2000). The pulsewidth of the laser must be smaller than the TRT; this will ensure that the heat generated in the target chromophore does not dissipate until the target is damaged (Altshuler et al. 2001). On the other hand the target may not contain an appreciable amount of chromophore and the photons are absorbed by an absorber chromophore which transfers the heat to the target chromophore, e.g. in permanent hair removal the photons are absorbed by the melanin in the hair shaft and is transferred to and destroys the stem cells and blood vessels in the hair follicle (Stewart et al. 2013; Altshuler et al. 2001). Fractional photothermolysis (FPT) involves the heating of narrow columns of tissue which causes cylindrical areas of tissue damage surrounded by intact skin which serves to support the recovery of the damaged tissue (Tournas and Zachary 2010).

❑ Laser-tissue Interaction

The effect of laser light on target tissue is influenced by the physical properties of the skin, including optical, chemical and mechanical properties, as well as the distribution and concentration of the components that make up the tissue. The effect is also influenced by the manner in which the light is applied and the characteristics of the incident laser beam. When the photons come into contact with the skin, it may be reflected, transmitted, scattered or absorbed (Stewart et al. 2013; Peavy 2002). When the light is absorbed photon energy is transferred to the absorbing chromophore, however when the light is transmitted or reflected the photon retains its energy. Four main targets/chromophores in the skin include melanin, water, haemoglobin and exogenous pigments.

The penetration depth at which a laser beam penetrates into target tissue is dependent on the wavelength, with longer wavelengths having a deeper penetration depth. The optical window of skin typically extends from 620 to 1,200 nm (Stewart et al. 2013). Blue-green light, below 600 nm, is absorbed by biologic pigments such as melanin and haemoglobin, while wavelengths above 1,200 nm are predominantly absorbed by water, such as in the case of the carbon dioxide (CO_2) laseror erbium: yttrium-aluminum-garnet (Er:YAG) laser. Light from the Nd:YAG laser is generally absorbed by protein (Ohshiro 1991; Stewart et al. 2013). Thus the choice of a laser is dependent on the penetration depth required. Haemoglobin is a commonly selected chromophore as it has several absorption peaks at 532, 585, 595 and 1064 nm (Stewart et al. 2013). Dermal water is heated by infrared light, leading to the contraction and tightening of collagen fibres, there is also a migration and reinforcement of fibroblasts in the area (Civas et al. 2010).

The mechanism of action for PBM is not yet fully understood. What is known is that light in the visible red spectrum and infrared (IR) light is directly absorbed by the mitochondria and more specifically the respiratory chain enzyme cytochrome c oxidase. This leads to an increase in adenosine triphosphate (ATP) and subsequent secondary messengers which activate a cascade of cellular events (Houreld 2013, 2014; Avci et al. 2013). Another theory is the photodissociation of nitric oxide (NO) from reduced cytochrome c oxidase, thus reversing the inhibition of cytochrome coxidase which is now free to bind with oxygen and carry out its function (Houreld 2013, 2014).

❑ Lasers for Skin Rejuvenation

Skin aging can be defined as a disease in which cell functions are degenerated through exposure to harmful factors on the skin surface and can present at any time, but is usually noticeable in the early thirties and is associated with wrinkles, dyspigmentation, telangiectasia and reduced tissue elasticity (Park et al. 2013; Sawhney and Hamblin 2014; Civas et al. 2010). Skin aging can be classified as intrinsic aging caused by natural aging irrespective of external factors and photoaging, which is caused due to long-term exposure to ultraviolet (UV) light, which superimposes on the intrinsic aging process (Gu et al. 2011). Intrinsic aging manifests itself as an increase in fine wrinkles and decreased elasticity, while photoaging induces atrophia cutis, dyspigmentation, surface furrows and surface roughness (Park et al. 2013), with reduced collagen and elastic fibres leading to decreased elasticity and skin tenacity (Gu et al. 2011). The development of new technologies has introduced many therapeutic modalities to address the issue of skin aging, including dermabrasion, chemical peels and lasers. Lasers are typically used in facial rejuvenation and include ablative and non-ablative lasers (Fig. 4). Both ablative and non-ablative lasers provide a means for treatment, however they are not without their limitations and as a result FPT was developed and is gaining popularity. FPT has desirable effects and reduced recovery time and bridges the gap between ablative and non-ablative modalities (Sawhney and Hamblin 2014).

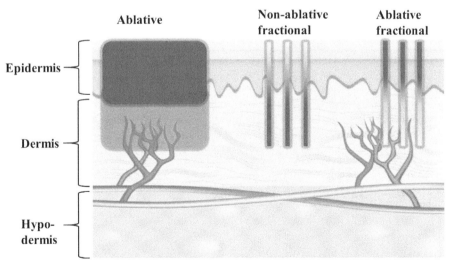

FIG. 4 *Lasers typically used in skin rejuvenation include ablative, non-ablative and fractional lasers, or a combination of these. Ablative lasers destroy and coagulate the epidermis and simultaneously heat the dermis, inducing wound healing and collagen deposition. Non-ablative lasers destroy coagulate the dermis, while the epidermis is protected through the simultaneous cooling of the skin. Fractional lasers destroy narrow cylindrical areas of tissue which is repaired by cells from the undamaged surrounding tissue. Fractionated lasers can be either ablative, causing full-thickness destruction, or non-ablative which leaves an intact epidermis.*

❑ Ablative Lasers

These lasers are high powered and destroy the epidermis and simultaneously heat the dermis causing collagen to shrink. The resultant wound inflicted in the skin heals with remodelling of the ECM and new smoother, tighter skin is formed. The superficial dermis and entire epidermis is coagulated and ablated to a depth of around 150 – 300 microns (Tournas and Zachary 2010; Stewart et al. 2013). The most commonly used ablative lasers include the CO_2 (10,600 nm) laser, Er:YAG laser (2,940 nm) and erbium-doped yttrium scandium gallium garnet (Er:YSGG) laser (2,790 nm). The CO_2 laser results in rapid heating and vaporization. Localized tissue coagulation and protein denaturation results in haemostasis and later on skin tightening. It could take up to several months to achieve the desired effects, but the improvements in wrinkles and scarring is clinically significant (Stewart et al. 2013). The Er:YAG laser is absorbed 10-16 times more by water than the CO_2 laser, resulting in more superficial ablation which reduces healing time as well as patients tolerance. However associated with this is reduced haemostasis and a reduction in tissue remodelling and skin tightening due to loss of dermal heating (Stewart et al. 2013).

This technique is invasive and due to the tissue destruction, this therapy requires intensive post-treatment care and has prolonged downtime. Side effects and complications include burns, pain, long-lasting erythema, scarring, infections, bleeding, oozing and hyper- or hypopigmentation, milia as well as clear demarcation lines between treated and untreated skin (Sawhney and Hamblin 2014; Stewart et al. 2013). Individuals may also be prohibited from going into sunlight (Trobonjaca and Simunovic 2000). This technology is typically used to treat rhytides, dyspigmentation (in lighter skins) and scarring (Stewart et al. 2013). Wanitphakdeedecha and colleagues (2009) used an ablative variable square pulse Er:YAG laser (300 micros, short pulse or 1,500 micros, extra-long pulse) to treat acne scars in 24 patients. Patients treated with the extra-long pulse showed a significant improvement in skin smoothness and scar volume, with minimal side effects (Wanitphakdeedecha et al. 2009).

❑ Non-ablative Lasers

Due to the limitations associated with ablative lasers, such as prolonged and unpleasant post-operative recovery time, newer rejuvenating lasers were developed and introduced and lead to the use of non-ablative lasers. This technology is less invasive and provides aesthetic improvement without inducing tissue damage. Non-ablative lasers tighten the skin by stimulating collagen production; the epidermis is protected through skin cooling and there is dermal collagen denaturation and remodelling (Tournas and Zachary 2010; Berlin and Goldberg 2010). The weak hydrogen bonds between the hydroxyl groups and the hydroxyproline residues in collagen type I and III are broken upon laser irradiation and dermal heating of the water found in surrounding tissue. This results in a random-coil configuration of the alpha-chains and subsequent shortening and thickening of the fibrils. The epidermis is spared from the heating by simultaneous cooling. The damage inflicted in the dermis triggers the wound healing response and new collagen fibres are laid down (Berlin and Goldberg 2010). A disadvantage of these lasers is that patients who exhibit both epidermal and dermal changes have limited benefits from this type of treatment.

There is little to no downtime associated with these lasers, with decreased scarring, dyspigmentation and infection and modest edema and erythema, however they show reduced efficacy as compared to ablative lasers (Sawhney and Hamblin 2014; Tournas and Zachary 2010; Stewart et al. 2013). Subtle clinical improvements are typically seen with this treatment and is aimed at patients with moderate photoaging and realistic expectations (Berlin and Goldberg 2010). Typical non-ablative lasers include intense pulsed light (IPL) sources (550 – 1,200 nm), high-dose (585/595 nm) pulsed dye lasers (PDL), low-dose (589/595 nm) PDLs, pulsed potassium titanyl phosphate (KTP) lasers (532 nm), Nd:YAG lasers (1,064 nm and 1,320 nm), diode lasers (1,450 nm), erbium glass lasers (1,540 nm), Alexandrite lasers, Er:YAG lasers and a combination of these (Sawhney and Hamblin 2014; Tournas and Zachary 2010; Lee et al. 2014). Lasers of longer wavelengths are more popular due to the deeper penetration depth and effective target of the mid dermis resulting in improved results (Alexiades-Armenakas et al. 2008). PDLs have shown modest results in skin rejuvenation and is likely due to the superficial penetration of the light into the papillary dermis and predominantly vascular targeting. IPLs are able to target both melanin and haemoglobin which results in an improvement in dyspigmentation and vascularity (Alexiades-Armenakas et al. 2008). Non-ablative lasers in the infrared spectrum are best suited for the treatment of rhytids and acne scarring.

Although not a laser in the true sense, IPL has shown significant photorejuevantion effects. It makes use of non-coherent, high-intensity, polychromatic light (filtered flash lamp) with a broad wavelength spectrum of 550-1,200 nm and is non-ablative and causes controlled thermal damage. Filters may be used to omit shorter wavelengths. The lower risk of post-inflammatory hyperpigmentation and decreased downtime have made IPL a popular choice in the treatment of skin aging (Gu et al. 2011). At longer wavelengths, IPL devices combine the targeting of dyspigmentation and vascularity leading in improvement in the treatment of photodamage (Alexiades-Armenakas et al. 2008). IPL is used for a range of conditions and is due to the use of filters that allow light of a selected wavelength to be used. Cao and colleagues (2011) irradiated human skin fibroblasts *in vitro* with IPL (20 ms pulse interval, 18, 23, 28 and 33 J/cm^2) and noted that there was a considerable increase in mRNA levels of collagen type I and III. There was also an increase in the number of cells in the S phase and hence proliferation and increased cell viability. This occurred in a dose dependent manner up to 28 J/cm^2 (Cao et al. 2011). IPL irradiation is accompanied by an increase in proteinases, resulting in a dynamic repair process. Gu et al. (2011) treated human photoaged skin with IPL and UVA and assessed the protein expression levels of matrix metalloproteases (MMP), proteases which degrade collagen and other elastic fibres, as well as its inhibitor, tissue inhibitor of metalloproteinase (TIMP). Both IPL and UVA irradiation resulted in an increase in MMP-1, -3, -9 and -12 and TIMP-1, however the expression pattern between the two differed; an increase in MMP-1, -3 and -12 was seen in UVA treated skin and lower MMP-1, -3 and -12 and higher MMP-9 was seen in IPL treated skin. There was an increase in collagen type I in IPL treated skin and more elastic fibre fragments seen in UVA treated skin (Gu et al. 2011).

Lee et al. (2014) irradiated pig skin with different spot diameters (5, 8 and 10 mm) and fluencies (26, 30 and 36 J/cm^2) with a 1,064 nm Nd:YAG or Alexandrite (755 nm) laser (pulse duration 30 ms) and assessed epidermal and dermal changes via histology. Dermal temperature was higher in Nd:YAG irradiated skin, while the opposite was seen in the epidermis, which higher temperatures see in skin irradiated at 755 nm. This is due to the different penetration depths of the two wavelengths. Epidermal temperatures were more effected by fluence rather than spot size, while the opposite was seen in the dermis. Irradiation conditions of spot size 10 mm and a fluence of 36 J/cm^2 were not optimal as the epidermal and dermal temperatures increased to >47°C and 80°C respectively. All other irradiation combinations showed epidermal temperatures below 47°C and thus did not cause epidermal damage. The optimal treatment parameters for skin rejuvenation was 8 mm with 30 J/cm^2 and 10 mm with 26 J/cm^2 for the 1,064 nm laser; and 8 mm with 36 J/cm^2 and 10 mm with 26 J/cm^2 for the 755 nm laser (Lee et al. 2014). Similar results were seen in an irradiated phantom skin model and pig skin (Park et al. 2013). In this study optimum conditions for skin rejuvenation using a 1,064 nm Nd:YAG laser was determined at a spot diameter of 5 mm and a fluence of 36 J/cm^2, as well as a spot diameter of 10 mm and a fluence of 26 J/cm^2. Civas et al. (2010) made use of a three dimensional (3D) procedure whereby three different laser devices and technologies were simultaneously used; broadband pulsed light (BBL, 560 – 1,200 nm) (Photogenesis) to treat superficial to mid-dermal damage, a 1,064 nm Nd:YAG laser (Laser Genesis) to treat vascular lesions and a 1100 – 1800 nm infrared light source (IRLS) (Titan®) to treat skin ptosis and laxity. Irradiation of the skin resulted in a more youthful and refreshed appearance, with prominent decreases in solar dyschromia and pore width, as well as a decrease in rhytids (Civas et al. 2010).

❑ Fractionated Lasers

Fractionated lasers provide a link between ablative and non-ablative lasers. They utilize water as the target chromophore and heat and vaporize narrow cylindrical areas of tissue, or microthermal zones (MTZ), to a depth of around 1 to 1.5 mm and a width of around $100 - 400$ μm and up to 6,400 MTZs per cm and there is no damage to the basement membrane (Sawhney and Hamblin 2014; Tournas and Zachary 2010; Stewart et al. 2013). These MTZs comprise about 15 to 25 percent of the skin surface area (Alexiades-Armenakas et al. 2008). The resultant micro-lesions are separated by undamaged tissue, which can account for up to about 15 to 85 percent of the treated surface area (Stewart et al. 2013). The healing rate of these MTZs is rapid in comparison to lesions created by traditional ablative lasers and is supported by the undamaged surrounding tissue. The ablated tissue is repopulated with cells from the undamaged surrounding tissue. This modality not only produces resurfacing but also volumetric tissue reduction with horizontal contraction, thereby reducing the surface area of the skin (Tournas and Zachary 2010). Fractionated lasers can be either ablative, causing full-thickness destruction, or non-ablative which leaves an intact stratum corneum. Fractional ablative lasers are more effective with an increased recovery time (Stewart et al. 2013). Some side effects of this treatment include oozing and crusting, edema, occasional acneiform lesions, post-inflammatory hyperpigmentation in darker skin types and on occasion scarring (Tournas and Zachary 2010). Mild to moderate results are seen with fractional lasers and multiple treatments, up to six, every one to four weeks may be necessary (Alexiades-Armenakas et al. 2008).

Fractional non-ablative lasers typically have a wavelength between 1,320 – 1,927 nm (e.g. Nd:YAG. Er: glass, Er: fibre, Er: thallium), while fractional ablative lasers have wavelengths between 2,940 – 10,600 nm (e.g. Er: YAG, Er: YSGG, CO_2) (Stewart et al. 2013). Some typical fractional ablative devices include: the Fraxelre:pair laser system (Solta Medical, Hayward, CA), a CO_2 laser; the LumenisDeepFX/ActiveFX (Lumenis Inc., Santa Clara, CA), a CO_2 laser; Lutronic eCO_2 laser (Lutronic USA, Princeton Junction, NJ), a CO_2 laser; the SmartXide DOT laser (Eclipsemed, Inc., Dallas, TX), a continuous wave CO_2 laser; the Mixto SX (Lasering USA Inc., San Ramon, CA), a CO_2 laser; the Pixel CO_2 device (Alma Lasers, Inc., Buffalo Grove, IL); the ScitonProFractional device (Sciton, Inc., Palo Alto, CA), a Er: YAG laser; the Palomar Lux2940 device (Palomar Medical Technologies, Burlington, MA), a Er:YAG laser; the Alma Pixel 2940 device (Alma Lasers, Inc., Buffalo Grove, IL), a Er: YAG laser; and the Cultura Pearl Fractional device (Cultura, Inc., Brisbane, CA), a Er:YAG laser (Tournas and Zachary 2010).

Ablative fractional lasers have been successfully used in the treatment of hypertrophic, atrophic and restrictive scars. Fractional CO_2 and Er: YAG lasers have shown improvements in treating these scars with respect to improvement in vascularity, pigmentation, scar thickness and improvement in pliability and patient satisfaction and has been shown to be safe for use in darker Fitzpatrick skin types (Giordano and Ozog 2015). However the mechanism of action still seems somewhat elusive and future work on the biologic mechanisms is still required. Tierney and colleagues (2011) conducted a prospective, single blinded study in 25 subjects on the use of an ablative fractionated CO_2 laser for the treatment of lower eyelid rhytids and laxity. Subjects were treated on two or three occasions with six to eight weeks between treatments and improvement was assessed via photographs six months following the last treatment. Patients reported minimal pain and noted moderate post-treatment erythema and edema and minor crusting and oozing. There was a significant improvement in the skin texture and tightening of the eyelids (Tierney et al. 2011). Tan and co-workers (2014) showed that fractional CO_2 laser for the treatment of photoaging in Asians was safe and effective for up to five years, with minimal, non-clinical-significant adverse effects. Similar results were obtained by Marmon et al. (2014) using a 1,440 nm diode-based fractional laser. Kohl et al. (2015) conducted a prospective clinical study on patient expectation before and satisfaction following three fractional CO_2 laser treatments for rhytids. There was a significant reduction in wrinkle size and depth and patient satisfaction was substantially improved following treatment with regards to overall skin appearance. Expectations prior to treatment were high and a fresher look and even complexion had higher priority than wrinkle reduction. These expectations were met or exceeded in some instances, while expectations of wrinkle reduction were not completely fulfilled (Kohl et al. 2015). Treatment of photodamage of chest skin is complicated due to the thin nature of the skin. Grunebaum et al. (2015) treated photodamaged skin on the chest with a 2,790 nm Er:YSGG laser in 12 patients with Fitzpatrick skin types I-III. It was found that a single pass with a fluence greater than or equal to 3 mJ lead to an unacceptable rate of hyperpigmentation and a double pass with a fluence less than or equal to 2.5 mJ resulted in a mild improvement without any significant unfavourable effects. Further studies need to be conducted in the resurfacing of chest skin to better define therapeutic settings and laser safety (Grunebaum et al. 2015).

Fractional non-ablative lasers, fractional ablative lases and ablative lasers have all shown positive results in the treatment of acne scarring. Of all the skin conditions which fractional lasers are able to improve, the treatment of acne scarring shows the most improvement and the procedure appears to be as effective as ablative lasers (Sebaratnam et al. 2014). Hedelund et al. (2010) treated ten patients for acne scarring with a 1,540 nm non-ablative fractional laser. One intra-individual area was randomly treated 3-monthly, while another similar area received no treatment. Overall scar texture, adverse effects, skin colour and patient satisfaction were evaluated at four and 12 weeks. Following treatment, scars were smoother than untreated scars, with no difference in skin redness and half the patients evaluated their scars as moderately to significantly improved. Minimum side effects of moderate pain, erythema, edema, bullae and crusts were observed (Hedelund et al. 2010). Cho et al. (2010) treated one half of the face of eight patients with acne scarring with a non-ablative 1,550 nm Er-glass laser (FPS) and the other side of the face with a fractional ablative 10,600 nm CO_2 laser (CO_2 FS). They showed that a single session of treatment using both the FPS and CO_2 FS was beneficial in the treatment of acne scars. Suh et al. (2015) treated 15 patients with dilated facial pores with an Er-doped fiber laser (1,410 nm) on three occasions, with three weeks between treatments. There was a 51 percent improvement in dilated pores in 14 of the patients, with improvements in skin texture, tone and smoothness in all patients. There were no unanticipated side effects and this treatment regime was suitable for patients with Fitzpatrick skin types III-IV (Suh et al. 2015).

❑ Low-level Light Therapy (LLLT)/ Photobiomodulation (PBM)

Low-level light (laser) therapy (LLLT), or photobiomodulation (PMB), is a non-invasive, non-thermal, novel treatment modality for skin rejuvenation and is an alternative to ablative and non-ablative lasers. PBM typically includes wavelengths of between 500 and 1,100 nm, a fluence of 1 to 4 J/cm² and an output power of 10 to 90 mW (Basford 1995), however higher outputs up to 500 mW can be used (Joensen et al. 2011). A wavelength of 633 nm/830 nm is most commonly used in skin rejuvenation (Sawhney and Hamblin 2014). PBM differs greatly from ablative and non-ablative skin rejuvenation in that PBM does not cause tissue destruction (to stimulate healing) but rather stimulates the cells directly in a non-thermal manner; there is an improvement in aged skin with no destruction of the epidermis or dermis. Irradiation of cells using PBM results in an increase in cellular viability, proliferation, migration, collagen production and the release of various cytokines and growth factors (Fig. 5). It also has an effect on matrix metalloproteinases (MMP), which degrade collagen and their tissue inhibitors (TIMPs), as well as an anti-inflammatory and analgesic effect (Hersant et al. 2015; Avci et al. 2013). Photo energy, from a laser or LED source, is directly absorbed by chromophores in the cell (mitochondrial respiratory chain in the case of red and infrared light) which stimulates cell signalling cascades (Houreld et al. 2012). Light parameters which play a very important role in PBM includes the wavelength, fluence and irradiance and these can greatly influence the results obtained. Use of these light sources has shown improvements in wrinkles and skin laxity.

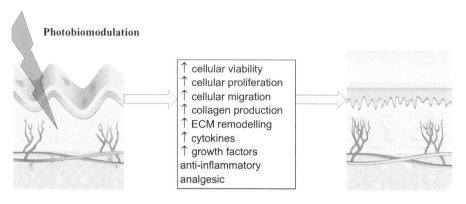

FIG. 5 *Photobiomodulation makes use of low-powered lasers which are non-thermal for skin rejuvenation. Photons are absorbed by chromophores in the cells which leads to an increase in secondary messengers which activate a cascade of cellular events. There is an increase in collagen deposition and remodelling of the extracellular matrix (ECM), resulting in less wrinkles and tighter skin.*

Joensen and colleagues (2011) conducted a study on the thermal effects of a 200 mW, 810 nm laser and a 60 mW, 904 nm laser, using four irradiation doses of 2, 6, 9, 12 J and two placebo irradiations (same duration as 2 J and 12 J respectively) in patients of different skin colour, age and gender. It was concluded that at low doses thermal effects are negligible (<1.5°C) in light- and medium-coloured skin, however at higher doses using the class 3B 200 mW laser a significant increase in skin temperature was seen, which may cause pain in persons of a darker skin colour. Wunsch and Matuschka (2014) conducted a randomized control clinical trial on 113 patients which received PBM twice a week for 15 weeks using polychromatic light (611-650 nm or 570-850 nm). Patients experienced significant improvements in skin feeling and complexion, increased collagen density and a reduction in fine lines and wrinkles. Weiss and colleagues (2005) used LED alone (590 nm) or in combination with other therapies including IPL, pulsed dye lasers, KTP and infrared lasers, radiofrequency as well as ablative lasers for skin rejuvenation in 900 patients. They concluded that the use LED reduced the appearance of fine lines and reversed the signs of aging and that the combined use of LED with other thermal-based procedures resulted in a decrease in erythema post-treatment. They further stated that the anti-inflammatory effect of LED improved the outcome of thermal-based rejuvenation therapies (Weiss et al. 2005). Barolet et al. (2009) irradiated a 3D skin model with 660 nm LED and showed an increase in collagen and a decrease in MMP-1. They also treated 40 patients three times a week for four weeks in a split-face, single-blinded study. Patients reported no adverse effects or downtime and there was no significant increase in skin temperature, with temperatures remaining stable or not more than 0.5°C. Eighty seven percent of participants showed a reduction in rhytids (Barolet et al. 2009). Lask and colleagues (2005) treated

30 patients with a laser device emitting blue (405-425 nm)/near infrared (850-890 nm) light. Ninety percent of the patients showed a decrease in pore size and enhancement in skin vitality and radiance. It was concluded that the combination of wavelengths has a wide application in aesthetic procedures (as seen by the treatment of other skin conditions such as post skin resurfacing and removal of skin lesions, post face-lift and post breast augmentation) and the treatments were free from side effects (Lask et al. 2005).

❑ Photodynamic Therapy (PDT)

PDT is typically used in the treatment of cancer and makes use of a photosensitizer (PS) which is activated upon exposure to light of a specific wavelength. The use of topical PSs, such as FDA approved 5-Aminolevulinic acid (5-ALA), for short periods of time with non-ablative photorejuvenation lasers has been shown to be safe and effective, with minimal side effects (Alexiades-Armenakas et al. 2008). Blue light IPL, PDL and long pulsed PDLs are typically used. Piacquadio and colleagues (2004) used 5-ALA in a phase III clinical study. Eighty nine percent of patients showed an improvement and it was concluded that 5-ALA was an effective and safe treatment for multiple actinic keratoses of the face and scalp (Piacquadio et al. 2004). Zhang and colleagues (2014) evaluated the effect of combined red light, or IPL with 5-ALA for the photorejuvenation of neck skin. They showed that IPL-PDT and red-light-PDT using 5-ALA was better than using IPL or red light alone.

❑ Conclusion

Aging causes a decline in cellular activity and these changes are accompanied by diminished cellular structural and functional integrity. Aging is associated with wrinkles, dyspigmentation, telangiectasia and reduced tissue elasticity and has a negative impact on ones self-esteem and body image. There is thus an everlasting demand for improvement in skin appearance and as a result aesthetic procedures such as phototherapy are becoming increasingly popular. Lasers and various other light sources have been extensively used to treat a myriad of dermatological conditions and have had a tremendous impact on the treatment of skin aging. Ablative lasers give better results, however the technology is associated with far more severe side-effects and increased patient downtime. Ablative lasers are no longer the mainstay in skin rejuvenation and their popularity is waning. Non-ablative laser technologies for skin rejuvenation repairs the signs of aging by causing thermal damage to the dermis while the epidermis is unharmed. This technology is less invasive with minimal side-effects and decreased patient downtime following irradiation. However the clinical results are often subtle. Driven by the need for more effective, safer technologies with a shorter downtime, fractional lasers were developed. The use of fractional lasers allows for the treatment of skin aging and other conditions, is easier to administer and has a decreased recovery time, however it is not free from side-effects. Fractional lasers deliberately induce microscopic, thermal-induced wounds, which stimulates the wound healing process. Fractional lasers are considered by many as the gold standard for skin rejuvenation due to their favourable efficacy to adverse effect profile (Stewart et al. 2013). PBM is a new treatment for skin rejuvenation with no reported side effects, however in order to broaden its applications in plastic surgery more research needs to be conducted and high quality, randomized placebo controlled clinical publications to validate its use in this field is required. *In vitro* studies making use of PBM has shown an increase in collagen production, angiogenesis, cellular viability, proliferation and migration and effects on the extracellular matrix, as well as speeding up the process of wound healing. Practitioners making use of any of these modalities must have experience in the treatment protocols and have a broad understanding of the treatment and be aware of the safety concerns surrounding these devices. The use of these devices in individuals of colour, with Fitzpatrick skin phototypes IV-VI, needs further research to investigate the safety and efficacy of such treatments (Alexis 2013). Another point to consider is the safety and efficacy of light-based treatments in the elderly and additional thought and investigation should be given when treating such individuals (Powell and Gach 2015).

There is an ever increasing demand from patients for better technologies to address the issues and treatment of skin aging and if current treatments can be improved upon with better results and less side effects patient expectations would be better met. Existing light therapies continue to change and evolve with ongoing research and clinical studies. Practitioners need to critically evaluate all the available data and ensure that devices are used appropriately and as more and more light devices come onto the market and are used by such a wide scope of practitioners, stricter control and better government legislation on its use should be enforced.

❏ References

Acland, K.M. and R.J. Barlow. 2000. Lasers for the dermatologist. B J Dermatol 143: 244-255.

Alexiades-Armenakas, M.R., J.S. Dover and K.A. Arndt. 2008. The spectrum of laser skin resurfacing: Nonablative, fractional and ablative laser resurfacing. J Am Acad Dermatol 58: 719-737.

Alexis, A.F. 2013. Lasers and light-based therapies in ethnic skin: treatment options and recommendations for Fitzpatrick skin types V and VI. B J Dermatol 169 (suppl. 3): 91-97.

Altshuler, G.B., R.R. Anderson, D. Manstein, H.H. Zenzie and M.Z. Smirnov. 2001. Extended theory of selective photothermolysis. Lasers Surg Med 29: 416-432.

Avci, P., A. Gupta, M. Sadasivam, D. Vecchio, Z. Pam, N. Pam, et al. 2013. Low-level laser (light) therapy (LLLT) in skin: stimulating, healing, restoring. Semin Cutan Med Surg 32: 41-52.

Barolet, D., C.J. Roberge, F.A. Auger, A. Boucher and L. Germain. 2009. Regulation of skin collagen metabolism In Vitro using a pulsed 660 nm LED light source: clinical correlation with a single-blinded study. J Invest Dermatol 129: 2751-2759.

Basford, J.R. 1995. Low intensity laser therapy: still not an established clinical tool. Lasers Surg Med 16: 331-342.

Berlin, A.L. and D.J. Goldberg. 2010. Non-ablative resurfacing. pp 20-37. *In*: Goldberg, D.J. [ed.]. Facial Resurfacing. Wiley-Blackwell, Hoboken, NJ, USA.

Cao, Y., R. Huo, Y. Feng, Q. Li and F. Wang. 2011. Effects of intense pulsed light on the biological properties and ultrastructure of skin dermal fibroblasts: Potential roles in photoaging. Photomed Laser Surg 29: 327-332.

Cho, S.B., S.J. Lee, S. Cho, S.H. Oh, W.S. Chung, J.M. Kang, et al. 2010. Non-ablative 1550-nm erbium-glass and ablative 10,600-nm carbon dioxide fractional lasers for acne scars: a randomized split-face study with blinded response evaluation. J Eur Acad Dermatol Venereol 24: 921-925.

Civas, E., B. Aksoy, E. Surucu, E. Koc and H.M. Aksoy. 2010. Effectiveness of non-ablative three dimensional (3D) skin rejuvenation: a retrospective study involving 46 patients. Photomed Laser Surg 28: 685-692.

Giordano, C.N. and D. Ozog. 2015. Microstructural and molecular considerations in the treatment of scars with ablative fractional lasers. Semin Cutan Med Surg 34: 7-12.

Grunebaum, L.D., J. Murdock, P. Cofnas and J. Kaufman. 2015. Safety and efficacy of 2,790-nm laser resurfacing for chest photoaging. Lasers Med Sci 30: 355-361.

Gu, W., W. Liu, X. Yang, X. Zhao, X. Yuan, H. Ma, et al. 2011. Effects of intense pulsed light and ultraviolet A on metalloproteinases and extracellular matix expression in human skin. Photomed Laser Surg 29: 97-103.

Hedelund, L., K.E. Moreau and D.M. Beyer. 2010. Fractional nonablative 1,540-nm laser resurfacing of atrophic acne scars. A randomized controlled trial with blinded response evaluation. Lasers Med Sci 25: 749-754.

Hersant, B., M. SidAhmed-Mezi, R. Bosc and J.P. Meningaud. 2015. Current indications of low-level laser therapy in plastic surgery: a review. Photomed Laser Surg 33: 283-297.

Kohl, E., J. Meierhöfer, M. Koller, F. Zeman, L. Groesser, S. Karrer, et al. 2015. Fractional carbon dioxide laser resurfacing of rhytids and photoaged skin – a prospective clinical study on patient expectations and satisfaction. Lasers Surg Med 47: 111-119.

Houreld, N.N. 2013. Visible red and near infra-red light is absorbed by cytochrome c oxidase and stimulates the production of ATP. pp 161-176. *In:* Kuester, E. and G. Traugott [eds.]. Adenosine Triphosphate: Chemical Properties, Biosynthesis and Function in Cells. Nova Science Publishers Inc., New York, NY, USA.

Houreld, N.N. 2014. Shedding light on a new treatment for diabetic wound healing: a review on phototherapy. The Scientific World Journal. 2014: http://dx.doi.org/10.1155/2014/398412.

Houreld, N.N., R.T. Masha and H. Abrahamse. 2012. Low-Intensity Laser irradiation at 660 nm stimulates cytochrome c oxidase in stressed fibroblast cells. Lasers Surg Med 44: 429-434.

Joensen, J., J.H. Demmink, M.I. Johnson, V.V. Iversen, R.A.B. Lopes-Martins and J.M. Bjordal. 2011. The thermal effects of therapeutic lasers with 810 and 904 nm wavelengths on human skin. Photomed Laser Surg 29: 145-153.

Lask, G., N. Fournier, M. Trelles, M. Elman, M. Scheflan, M. Slatkine, et al. 2005. The utilization of nonthermal blue (405-425 nm) and near infrared (850-890 nm) light in aesthetic dermatology and surgery – a multicentre study. J Cosmet Laser Ther 7: 163-170.

Lee, J.H., S.R. Park, J.H. Jo, S.Y. Park, Y.K. Seo and S.M. Kim. 2014. Comparison of epidermal/dermal damage between the long-pulsed 1064 nm Nd:YAG and 755 nm alexandrite lasers under relatively high fluence conditions: quantitative and histological assessments. Photomed Laser Surg 32: 386-393.

Marmon, S., S.Y.N. Shek, C.K. Yeung, N.P.Y. Chan, J.C.Y. Chana and H.H.L. Chan. 2014. Evaluating the safety and efficacy of the 1,440-nm laser in the treatment of photodamage in Asian skin. Lasers Surg Med 46: 375-379.

Ohshiro, T. 1991. An introduction to LLLT. pp 36-47. *In*: Ohshiro, T. and R.G. Calderhead [eds.]. Progress in Laser Therapy. Selected Papers from the October 1990 ILTA Congress. John Wiley and Sons, West Sussex, England.

Park, S.R., J.H. Lee, J.H. Jo, Y.K. Seo and S.M. Kim. 2013. The effects of 1064 nm Nd:YAG laser irradiation under the different treatment conditions for skin rejuvenation: quantitative and histologic analyses. Photomed Laser Surg 31: 283-292.

Peavy, G.M. 2002. Lasers and laser-tissue interaction. Vet Clin Small Anim 32: 517-534.

Piacquadio, D.J., D.M. Chen, H.F. Farber, J.F. Fowler, S.D. Glazer, J.J. Goodman, et al. 2004. Photodynamic therapy with aminolevulinic acid topical solution and visible blue light in the treatment of multiple actinic keratoses of the face and scalp: investigator-blinded, phase 3, multicenter trials. Arch Dermatol 140: 41-46.

Powell J.B. and J.E. Gach. 2015. Phototherapy in the elderly. Clinical and Experimental Dermatology 40: 605-610.

Sawhney, M.K. and M.R. Hamblin. 2014. Low level laser (light) therapy (LLLT) for cosmetic medicine and dermatology. *In*: Smith, K.C. [ed.]. Photobiological Sciences Online. American Society for Photobiology, http://www.photobiology.info/.

Sebaratnam, D.F., A.C. Lim, P.M. Lowe, G.J. Goodman, P. Bekhor and S. Richards. 2014. Lasers and laser-like devices: Part two. Australas. J Dermatol 55: 1-14.

Stewart, N., A.C. Lim, P.M. Lowe and G. Goodman. 2013. Lasers and laser-like devices: part one. Australas. J Dermatol 54: 173-183.

Suh, D.-H., K.-Y. Chang, S.-J. Lee, K.-Y. Song, J.H. Choi, M.K. Shin, et al. 2015. Treatment of dilated pores with 1410-nm fractional erbium-doped fiber laser. Lasers Med Sci 30: 1135-1139.

Tan, J., Y. Lei, H.-W. Ouyang and M.H. Gold. 2014. The use of fractional CO_2 laser resurfacing in the treatment of photoaging in Asians: five years long-term results. Lasers Surg Med 46: 750-756.

Tierney, E.P., W. Hanke and L. Watkins. 2011. Treatment of lower eyelid rhytids and laxity with ablative fractional carbon-dioxide laser resurfacing: Case series and review of the literature. J Am Acad Dermatol 64: 730-740.

Tournas, J.A. and C.B. Zachary. 2010. Fractional ablative resurfacing. pp 38-59. *In*: Goldberg, D.J. [ed.]. Facial Resurfacing. Wiley-Blackwell, Hoboken, NJ, USA.

Trobonjaca, T. and Z. Simunovic. 2000. Aesthetic treatments with low level laser therapy. pp 361-371. *In*: Simunovic, Z. [ed.]. Lasers in Medicine and Dentistry: Basic Science and Up-To-Date Clinical Applications of Low Energy-Level Laser Therapy- LLLT. Vitagrafd.o.o.o. Rijeka, Croatia.

Tunér, J. and L. Hode. 2002. Laser Therapy. Clinical Practice and Scientific Background. Prima Books, Grängesberg, Sweden.

Wanitphakdeedecha, R., W. Manuskiatti, S. Siriphukpong and T.M. Chen. 2009. Treatment of punched-out atrophic and rolling acne scars in skin phototypes III, IV and V with variable square pulse erbium:yttrium-aluminium-garnet laser resurfacing. Dermatol Surg 35: 1376-1383.

Weiss, R.A., D.H. McDaniel, R.G. Geronemus, M.A. Weiss, K.L. Beasley, G.M. Munavalli et al. 2005. Clinical experience with light-emitting diode (LED) photobiomodulation. Dermatol Surg 31: 1199-1205.

Wunsch, A. and K. Matuschka. 2014. A controlled trial to determine the efficacy of red and near-infrared light treatmentin patient satisfaction, reduction of fine lines, wrinkles, skin roughness and intradermal collagen density increase. Photomed Laser Surg 32: 93-100.

Zhang, H.Y., J. Ji, Y.M. Tan, L.L. Zhang, X.J. Wang, PR. Wang, et al. 2014. Evaluation of 5-aminolevulinic acid-mediated photorejuvenation of neck skin. Photodiagnosis Photodyn Ther 11: 498-509.

11
CHAPTER

Aging Skin: A Window to the Body

Dr. med. Georgios Nikolakis,[1,*] *Dr. med. Evgenia Makrantonaki*[1,2,3,a] and
Prof. Dr. med. Prof. h.c. Dr. h.c. Christos C. Zouboulis[1,b]

❑ Introduction

Aging is defined as a natural, gradual process of biochemical events, leading to gradual damage accumulation and resulting in disease and death (Vina et al. 2007). Such changes are hidden as far as the inner organs are concerned and therefore, the skin appears as the first and main teller of these gradual alterations (Nikolakis et al. 2013). Moreover, the easy and cost-effective accessibility of this organ, as well as the detection or isolation of its main cellular (keratinocytes, fibroblasts, hair follicle and sebaceous cells, mast cells, Langerhans cells etc.) and non-cellular components (extracellular matrix, collagen, elastin) provides a model for the assessment and determination of the involved molecular mechanisms (Ganceviciene et al. 2012). For this, it can be considered the "key hole" to observe the aging process of the whole organism.

Skin has long been recognized to protect organisms against deleterious environmental factors and is important for the homeostasis of temperature, electrolyte and fluid balance of the body (Makrantonaki et al. 2012a; Makrantonaki et al. 2015).

[1] Departments of Dermatology, Venereology, Allergology and Immunology, Dessau Medical Center, 06847 Dessau, Germany.
[2] Geriatry Research Group, Charité Universitaetsmedizin, Berlin, 13347 Berlin, Germany.
[3] Department of Dermatology and Allergology, University Medical Center Ulm, 89081 Ulm, Germany.
[a] E-mail: evgenia.makrantonaki@uni-ulm.de
[b] E-mail: christos.zouboulis@klinikum-dessau.de
[*] Corresponding author: georgios.nikolakis@klinikum-dessau.de

❑ Skin Aging: Different Pathophysiology Leads to Different Phenotype

Aged skin is characterized by a phenotype of a disturbed lipid barrier, angiogenesis, production of sweat, gradual deterioration of the epidermal immune response and production of calcitriol, cellular heterogeneity, as well as the tendency towards development of various benign or malignant diseases (Kinn et al. 2015; Zouboulis and Makrantonaki 2011). These biological processes include endogenous variables such as genetic predisposition, impairment of cellular metabolic pathways, qualitative and quantitative hormonal alterations, termed intrinsic aging. At the other end of the spectrum, exogenous factors, such as ultraviolet (UV) irradiation, chemicals and toxins, pollution, lead to extrinsic aging (Cevenini et al. 2008). Based on this knowledge, two experimental models of human skin were developed and utilized in order to express the two main axes of skin aging (patho) physiology: The model for intrinsic aging is skin deriving from areas which are not sun-exposed, such as the inner side of the upper arm and the gluteal region, whilst for the model for extrinsic aging involves constantly UV-exposed skin regions, such as facial skin. The phenotype of intrinsically aged skin appears macroscopically thin and atrophic, exhibits fine wrinkles, subcutaneous fat loss, prominent dryness and reduced elasticity (Callaghan and Wilhelm 2008). In contrast, extrinsically photoaged skin exhibits deeper wrinkles, thickening of the epidermis, dullness, roughness and mottled discoloration. Telangiectasias and pigmentary discoloration might also be observed in advanced and severe degrees of photoaging (Callaghan and Wilhelm 2008; El-Domyati et al. 2002; Kligman 1989; Lock-Andersen et al. 1997; Makrantonaki and Zouboulis 2007; Moragas et al. 1993).

The phenotype of aging shows considerable variations between different ethnical groups. Caucasians have greater skin wrinkle formation and sagging in comparison to other skin phenotypes, while the manifestations have an earlier onset (Rawlings 2006). Furthermore, Caucasians are more prone to skin desquamation, which is dependent of age (Chu and Kollias 2011). Afro-American and Caucasian women are both having a higher prevalence of age-related dryness compared to other ethnicity groups (Diridollou et al. 2007). Chinese women have more severe periorbital wrinkles in comparison to women from Japan, while Thai women were characterized by severe wrinkling of the lower half of their faces (Tsukahara et al. 2004). Caucasian females have a higher prevalence of sagging in the subzygomatic area (Rawlings 2006). Wrinkling in each facial area has a later onset in Chinese women in comparison to French women, although age-related pigment spot intensity is the cardinal sign of aging in Chinese women (Nouveau-Richard et al. 2005). Lastly, although Asian skin seems to have similar transepidermal water loss and ceramide levels to Caucasian skin, the stratum corneum barrier appears to be more susceptible to mechanical stimuli. Asian skin is more sensitive to exogenous chemicals because of the thinner stratum corneum barrier, higher eccrine gland intensity and smaller pore areas in comparison to other ethnic groups, indicating the correlation of the latter to the sebaceous gland activity (Rawlings 2006). Since skin aging phenotype varies according to the population, not universal but ethnicity specific aging characteristics could only be correlated with age-associated diseases. Photographic severity scales and other clinical methods are developed to assess the severity of skin aging features (Callaghan and Wilhelm 2008; Valet et al. 2009).

❑ Intrinsic Aging

Current experimental research led to the development of different theories in order to determine different pathophysiological key aspects of aging. Among them are the theory of cellular senescence, telomere shortening and decreased proliferative capacity, the inflammation theory, mitochondrial DNA single mutations and the free radical theory (Allsopp et al. 1992; Dimri et al. 1995; Harman 2003; Makrantonaki et al. 2010; Medvedev 1990; Michikawa et al. 1999).

Cellular Senescence

Senescence is the term used to describe the decrease of regenerative potential of cells or tissues through an individual´s lifetime. The mechanisms involved in these processes involve response to numerous cellular stresses, including production of reactive oxygen species and telomere shortening. Lately, the role of microRNAs has been highlighted as fine tuners of the balance between proliferative capacity and replicative senescence of skin key cellular components, such as keratinocytes and fibroblasts (Mancini et al. 2014).

Human dermal fibroblasts were shown to exhibit enlarged cell bodies after many series of passages *in vitro*. Furthermore, they were more often stained positive for the myofibroblast marker α-smooth actin, the senescence markers β-galactosidase and p16, in comparison to early passage fibroblasts. The fibroblasts were in a subsequent step involved in the creation of *in vitro* reconstructed skin or human skin equivalents (HSE). HSE formation with late passage fibroblasts resulted in an altered phenotype mimicking intrinsic aging *in vivo* with thinner dermis and reduced matrix formation, weaker expression of the differentiation marker keratin 10 (Janson et al. 2013a), highlighting the effects of aging in ECM quality, keratinocyte differentiation and strata formation. However, the changes regarding epidermal proliferation and the basement membrane, which are observed *in vivo*, were missing (Gilhar et al. 2004).

Both matrix degradation and proinflammatory responses are involved in skin aging. Recent studies compared the genome of human sebocytes and whole skin and the secretome of normal human fibroblasts isolated from intrinsically aged skin of young, middle aged and old donors. Thirty nine genes and 70 proteins depicted an age-dependent pattern. Twenty-seven of the proteins were isolated exclusively from intrinsically aged skin and are associated with processes such as metabolism and adherence junction interactions. These present a distinct pattern related to intrinsic aging mechanisms, thus differing from the classical senescent-associated secretory phenotype of cellular senescence, mentioned later in "immunological impairment" (Makrantonaki et al. 2006; Makrantonaki et al. 2012b; Waldera Lupa et al. 2015).

High passage fibroblasts deriving from the papillary and reticular dermis were utilized for the reconstruction of artificial skin *in vitro* (Janson et al. 2013b). The HSE which were formed from reticular fibroblasts showed impaired differentiation patterns and areas of impaired epidermal strata formation. More specifically, a more prominent expression of the epidermal differentiation markers loricrin, filaggrin and small proline-rich protein 2 in the stratum granulosum and corneum of the HSE deriving from papillary fibroblasts in comparison to reticular fibroblast derived ones was observed. In addition, the presence of papillary fibroblasts resulted in a higher number of Ki67-positive basal keratinocytes. Papillary fibroblast senescence led to a more reticular-like fibroblast phenotype (Janson et al. 2013b).

Another approach to assimilate intrinsic aging is to use normal human fibroblasts and prolong the culture time of HSEs for up to 120 days. The phenotypic changes resembled the ones of *in vivo* intrinsic aging with a significant decrease of the epidermis thickness and the number of basal keratinocytes expressing the proliferation marker Ki67. Moreover, differentiation markers were also strongly decreased, while as the senescence marker p16INK4a was significantly increased (Dos Santos et al. 2015).

Immunological Alterations

Aging is usually associated with a gradual deterioration of the immune system and immunological swifts named immunosenescence. In contrast, it is also reported to correlate to a hyper-inflammatory state, termed inflammaging (Franceschi et al. 2000; Nikolakis et al. 2013). The impairment of the aged immune system makes it susceptible to certain infections, autoimmune diseases and malignancies. The age-relating processes in this case are not exclusively intrinsic, but extrinsic factors such as UV-damage are also being involved (Giacomoni et al. 2000). Damaged cells secrete inflammatory mediators, such as prostaglandins and leukotrienes, inducing the release of tumor necrosis factor-α (TNF-α) and histamine from resident mast cells. This leads to the release of P-selectins and the upregulation of adhesion molecules, as well as interleukin-1 dysregulation. Molecules which can promote the intercellular adhesion molecule-1 (ICAM-1) synthesis and the subsequent recruitment of circulating immune cells in the dermis are aging factors. On a subsequent step, these inflammatory cells release proteases and radical oxygen species, which provoke long-term damage in cutaneous cells (Giacomoni et al. 2000; Linton and Dorshkind 2004; Plackett et al. 2004; Plowden et al. 2004; Ye et al. 2002). Surface oxidative damage leads to formation of squalene peroxide, which correlates with extrinsic aging factors, mainly UV-damage (Giacomoni et al. 2000). Senescent cells are believed to force the surrounding cells in acquiring the so-called "senescent-associated secretory phenotype" by the secretion of various pro-inflammatory factors (Coppe et al. 2008). Furthermore, there is increasing evidence that chronic inflammation correlates with normal aging and impairs stem cell dysfunction (Freund et al. 2010).

Disruption of Epidermal Barrier

With advancing age, the epidermis develops an abnormality of the barrier homeostasis, which is even more prominent in photoaged skin (Elias and Ghadially 2002; Nikolakis et al. 2013). This is due to an overall reduction of stratum corneum lipids and a disturbance regarding the cholesterol and fatty acid synthesis (Tsutsumi and Denda 2007). Alterations in the cell membrane lipids are observed with human cell aging, such as the decrease in the polyunsaturated fatty acid content of phospholipids and the increase in cholesterol levels. Modulation of peroxisome proliferator-activated receptor gamma (PPARγ) in human dermal fibroblasts partially reduces the effects of stressed induced senescence through 8-methoxypsoralen plus UVA-irradiation, such as such cytoplasmic enlargement, the expression of senescence-associated-beta-galactosidase, matrix-metalloproteinase-1, cell cycle proteins and cell membrane lipid alterations (Briganti et al. 2014). Not only the "mortar" of the skin barrier, but the bricks as well are affected by aging: Genes associated with keratinocyte differentiation, including keratins and cornified envelope components, undergo an age-related downregulation (Robinson et al. 2009). Sebaceous lipids are also implicated in skin aging. The potential release of sebaceous lipids was highlighted in the recent development of a co-culture model of *ex vivo* skin with immortalized sebocytes. Although the sebaceous glands of the *ex vivo* skin were rapidly degenerated, co-culture of the latter with immortalized sebocytes led to a partial prevention of age-related events of the explant epidermis, namely basal keratinocyte proliferation and apoptosis of epidermal cells (Nikolakis et al. 2015).

Intrinsic Aging of other Skin Cell Types

Not only the major components composing the skin, but other cell types, such as the ones comprising the skin appendages undergo age-related changes through intrinsic and/or extrinsic aging. A premium example is the sebaceous gland. Sebaceous gland cells also show a profound decrease of sebaceous lipid release, which is age-related as well as a decrease of the size of sebaceous cells (Engelke et al. 1997; Pochi et al. 1979), after an initial increase, i.e. senile sebaceous gland hyperplasia, in order to compensate the reduction of the single cell capacity to produce lipids (Zouboulis and Boschnakow 2001). These particular *in vivo* observations were confirmed after *in vitro* treatment of human sebocytes with a hormone mixture of androgens, estrogens and growth factor levels correlating to the average serum levels of 20-year old and 60-year old women. Significant reduction of sebaceous lipogenesis was the result of the treatment with the 60-year old hormone mixture in comparison to the former, showing remarkable correlation to the phenotypical changes observed *in vivo*. Differences in gene expression were reported, according to the age-correspondence of the mixture used. These differences included the regulation of genes, which were shown to be regulated were implicated in DNA repair and stability, oxidative stress, mitochondrial processes, ubiquitin-induced proteolysis, cell cycle and apoptosis and other pathways. The most significantly altered pathway was that of tumor growth factor-β, known for its association with malignancies (Makrantonaki et al. 2006). Moreover, genes which are associated with the development of neurodegenerative diseases were reported to be expressed in human sebaceous cells, also prone to regulation through hormone treatment. These results are supported from the common embryogenic origin of the skin and the neuronal tissue and suggests interesting perspectives for the skin and rejuvenation research: Taking into account the fact that the skin and the nervous system both derive from the ectoderm, this finding led to the logical assumption that skin may be used as a tool for investigating aging of the nervous system. Additional experiments, in which the whole genome of human skin biopsies from young and elderly males and females was investigated, confirmed this hypothesis. Skin expresses several genes associated with age-associated diseases of the nerve system and these genes are regulated with increasing age, may be due to the accompanying hormone decline (Makrantonaki et al. 2012b).

The hair follicle is also susceptible to intrinsic and extrinsic aging mechanisms. There is a specialized mesenchymal population, called the dermal papilla, the number and senescence of which is correlated with follicular decline (Chi et al. 2013). The dermal papilla, located in the hair follicle, is capable to express androgen receptors and plays an important role in hair growth. Dermal papilla cells deriving from patients with androgenetic alopecia were reported to have an increased expression of senescence marker p16INK4a. The fact that the treatment of these cells with androgens led to p16INK4a upregulation suggests a major role of the androgen/androgen receptor complex in the pathogenesis of hair follicle aging. Interestingly, these effects are observed from non-balding frontal and transitional zone of balding scalp follicles but not in beard follicles (Yang et al. 2013). Hair greying is known also a hallmark of aging, with a pathophysiology ranging from follicular melanocyte stem cell defects to follicular melanocyte death (Arck et al. 2006; Peters et al. 2011). Oxidative damage leads to selective apoptosis of melanocyte stem cells, through depletion of the antiapoptotic B-cell lymphoma 2 gene (BCL-2). BCL-2 is known to be expressed in order for melanocytes to evade UVA-induced ROS damage (Seiberg 2013). Aging hair follicle stem cells of the mouse epidermis showed increased amounts of 53BP1-foci, independent of telomere shortening, suggesting increased number of double-stand breaks in these cells (Schuler and Rube 2013).

Dermal Aging

The number and composition of skin glycosaminoglycans (GAGs) change, as it was depicted in corneal keratinocytes and skin-derived fibroblasts. Hyaluronan appears to have a prominent role among the different components involved (Inoue and Katakami 1993; Toole 1997). Hyaluronan is a GAG which has the ability to bind and retain water molecules (Baumann 2007), contributing direly to skin hydration (Papakonstantinou et al. 2012). It was shown to affect the expression of metalloproteinases (MMPs). MMPs are special proteases implicated in physiological and pathological skin processes, prime examples of which are skin morphogenesis, tissue remodeling, wound healing and tumorigenesis (Shapiro 1998). Different proteases such as trypsin and plasmin regulate the MMP activity in the level of transcription and level of activation of the inactive zymogen forms. Hyaluronan increases expression and activation of MMP-2 and MMP-9 of skin explant cultures (Isnard et al. 2002). Epidermal hyaluronan disappears from aged skin, while reduction of the size of polymers may result in an overall reduction of skin moisture (Longas et al. 1987; Meyer and Stern 1994). The expression of hyaluronan and its surface receptor drastically decreases after prolonged culture *ex vivo* in an HSE (Dos Santos et al. 2015). miR-23a-3p microRNA, which targets the enzyme hyaluronan synthase-2, was upregulated in the skin of old mice compared to young ones. (Rock et al. 2015). As far as skin explant cultures are concerned, other ECM components, such as dermatane sulfate, keratane sulfate and chondroitin sulfate can upregulate MMP-9 activation, thus being of pathophysiological significance for skin remodeling (Isnard et al. 2003).

The ECM of the skin comprises different complex components such as collagen proteins, glycosaminoglycan-rich proteoglycans and elastic fibers. The ECM is constantly under structural modification and remodeling, with main components the collagen I and III, which offer skin its tensile strength (Nikolakis et al. 2013). Skin elasticity is due to various other ECM molecules with slow turnover rate, mainly elastin and fibrillin-1, which form an elastin core and a microfibrillar scaffold. Fibrillin-1 is one of the potential biomarkers for the objective assessment of aging (Langton et al.

2010; Naylor et al. 2011). The fact that many ECM molecules are not rapidly regenerating makes them excellent potential immunohistochemical targets for quantifying dermal aging.

Glycation

Glycation is the non-enzymatic reaction between sugars and proteins, lipids and nucleic acids. A long-standing high level of sugar in rats was shown to decrease epidermal lipid synthesis, lamellar body production and antimicrobial peptide expression (Park et al. 2011). The impact of advanced glycation end products (AGEs) and in aging has been highlighted over the recent years. Their formation is a stepwise process and starts with the Maillard reaction, which ends to the production of a non-stable Schiff base (or an Amadori product after further rearrangements) after reaction of the sugar carbonyl groups with amino groups of protein amino acid residues (Paul and Bailey 1996). Stable products might result also after protein adduct formation or cross-linking of Schiff base or Amadori products. AGEs exert their actions both per se and through interaction with specific receptors (receptor for AGEs – RAGE). This is a pattern recognition receptor, binding also various other molecules such as S100, β-amyloids and β-sheet fibrils (Bierhaus et al. 2005; Fleming et al. 2011). Binding of AGEs leads to activation of NFκB and transcription of various inflammatory genes (Gkogkolou and Bohm 2012). AGEs are accumulated gradually with aging. Increased levels of AGEs are the result of diseases such as diabetes mellitus, the excessive production of ROS, dietary factors and smoking (Cerami et al. 1997; Fleming et al. 2011). AGEs deposition in peripheral tissues is implicated in many diseases, such as diabetes-related macular degeneration, osteoarthritis and diabetic angiopathy (Glenn et al. 2007; Sell et al. 1993; Stitt 2001; Vlassara et al. 2002). AGEs contribute to the impairment of the arterial wall content, through their accumulation together with gradual elastin reduction (Thijssen et al. 2015; Wang et al. 2015). AGEs significantly increased TGF-β1 and metalloproteinase-2 expression in cardiac fibroblasts, which are implicated in aging and ECM remodeling respectively (Fang et al. 2015). Total content of AGEs accumulated in the organism is also defined from their removal rate, in which the glutathione-dependent system of glyoxalase I and II, as well as the fructosyl-amine oxidases and the fructosamine kinases (Wu and Monnier 2003; Xue et al. 2011). Proteins with a slow turnover rate, like collagen types I and IV, are mainly susceptible to glycation during intrinsic aging (Dyer et al. 1993; Jeanmaire et al. 2001). Collagen glycation leads to intermolecular crosslink formation of adjacent collagen fibers, leading to decreased flexibility and stiffness (Avery and Bailey 2006). Moreover, AGE-induced collagen modification makes collagen resistant to MMP proteolysis, thus hindering its degradation and substitution with new and functional fibers (DeGroot et al. 2001). Other ECM protein targets are elastin and fibronectin (Dyer et al.

1993; Jeanmaire et al. 2001; Mizutari et al. 1997). AGEs mediate their effects also direct on cells, by reducing the proliferation and inducing apoptosis of dermal fibroblasts (Alikhani et al. 2005), decrease keratinocyte cell viability and migration (Zhu et al. 2011) and the premature cellular senescence of both (Berge et al. 2007; Ravelojaona et al. 2009; Sejersen and Rattan 2009). In a recent study AGE-associated skin autofluorescence was reported to mirror the vascular function. The authors analysed the AGE-modifications in collagens obtained from residual bypass graft material via hydroxyproline assay and AGE intrinsic fluorescence and correlated their findings with skin autofluorescence measured by an autofluorescence reader. In addition, they measured pulse wave velocity which reflects vessel stiffness and correlated the findings. They found that skin autofluorescence and pulse wave velocity significantly correlate with the content of AGE in graft material so that both methods could be utilized as predictive markers of vessel function in patients suffering from coronary heart disease (Hofmann et al. 2013; Yamagishi et al. 2015). Recently, a glycated reconstructed skin equivalent was assembled from glycation induced extracellular matrix, in order to facilitate the investigation (Pennacchi et al. 2015).

Furthermore non-enzymatic glycation substantially affects collagen's ability to dissipate energy in bony tissue. Glycation-related alterations of bone's organic matrix, mostly collage type I, reduce its capacity to withstand strain forces typically associated with fall (3000-5000 µstrain) (Poundarik et al. 2015). Moreover, there is evidence that it leads to age-related anemia and hematopoietic stem cell exhaustion (Sestier 2015), ocular veovascularization (Kandarakis et al. 2015), compromised lymph flow (Zolla et al. 2015), etc. Series of experiments are needed to correlate skin AGE accumulation with the previously mentioned comorbidities, in order to provide robust models of global aging in the near future.

❑ Skin Stem Cell Aging

Stem cells are cells able to undergo self-regeneration by multiple cycles of division, while retaining their undifferentiated phenotype (Fuchs and Chen 2013; Thomson et al. 1998). Embryonic stem cells are multipotent cells and are able to give rise to all other cell types, while adult stem cells have more restricted potentials. The latter have also high proliferative capacity and are required for tissue renewal throughout the organism lifespan (Zouboulis et al. 2008). As far as the skin is concerned, epidermal stem cells are located in the stratum basale and differentiate to transient amplifying cells (TA-cells) and differentiating progenitors, forming functional epidermal proliferative units (EPUs), extending from the basal to the corneal layer (Potten 1974). Furthermore, dermal stem cells are also of great importance for skin homeostasis, since they produce the progeny responsible for ECM synthesis and growth factors. Although they are of mesodermal origin, they can give rise to endodermal liver cells and ectodermal nerve cells, suggesting the potential for giving birth to a broader palette of cell type progenitors (Biernaskie et al. 2006; Chen et al. 2007; Zouboulis et al. 2008). Since they comprise the pool of tissue regeneration, stem cells also came in focus of the aging research as a potential target of intrinsic and extrinsic aging factors, which could potentially affect the number and the function of these cells. On the other hand, the potential therapeutic effects of utilization of stem cells and especially the abundant and easy way to access adipose-derived stem cells, are also being examined (Kim et al. 2011; Yang et al. 2010).

The epidermal turnover rate is 28 days in young individuals, while it varies between 40-60 days in the elderly (Grove and Kligman 1983). Epidermal stem cells are considered unique in comparison to other adult stem cells in their ability to resist aging. They show no effects associated with increased ROS levels, perhaps as a result of maintaining high levels of superoxide dismutase (Racila and Bickenbach 2009). Interestingly, stem cell numbers do not necessarily decline with age (Conboy et al. 2005). However there are studies suggesting a functional deficit to produce differentiated progeny (Sharpless and DePinho 2007). Wound healing is a prime example, since keratinocytes isolated from older donors give rise to a lower proportion of holoclones, in comparison to younger ones (Barrandon and Green 1987). Higher levels of the senescence marker p16[INK4A] in human epidermal cells of senior individuals (Ressler et al. 2006) suggests an impairment of stem cell mobilisation with age, as well the inability to respond to proliferating signals. Furthermore, epidermal stem cells of older individuals express lower levels of the stem cell markers β1-integrin and melanoma chondroitin sulfate proteoglycan (MCSP), which are correlated with the higher self-renewal capacity (Giangreco et al. 2010).

Multiple mechanisms are involved in stem cell exhaustion. DNA repair mechanism deficits are considered one of the main causes. Deletion of the DNA repair gene ataxia–telangiectasia and Rad3-related (ATR) resulted in progeroid phenotypes in adult mice, involving alopecia, kyphosis, osteoporosis, thymic involution and fibrosis (Ruzankina et al. 2007). Experiments with mouse skin have shown that epidermal stem cells are resistant to cellular aging (Giangreco et al. 2008; Stern and Bickenbach 2007), highlighting the role of the microenvironment (stem cell niche) in age-related stem cell exhaustion (Asumda 2013; Conboy et al. 2005; Zouboulis et al. 2008). Accumulation of 53BP1-foci throughout the highly compacted heterochromatin of aged hair-follicle stem cells confirmed that DNA damage is between the primary mechanisms of stem cell exhaustion (Schuler and Rube 2013).

Jak-Stat and Notch pathways are involved to age-associated epidermal stem cell alterations (Doles et al. 2012). More specifically, cells of the aging epidermis as well as the epidermal stem cell population express high levels of phosphorylated Stat3, which is also involved in tumour progression

(Bromberg et al. 1999; Demaria et al. 2012; Demaria and Poli 2012; Doles et al. 2012), whereas skin was used as a model to provide insights in the way that aging is linked with age-associated pathophysiologic events, including inflammation and tumourigenesis. The Wnt and mTOR pathway are also involved in skin aging. Persistent expression of Wnt1 led to rapid growth of hair follicles, followed by epithelial stem cell senescence, apoptosis and epidermal stem cell exhaustion (Castilho et al. 2009). Lastly, the PI3K-Akt pathway is involved in the senescence of embryonic neural crest- or somite-derived multipotent progenitor cells with properties of stem cells of the dermal compartment, termed skin-derived precursors. These cells were shown to contribute to wound healing, maintenance of the dermis and hair follicle morphogenesis (Biernaskie et al. 2009). Separation of these cells from their niche led to accelerated senescence together with a profound decrease of Akt activity. Similar cell phenotypes were obtained after blocking the aforementioned pathway with several inhibitors (Liu et al. 2011).

The p63 protein in both its isoforms, with (TAp63) and without (ΔNp63) in its transactivation domain, was demonstrated to have multiple functions during skin development and a protective role against premature aging through maintenance of SKPs, as well as a fundamental role in cardiac development. TAp63-/- mice display a phenotype with severe ulcerations, kyphosis, hair loss and impaired wound healing. Interestingly, siRNA-specific knockdown of Tap63 prevented the formation of beating cardiomyocytes in mice (Beaudry and Attardi 2009; Paris et al. 2012; Su and Flores 2009).

Although mechanisms related to age-related defects in stem cell polarity and asymmetrical damage protein segregation have been described in bacteria and yeast, data from humans are still lacking (Bufalino et al. 2013; Florian and Geiger 2010).

❏ Extrinsic Aging

Chronic Photodamage

Chronic photodamage of the skin is the prime factor leading to skin aging, exerting its manifestations through induction of DNA damage and UV-mediated ROS. ROS formation facilitates the expression of the transcription factor c-Jun via mitogen-activated protein kinases, leading to an overexpression of MMP-1, MMP-3 and MMP-9 and inhibition of procollagen-1 (Chung et al. 2000). The cutaneous manifestations of this process are pigmentary changes and wrinkling (Baumann 2007). A main difference in the phenotype of extrinsic from intrinsically aged skin is the thickened epidermis and the hyperplasia of the elastic tissue, termed solar elastosis (Makrantonaki and Zouboulis 2007; Zouboulis and Makrantonaki 2011). The level of sun exposure determines the level of hyperplastic response, with the accumulation of abundant dystrophic elastotic material in the dermis considered to be pathognomonic for this condition (Bernstein et al. 1994; Mitchell 1967). Photoaged skin accumulates more mutations of mitochondrial DNA in comparison to photoprotected skin (Berneburg et al. 1997). The role of the 1000-fold repeats of TTAGGG sequences, termed telomeres, has been implicated in photoaging, since the photo-exposed epidermis exhibits shorter telomere length in the epidermis than in the dermis (Sugimoto et al. 2006).

UV radiation interferes with the cutaneous immune system, action, which has also therapeutic implications in many cases in dermatology. On the other hand, inhibition of action of certain immune cells (Langerhans cells, T cells) might hinder the blocking mechanisms of early cell tumorigenic progression (Gilchrest 1996).

Smoking

Smoking is a widely accepted factor, which accelerates extrinsic aging (Ernster et al. 1995; Kadunce et al. 1991; Yin et al. 2001), targeting mainly the elastin network of the skin (Just et al. 2007). Cigarette smokers wrinkle formation depict a distinctive pattern with prominent perioral lines and sharply contoured crow's feet, termed the 'smoker's face'. The physical movement of the lips and face while inhaling the smoke is the natural explanation for their formation. Facial wrinkles radiate typically at right angles from the lips and eyes and a thinning of the facial features are also observed (Kadunce et al. 1991; Model 1985).

Glycation

The development of AGEs is also a result of extrinsically aged skin. In young individuals, AGE accumulation is mainly co-localised with solar elastosis, indicating that UV irradiation affects AGE precipitation *in vivo* (Gkogkolou and Bohm 2012; Jeanmaire et al. 2001; Mizutari et al. 1997). Using photo-exposed and photo-protected skin specimens, a significant increase of lower molecular mass of hyaluronan was observed in photo-exposed skin, with a concomitant downregulation of its receptors CD44 and RHAMM (Tzellos et al. 2009; Tzellos et al. 2011).

❑ Age-associated Skin Diseases

Aging, both intrinsic and extrinsic, comprises a major variable of many cutaneous manifestations. There is a number of important skin functions, which deteriorate with increasing age, like epidermal regeneration capacity, synthesis of sebum and sweat, dermoepidermal adhesion, wound healing, thermoregulation and the speed of natural elimination of potentially hazardous chemical factors (Makrantonaki et al. 2012c). In addition, several age-associated diseases such as diabetes, arterial hypertension and malignancies indicate their subtle manifestation through skin, e.g. through disturbance of wound healing processes and chronic ulcerations or paraneoplastic syndromes.

Based on these characteristics, we present below some common age-associated skin diseases or diseases whose prevalence and manifestation have specific characteristics when appearing in elderly patients.

Wound Healing

The prevalence of leg ulcers, as a result of an end-stadium venal insufficiency affects a great number of elderly patients, with 4% of the population suffering from healed or active venous ulcers. Apart from the chronic pain, immobility of the patients, depression and decreased quality of life characterize the disease (Eklof et al. 2009; Nicolaides et al. 2008; Rabe et al. 2012). Multi-medication of the elderly can be also the cause for their development (Dissemond 2011). Leg ulcers and decubital ulcers consist a major financial problem for the health system, since they require a longer inpatient care, until they are sufficiently treated, compared to other age-related skin disorders (Theisen et al. 2012).

Skin Infections

Skin and soft tissue infections are frequent in senior patients, also because of the impaired epidermal skin barrier. *Staphylococcus aureus* and β-haemolytic streptococci are often the causative organisms leading to infections such as impetigo, folliculitis, furunculosis, carbunculosis and erysipelas. Comorbidities such as lymphedema and deep vein thrombosis play an important role in facilitating skin infections. Excoriations caused from pruritus of the elderly as a result of the barrier impairment or underlined conditions such as renal disease or diabetes mellitus might provide the ground for bacterial superinfections (Laube and Farrell 2002). Zoster manifests itself after reactivation of the Varicella zoster virus, usually following a "blow" to the immune system (e.g. infection, operation) on a basis of already existing age-related immune alterations (Na et al. 2012).

Immunological Diseases

The increase of certain immunologic skin disorders, correlated to age-related immune system alterations, is a possible explanation for the prevalence of such diseases. A prime example is the T cell mediated shift from the naïve to the memory phenotype, their reduced proliferation following activation, Langerhans cell number reduction and the cytokine profile alterations, which make skin cells more susceptible to endotoxins (Gilchrest et al. 1982; Sunderkotter et al. 1997). Bullous pemphigoid is clinically characterized by tense skin blistering and crusts usually on erythematous skin (Schmidt and Zillikens 2009) and pemphigus vulgaris is a chronic blistering disease characterized histologically by intraepidermal bulla formation. Pemphigus vulgaris mostly affects older adults of 40 to 70 years, while bullous pemphigoid peaks at 80 years (Ingen-Housz-Oro et al. 2012; Langan et al. 2008; Makrantonaki et al. 2012c). On the other hand, immunological skin senescence might explain why the manifestations of inflammatory skin diseases such as psoriasis or lupus erythematosus of the elderly are mild in comparison to young patients. Erythrodermic psoriasis has a higher prevalence in those patients, while the scalp skin of the elderly patients with plaque psoriasis is more frequently affected. In contrast, younger patients usually present with erythematosquamous plaques on the knees and elbows (Ejaz et al. 2009; Ferrandiz et al. 2002; Kwon et al. 2012; Makrantonaki et al. 2012c).

Pigmentary Disorders

Vitiligo is a disorder of progressive loss of melanocytes from the skin and hair follicle. It was recently shown that melanocytes in vitiligo are accumulating an increased number of p16, which does not correlate to the age of the donor and several active proteins of the senescence-associated secretory phenotype, implying a pathophysiologic mechanism of premature cellular senescence (Bellei et al. 2013).

Skin Tumors

A high rate of skin cancers (90%) is attributed to sun exposure (Gallagher 2005). Among them, a common form of non-invasive intraepithelial skin neoplasm, namely actinic keratosis, is characterized by atypical proliferation of suprabasal keratinocytes and a frequent reason for dermatological consultation. This lesion might evolve to squamous cell carcinoma (SCC) and is currently defined as an in-situ SCC (Goldberg and Mamelak 2010). Actinic keratoses occur in UV-exposed skin and develop in older, fair skin individuals (Schmitt and Miot 2012). The frequency of actinic keratosis correlates with lighter skin phototypes. Apart from sun exposure, drugs, such as thiazide diuretics, are also contributing to the genesis of the lesions (Traianou et al. 2012).

Basal cell carcinoma (BCC) and SCC appear on sun-exposed skin and Fitzpatrick type II and III skin types are more prone to their development (Gilchrest 1996). BCC is the most common skin cancer of the Caucasians and comprises a usually only locally invasive cancer, deriving from the basaloid cells, resembling the undifferentiated basal cells of the epidermis and its appendages. 85% of all BCCs are localised on the head and neck area (Baxter et al. 2012). Its prevalence is increasing with age and sun exposure (Bath-Hextall et al. 2007). SCC is the second most common non-melanoma skin cancer, occurring more often in men in comparison to women. It is characterized by the malignant transformation of suprabasal keratinocytes. It shows a higher metastatic potential than the BCC and its incidence rises after the age of 40. Factors correlated with UV-exposure, such as agricultural work, sun burns, solarium, PUVA therapy play an important role in its pathogenesis, as well as factors, such as ionizing radiation, chemical carcinogens, immunosuppression/immunosenescence (Perrotta et al. 2011) and human papilloma virus infection (Makrantonaki et al. 2012c; Samarasinghe and Madan 2012).

Malignant melanoma is a tumor deriving from the epidermal melanocytes. Melanoma is also more prevalent in senior patients, since half of the patients with the disease in Europe, USA and Australia are over 65 years old (Chamberlain et al. 2002; Chang et al. 1998; Lasithiotakis et al. 2006). A retrospective study of 610 patients showed that patients over 70 years appear to have thicker melanomas, higher local/transit metastases and a higher mitotic ratio (Macdonald et al. 2011). For all histological subtypes except of lentigo maligna melanoma, men of more than 50 years of age were most likely to be diagnosed with thick (≥2.0 mm) tumors (Swetter et al. 2004). In contrast, younger women had fewer thick melanomas in all histological subtypes. In addition, ulceration is more common in the aged population. Interestingly, de novo melanomas are more common in the elderly, whereas it is more probable that a malignant tumor will develop on the basis of a pre-existing single nevus in the elderly, also due to the decrease of nevus counts in this population (Swetter et al. 2004). Older age is considered an independent poor prognostic factor, while it is unclear that conditions, such as impaired host defenses and a change in the disease's pathophysiology, have a confounding role (Tsai et al. 2010).

❑ Skin as a Tool for Understanding Global Aging

Apart from the skin-associated intrinsic and extrinsic alterations and the skin diseases usually related to the aging process, there is an ongoing interest of the utilization of the skin as a model for age-associated pathologic conditions of various systems, such as the nervous and endocrine system. The way that skin can efficiently mirror inner organ alterations or deficiencies coming with age is also highlighted by the prominent skin signs of genetic diseases, which resemble aspects of aging at a very early age.

Hormone Deficiency

Increasing age leads to decrease of insulin growth factor (IGF) and this has a reflection to the skin, since it affects sebaceous differentiation and epidermal thickness (Makrantonaki et al. 2008). Patients suffering from conditions of multiple hormone deficiency or IGF-1 deficiency present with a phenotype of premature aged skin. Important aspects of the growth hormone/IGF-1 deficiency are hyperglycemia, obesity, osteopenia, hypercholesterolemia, decrease of lean mass, cardiovascular diseases and premature mortality (Laron 2005; Makrantonaki et al. 2010; Tomlinson et al. 2001; Zouboulis et al. 2007).

Neurodegenerative Diseases

In addition to the common ectodermal origin of the nervous system and the skin, the use of the second as a model of detection of hormone-associated aging has been recently highlighted. cDNA microarray analysis of immortalized sebocytes treated with a hormonal mixture of growth factors and sex steroids resembling the one of 20 and 60-year old women resulted in the regulation of 899 genes, which have been related to significant metabolic pathways related to aging (Makrantonaki et al. 2012a; Makrantonaki et al. 2012b). Furthermore, specific genes associated with the pathomechanism of neurodegenerative diseases, such as Parkinson's disease, Huntington disease, Alzheimer's disease, dentatorubral pallidoluysian atrophy and amyotrophic lateral sclerosis were also documented to alter their expression. Amyloid precursor protein was expressed and found to play a role in human epidermis (Herzog et al. 2004), while the expression of β-amyloid and tau protein was detected in skin mast cells, bearing another proof of skin reflecting neural degeneration (Kvetnoi et al. 2003). Moreover, skin melanocytes undergo apoptosis after treatment of β-amyloid, while nerve growth factor attenuates the action of the latter and exerts a protective effect (Yaar 1997). Induction of pluripotent stem cell-derived neuronal cells from normal human fibroblasts of an 82-year old patient with Alzheimer´s disease led to expression of the p-tau and GSK3B, a physiological kinase of tau, which are involved in Alzheimer´s disease pathophysiology. This model could provide a useful skin-derived tool for a better understanding of Alzheimer´s disease and for the future development of therapeutic strategies against it (Hossini et al. 2015).

MMP regulation seems to play a very important role for neurodegenerative disorders, such as Alzheimer´s disease, Parkinson´s disease and Huntington's disease. MMPs and the tissue inhibitors of MMPs are highlighted in neuronal aging since they remodel the extracellular matrix of the central nervous system (Mukherjee and Swarnakar 2015). A possible correlation in the dysregulation of these remodeling mechanisms might provide valuable markers of skin ECM degradation or remodeling impairment as tools to assess age-related neural degeneration.

Progeria Syndromes: Disease Models for Aging

Hutchinson–Gilford progeria syndrome (HGPS) is a rare genetic disorder with clinical features of premature aging. Clinical symptoms of this syndrome include scleroderma-like skin changes, bone abnormalities, alopecia, lack of subcutaneous fat, growth retardation, bone abnormalities and joint stiffness. The average life span of HGPS patients is 13 years, with atherosclerotic heart disease being between the most common cause of death (DeBusk 1972; Merideth et al. 2008). The disease occurs due to a single nucleotide mutation, which results in the production of a truncated mRNA transcript encoding a prelamin A protein with an internal deletion of 50 amino acids, known as progerin. Surprisingly, the discovery of progerin in normal cells suggests mechanisms of progeria in normal aging (Scaffidi and Misteli, 2008; Wenzel et al. 2012). The way that progerin builds up in normal skin with age and is detected in the papillary dermis, spreading to reticular dermis with age and a few terminally differentiated keratinocytes in the elderly, confirms how skin can accurately function as a model, reflecting human aging (McClintock et al. 2007). *In vivo* and *in vitro* data implicate the premature exhaustion of stem cells as a major reason for the progeria phenotype. Skin was again the means to confirm stem cell impairment, since cells isolated from all known stem cell-rich skin areas of a progeria mouse model (bulge region, sebaceous gland) showed reduced clonogenic capacity in comparison to controls. In addition, progeria skin keratinocytes exhibited lower levels of the stem cell markers α6-integrin and CD34 (Rosengardten et al. 2011). HGPS skin fibroblasts exhibit nuclear defects, such as altered gene expression, nuclear blebbing, disorganization of the underlying heterochromatin, stem cell dysfunction, increased DNA damage, cellular senescence and high p16[INK4A] levels (Capell et al. 2009).

Werner syndrome is a premature aging disorder, associated with increased occurrence of inflammatory diseases, cataract, diabetes mellitus type II and atherosclerosis. Surprisingly, skin manifestations and hair graying precede the inner organ defects. Skin fibroblasts *in vitro* are characterized by premature cellular senescence correlated to genomic instability resulting in stress kinase activation, such as p38 (Davis et al. 2007). Restrictive respiratory disease, hyperuricemia, proteinuria and primary hypogonadism are also findings of premature aging syndromes (Winkelspecht et al. 1997).

These and several other syndromes associated with prematuge aging phenotypes (Bloom syndrome, Cockayne syndrome, trichothiodystrophy, ataxia-telangiectasia, Rothmund–Thomson syndrome and xeroderma pigmentosum) have contributed to important findings regarding aging and cancer (Capell et al. 2009).

Metabolic Diseases

Diabetes mellitus is a common disease affecting multiple organs of the elderly and skin can be an attractive model of combining the cutaneous manifestations of uncontrolled chronic hyperglycaemia with skin defects. Chronic hyperglycaemia leads to an increase of AGEs, thus enhancing the aging process (Gkogkolou and Bohm 2012). Specifically, the impairment of the skin barrier, namely decreased epidermal lipid synthesis and antimicrobial peptide expression, was shown to be correlated with haemoglobin A1c levels in a chronic hyperglycemia mouse model (Park et al. 2011). Diabetic mice exhibit a reduced hydration state of the stratum corneum and a decrease of the activity of the sebaceous gland, resembling senile xerosis (Sakai et al. 2005). Diabetic skin depicts abnormalities of the elastic cutaneous network, resulting in age-associated laxity (Braverman 1989). Diabetic skin, as well as aged skin showed reduction of blood flow in rest and in response to sustained heat (Petrofsky et al. 2010; Petrofsky et al. 2008). Skin autofluorescence as a measure of AGEs in skin is a marker, which was reported to correlate with hyperglycemia, age, adiposity, vascular damage and the metabolic syndrome (Monami et al. 2008), suggesting a promising non-invasive method for patients in risk for developing complications (Lutgers et al. 2006).

❏ Conclusion

This chapter presents key mechanisms involved in skin aging and confirms the fact that aging skin can reflect accurately age-related comorbidities. Proper correlation of age-related skin and inner organ defects can provide reproducible, easily accessible and cost-effective predictors of diseases such as cancer, coronary disease and diabetes. In a future step, it could determine the time points for the initiation of specific treatments for these diseases and lastly provide reproducible follow-up markers to monitor the patient's response.

❏ References

Alikhani, Z., M. Alikhani, C.M. Boyd, K. Nagao, P.C. Trackman and D.T. Graves. 2005. Advanced glycation end products enhance expression of pro-apoptotic genes and stimulate fibroblast apoptosis through cytoplasmic and mitochondrial pathways. J Biol Chem 280: 12087-95.

Allsopp, R.C., H. Vaziri, C. Patterson, S. Goldstein, E.V. Younglai, A.B. Futcher, et al. 1992. Telomere length predicts replicative capacity of human fibroblasts. Proc Natl Acad Sci USA 89: 10114-8.

Arck, P.C., R. Overall, K. Spatz, C. Liezman, B. Handjiski and B.F. Klapp, et al. 2006. Towards a "free radical theory of graying": melanocyte apoptosis in the aging human hair follicle is an indicator of oxidative stress induced tissue damage. FASEB J 20: 1567-9.

Asumda, F.Z. 2013. Age-associated changes in the ecological niche: implications for mesenchymal stem cell aging. Stem Cell Res Ther 4: 47.

Avery, N.C. and A.J. Bailey. 2006. The effects of the Maillard reaction on the physical properties and cell interactions of collagen. Pathol Biol (Paris) 54: 387-95.

Barrandon, Y. and H. Green. 1987. Three clonal types of keratinocyte with different capacities for multiplication. Proc Natl Acad Sci USA 84: 2302-6.

Bath-Hextall, F., J. Leonardi-Bee, C. Smith, A. Meal and R. Hubbard. 2007. Trends in incidence of skin basal cell carcinoma. Additional evidence from a UK primary care database study. Int J Cancer 121: 2105-8.

Baumann, L. 2007. Skin ageing and its treatment. J Pathol 211: 241-51.

Baxter, J.M., A.N. Patel and S. Varma. 2012. Facial basal cell carcinoma. BMJ 345: e5342.

Beaudry, V.G. and L.D. Attardi. 2009. SKP-ing TAp63: stem cell depletion, senescence and premature aging. Cell Stem Cell 5: 1-2.

Bellei, B., A. Pitisci, M. Ottaviani, M. Ludovici, C. Cota, F. Luzi, et al. 2013. Vitiligo: a possible model of degenerative diseases. PLoS One 8: e59782.

Berge, U., J. Behrens and S.I. Rattan. 2007. Sugar-induced premature aging and altered differentiation in human epidermal keratinocytes. Ann N Y Acad Sci 1100: 524-9.

Berneburg, M., N. Gattermann, H. Stege, M. Grewe, K. Vogelsang, T. Ruzicka, et al. 1997. Chronically ultraviolet-exposed human skin shows a higher mutation frequency of mitochondrial DNA as compared to unexposed skin and the hematopoietic system. Photochem Photobiol 66: 271-5.

Bernstein, E.F., Y.Q. Chen, K. Tamai, K.J. Shepley, K.S. Resnik, H. Zhang, et al. 1994. Enhanced elastin and fibrillin gene expression in chronically photodamaged skin. J Invest Dermatol 103: 182-6.

Bierhaus, A., P.M. Humpert, M. Morcos, T. Wendt, T. Chavakis, B. Arnold, et al. 2005. Understanding RAGE, the receptor for advanced glycation end products. J Mol Med (Berl) 83: 876-86.

Biernaskie, J., M. Paris, O. Morozova, B.M. Fagan, M. Marra, L. Pevny, et al. 2009. SKPs derive from hair follicle precursors and exhibit properties of adult dermal stem cells. Cell Stem Cell 5: 610-23.

Biernaskie, J.A., I.A. McKenzie, J.G. Toma and F.D. Miller. 2006. Isolation of skin-derived precursors (SKPs) and differentiation and enrichment of their Schwann cell progeny. Nat Protoc 1: 2803-12.

Braverman, I.M. 1989. Elastic fiber and microvascular abnormalities in aging skin. Clin Geriatr Med 5: 69-90.

Briganti, S., E. Flori, B. Bellei and M. Picardo. 2014. Modulation of PPARgamma provides new insights in a stress induced premature senescence model. PLoS One 9: e104045.

Bromberg, J.F., M.H. Wrzeszczynska, G. Devgan, Y. Zhao, R.G. Pestell, C. Albanese, et al. 1999. Stat3 as an oncogene. Cell 98: 295-303.

Bufalino, M.R., B. Deveale and D. van der Kooy. 2013. The asymmetric segregation of damaged proteins is stem cell-type dependent. J Cell Biol 201: 523-30.

Callaghan, T.M. and K.P. Wilhelm. 2008. A review of ageing and an examination of clinical methods in the assessment of ageing skin. Part 2: Clinical perspectives and clinical methods in the evaluation of ageing skin. Int J Cosmet Sci 30: 323-32.

Capell, B.C., B.E. Tlougan and S.J. Orlow. 2009. From the rarest to the most common: insights from progeroid syndromes into skin cancer and aging. J Invest Dermatol 129: 2340-50.

Castilho, R.M., C.H. Squarize, L.A. Chodosh, B.O. Williams and J.S. Gutkind. 2009. mTOR mediates Wnt-induced epidermal stem cell exhaustion and aging. Cell Stem Cell 5: 279-89.

Cerami, C., H. Founds, I. Nicholl, T. Mitsuhashi, D. Giordano, S. Vanpatten, et al. 1997. Tobacco smoke is a source of toxic reactive glycation products. Proc Natl Acad Sci USA 94: 13915-20.

Cevenini, E., L. Invidia, F. Lescai, S. Salvioli, P. Tieri, G. Castellani, et al. 2008. Human models of aging and longevity. Expert Opin Biol Ther 8: 1393-405.

Chamberlain, A.J., L. Fritschi, G.G. Giles, J.P. Dowling and J.W. Kelly. 2002. Nodular type and older age as the most significant associations of thick melanoma in Victoria, Australia. Arch Dermatol 138: 609-14.

Chang, A.E., L.H. Karnell and H.R. Menck. 1998. The National Cancer Data Base report on cutaneous and noncutaneous melanoma: a summary of 84,836 cases from the past decade. The American College of Surgeons Commission on Cancer and the American Cancer Society. Cancer 83: 1664-78.

Chen, F.G., W.J. Zhang, D. Bi, W. Liu, X. Wei, F.F. Chen, et al. 2007. Clonal analysis of nestin (–) vimentin (+) multipotent fibroblasts isolated from human dermis. J Cell Sci 120: 2875-83.

Chi, W., E. Wu and B.A. Morgan. 2013. Dermal papilla cell number specifies hair size, shape and cycling and its reduction causes follicular decline. Development 140: 1676-83.

Chu, M. and N. Kollias. 2011. Documentation of normal stratum corneum scaling in an average population: features of differences among age, ethnicity and body site. Br J Dermatol 164: 497-507.

Chung, J.H., S. Kang, J. Varani, J. Lin, G.J. Fisher and J.J. Voorhees. 2000. Decreased extracellular-signal-regulated kinase and increased stress-activated MAP kinase activities in aged human skin in vivo. J Invest Dermatol 115: 177-82.

Conboy, I.M., M.J. Conboy, A.J. Wagers, E.R. Girma, I.L. Weissman and T.A. Rando. 2005. Rejuvenation of aged progenitor cells by exposure to a young systemic environment. Nature 433: 760-4.

Coppe, J.P., C.K. Patil, F. Rodier, Y. Sun, D.P. Munoz, J. Goldstein, et al. 2008. Senescence-associated secretory phenotypes reveal cell-nonautonomous functions of oncogenic RAS and the p53 tumor suppressor. PLoS Biol 6: 2853-68.

Davis, T., F.S. Wyllie, M.J. Rokicki, M.C. Bagley and D. Kipling. 2007. The role of cellular senescence in Werner syndrome: toward therapeutic intervention in human premature aging. Ann N Y Acad Sci 1100: 455-69.

DeBusk, F.L. 1972. The Hutchinson-Gilford progeria syndrome. Report of 4 cases and review of the literature. J Pediatr 80: 697-724.

DeGroot, J., N. Verzijl, M.J. Wenting-Van Wijk, R.A. Bank, F.P. Lafeber, J.W. Bijlsma, et al. 2001. Age-related decrease in susceptibility of human articular cartilage to matrix metalloproteinase-mediated degradation: the role of advanced glycation end products. Arthritis Rheum 44: 2562-71.

Demaria, M. and V. Poli. 2012. Pro-malignant properties of STAT3 during chronic inflammation. Oncotarget 3: 359-60.

Demaria, M., S. Misale, C. Giorgi, V. Miano, A. Camporeale, J. Campisi, et al. 2012. STAT3 can serve as a hit in the process of malignant transformation of primary cells. Cell Death Differ 19: 1390-7.

Dimri, G.P., X. Lee, G. Basile, M. Acosta, G. Scott, C. Roskelley, et al. 1995. A biomarker that identifies senescent human cells in culture and in aging skin in vivo. Proc Natl Acad Sci USA 92: 9363-7.

Diridollou, S., J. de Rigal, B. Querleux, F. Leroy and V. Holloway Barbosa. 2007. Comparative study of the hydration of the stratum corneum between four ethnic groups: influence of age. Int J Dermatol 46 Suppl 1: 11-4.

Dissemond, J. 2011. Medications. A rare cause for leg ulcers. Hautarzt 62: 516-23.

Doles, J., M. Storer, L. Cozzuto, G. Roma and W.M. Keyes. 2012. Age-associated inflammation inhibits epidermal stem cell function. Genes Dev 26: 2144-53.

Dos Santos, M., E. Metral, A. Boher, P. Rousselle, A. Thepot and O. Damour. 2015. *In vitro* 3-D model based on extending time of culture for studying chronological epidermis aging. Matrix Biol 47: 85-97 [Epub ahead of print].

Dyer, D.G., J.A. Dunn, S.R. Thorpe, K.E. Bailie, T.J. Lyons, D.R. McCance, et al. 1993. Accumulation of Maillard reaction products in skin collagen in diabetes and aging. J Clin Invest 91: 2463-9.

Ejaz, A., N. Raza, N. Iftikhar, A. Iftikhar and M. Farooq. 2009. Presentation of early onset psoriasis in comparison with late onset psoriasis: a clinical study from Pakistan. Indian J Dermatol Venereol Leprol 75: 36-40.

Eklof, B., M. Perrin, K.T. Delis, R.B. Rutherford and P. Gloviczki. 2009. Updated terminology of chronic venous disorders: the VEIN-TERM transatlantic interdisciplinary consensus document. J Vasc Surg 49: 498-501.

El-Domyati, M., S. Attia, F. Saleh, D. Brown, D.E. Birk, F. Gasparro, et al. 2002. Intrinsic aging vs. photoaging: a comparative histopathological, immunohistochemical and ultrastructural study of skin. Exp Dermatol 11: 398-405.

Elias, P.M. and R. Ghadially. 2002. The aged epidermal permeability barrier: basis for functional abnormalities. Clin Geriatr Med 18: 103-20, vii.

Engelke, M., J.M. Jensen, S. Ekanayake-Mudiyanselage and E. Proksch. 1997. Effects of xerosis and ageing on epidermal proliferation and differentiation. Br J Dermatol 137: 219-25.

Ernster, V.L., D. Grady, R. Miike, D. Black, J. Selby and K. Kerlikowske. 1995. Facial wrinkling in men and women, by smoking status. Am J Public Health 85: 78-82.

Fang, M., J. Wang, S. Li and Y. Guo. 2015. Advanced glycation end-products accelerate the cardiac aging process through the receptor for advanced glycation end-products/transforming growth factor-beta-Smad signaling pathway in cardiac fibroblasts. Geriatr Gerontol Int 28: 12499.

Ferrandiz, C., R.M. Pujol, V. Garcia-Patos, X. Bordas and J.A. Smandia. 2002. Psoriasis of early and late onset: a clinical and epidemiologic study from Spain. J Am Acad Dermatol 46: 867-73.

Fleming, T.H., P.M. Humpert, P.P. Nawroth and A. Bierhaus. 2011. Reactive metabolites and AGE/RAGE-mediated cellular dysfunction affect the aging process: a mini-review. Gerontology 57: 435-43.

Florian, M.C. and H. Geiger. 2010. Concise review: polarity in stem cells, disease and aging. Stem Cells 28: 1623-9.

Franceschi, C., M. Bonafe and S. Valensin. 2000. Human immunosenescence: the prevailing of innate immunity, the failing of clonotypic immunity and the filling of immunological space. Vaccine 18: 1717-20.

Freund, A., A.V. Orjalo, P.Y. Desprez and J. Campisi. 2010. Inflammatory networks during cellular senescence: causes and consequences. Trends Mol Med 16: 238-46.

Fuchs, E. and T. Chen. 2013. A matter of life and death: self-renewal in stem cells. EMBO Rep 14: 39-48.

Gallagher, R.P. 2005. Sunscreens in melanoma and skin cancer prevention. CMAJ 173: 244-5.

Ganceviciene, R., A.I. Liakou, A. Theodoridis, E. Makrantonaki and C.C. Zouboulis. 2012. Skin anti-aging strategies. Dermatoendocrinol 4: 308-19.

Giacomoni, P.U., L. Declercq, L. Hellemans and D. Maes. 2000. Aging of human skin: review of a mechanistic model and first experimental data. IUBMB Life 49: 259-63.

Giangreco, A., M. Qin, J.E. Pintar and F.M. Watt. 2008. Epidermal stem cells are retained in vivo throughout skin aging. Aging Cell 7: 250-9.

Giangreco, A., S.J. Goldie, V. Failla, G. Saintigny and F.M. Watt. 2010. Human skin aging is associated with reduced expression of the stem cell markers beta1 integrin and MCSP. J Invest Dermatol 130: 604-8.

Gilchrest, B.A. 1996. A review of skin ageing and its medical therapy. Br J Dermatol 135: 867-75.

Gilchrest, B.A., G.F. Murphy and N.A. Soter. 1982. Effect of chronologic aging and ultraviolet irradiation on Langerhans cells in human epidermis. J Invest Dermatol 79: 85-8.

Gilhar, A., Y. Ullmann, R. Karry, R. Shalaginov, B. Assy, S. Serafimovich, et al. 2004. Ageing of human epidermis: the role of apoptosis, Fas and telomerase. Br J Dermatol 150: 56-63.

Gkogkolou, P. and M. Bohm. 2012. Advanced glycation end products: key players in skin aging? Dermatoendocrinol 4: 259-70.

Glenn, J.V., J.R. Beattie, L. Barrett, N. Frizzell, S.R. Thorpe, M.E. Boulton, et al. 2007. Confocal Raman microscopy can quantify advanced glycation end product (AGE) modifications in Bruch's membrane leading to accurate, nondestructive prediction of ocular aging. FASEB J 21: 3542-52.

Goldberg, L.H. and A.J. Mamelak. 2010. Review ofactinic keratosis. Part I: etiology, epidemiology and clinical presentation. J Drugs Dermatol 9: 1125-32.

Grove, G.L. and A.M. Kligman. 1983. Age-associated changes in human epidermal cell renewal. J Gerontol 38: 137-42.

Harman, D. 2003. The free radical theory of aging. Antioxid Redox Signal 5: 557-61.

Herzog, V., G. Kirfel, C. Siemes and A. Schmitz. 2004. Biological roles of APP in the epidermis. Eur J Cell Biol 83: 613-24.

Hofmann, B., A.C. Adam, K. Jacobs, M. Riemer, C. Erbs, H. Bushnaq, et al. 2013 Advanced glycation end product associated skin autofluorescence: a mirror of vascular function? Exp Gerontol 48: 38-44.

Hossini, A.M., M. Megges, A. Prigione, B. Lichtner, M.R. Toliat, W. Wruck, et al. 2015. Induced pluripotent stem cell-derived neuronal cells from a sporadic Alzheimer's disease donor as a model for investigating AD-associated gene regulatory networks. BMC Genomics 16: 84.

Ingen-Housz-Oro, S., M. Alexandre, C. Le Roux-Villet, C. Picard-Dahan, E. Tancrede-Bohin, N. Wallet-Faber, et al. 2012. Pemphigus in elderly adults: clinical presentation, treatment and prognosis. J Am Geriatr Soc 60: 1185-7.

Inoue, M. and C. Katakami. 1993. The effect of hyaluronic acid on corneal epithelial cell proliferation. Invest Ophthalmol Vis Sci 34: 2313-5.

Isnard, N., G. Peterszegi, A.M. Robert and L. Robert. 2002. Regulation of elastase-type endopeptidase activity, MMP-2 and MMP-9 expression and activation in human dermal fibroblasts by fucose and a fucose-rich polysaccharide. Biomed Pharmacother 56: 258-64.

Isnard, N., L. Robert and G. Renard. 2003. Effect of sulfated GAGs on the expression and activation of MMP-2 and MMP-9 in corneal and dermal explant cultures. Cell Biol Int 27: 779-84.

Janson, D., M. Rietveld, R. Willemze and A. El Ghalbzouri. 2013a. Effects of serially passaged fibroblasts on dermal and epidermal morphogenesis in human skin equivalents. Biogerontology 14: 131-40.

Janson, D., G. Saintigny, C. Mahe and A. El Ghalbzouri. 2013b. Papillary fibroblasts differentiate into reticular fibroblasts after prolonged in vitro culture. Exp Dermatol 22: 48-53.

Jeanmaire, C., L. Danoux and G. Pauly. 2001. Glycation during human dermal intrinsic and actinic ageing: an in vivo and in vitro model study. Br J Dermatol 145: 10-8.

Just, M., M. Ribera, E. Monso, J.C. Lorenzo and C. Ferrandiz. 2007. Effect of smoking on skin elastic fibres: morphometric and immunohistochemical analysis. Br J Dermatol 156: 85-91.

Kadunce, D.P., R. Burr, R. Gress, R. Kanner, J.L. Lyon and J.J. Zone. 1991. Cigarette smoking: risk factor for premature facial wrinkling. Ann Intern Med 114: 840-4.

Kandarakis, S.A., C. Piperi, D.P. Moschonas, P. Korkolopoulou, A. Papalois and A.G. Papavassiliou. 2015. Dietary glycotoxins induce RAGE and VEGF up-regulation in the retina of normal rats. Exp Eye Res 137: 1-10.

Kim, J.-H., M. Jung, H.-S. Kim, Y.-M. Kim and E.-H. Choi. 2011. Adipose-derived stem cells as a new therapeutic modality for ageing skin. Experimental Dermatology 20: 383-7.

Kinn, P.M., G.O. Holdren, B.A. Westermeyer, M. Abuissa, C.L. Fischer, J.A. Fairley, et al. 2015. Age-dependent variation in cytokines, chemokines and biologic analytes rinsed from the surface of healthy human skin. Sci Rep 5: 10472.

Kligman, L.H. 1989. Photoaging. Manifestations, prevention and treatment. Clin Geriatr Med 5: 235-51.

Kvetnoi, I.M., T.V. Kvetnaia, I. Riadnova, B.B. Fursov, H. Ernandes-Jago, J.R. Blesa. 2003. Expression of beta-amyloid and tau-protein in mastocytes in Alzheimer disease. Arkh Patol 65: 36-9.

Kwon, H.H., I.H. Kwon and J.I. Youn. 2012. Clinical study of psoriasis occurring over the age of 60 years: is elderly-onset psoriasis a distinct subtype? Int J Dermatol 51: 53-8.

Langan, S.M., L. Smeeth, R. Hubbard, K.M. Fleming, C.J. Smith and J. West. 2008. Bullous pemphigoid and pemphigus vulgaris–incidence and mortality in the UK: population based cohort study. BMJ 337: a180.

Langton, A.K., M.J. Sherratt, C.E. Griffiths and R.E. Watson. 2010. A new wrinkle on old skin: the role of elastic fibres in skin ageing. Int J Cosmet Sci 32: 330-9.

Laron, Z. 2005. Do deficiencies in growth hormone and insulin-like growth factor-1 (IGF-1) shorten or prolong longevity? Mech Ageing Development 126: 305-7.

Lasithiotakis, K.G., U. Leiter, R. Gorkievicz, T. Eigentler, H. Breuninger, G. Metzler, et al. 2006. The incidence and mortality of cutaneous melanoma in Southern Germany: trends by anatomic site and pathologic characteristics, 1976 to 2003. Cancer 107: 1331-9.

Laube, S. and A.M. Farrell. 2002. Bacterial skin infections in the elderly: diagnosis and treatment. Drugs Aging 19: 331-42.

Linton, P.J. and K. Dorshkind. 2004. Age-related changes in lymphocyte development and function. Nat Immunol 5: 133-9.

Liu, S., X. Wang, J. Zhou, Y. Cao, F. Wang and E. Duan. 2011. The PI3K-Akt pathway inhibits senescence and promotes self-renewal of human skin-derived precursors in vitro. Aging Cell 10: 661-74.

Lock-Andersen, J., P. Therkildsen, F. de Fine Olivarius, M. Gniadecka, K. Dahlstrom, T. Poulsen, et al. 1997. Epidermal thickness, skin pigmentation and constitutive photosensitivity. Photodermatol Photoimmunol Photomed 13: 153-8.

Longas, M.O., C.S. Russell, X.Y. He. 1987. Evidence for structural changes in dermatan sulfate and hyaluronic acid with aging. Carbohydr Res 159: 127-36.

Lutgers, H.L., R. Graaff, T.P. Links, L.J. Ubink-Veltmaat, H.J. Bilo, R.O. Gans, et al. 2006. Skin Autofluorescence as a Noninvasive Marker of Vascular Damage in Patients With Type 2 Diabetes. Diabetes Care 29: 2654-9.

Macdonald, J.B., A.C. Dueck, R.J. Gray, N. Wasif, D.L. Swanson, A. Sekulic, et al. 2011. Malignant melanoma in the elderly: different regional disease and poorer prognosis. J Cancer 2: 538-43.

Makrantonaki, E. and C.C. Zouboulis. 2007. Molecular mechanisms of skin aging: state of the art. Ann N Y Acad Sci 1119: 40-50.

Makrantonaki, E., J. Adjaye, R. Herwig, T.C. Brink, D. Groth, C. Hultschig, et al. 2006. Age-specific hormonal decline is accompanied by transcriptional changes in human sebocytes in vitro. Aging Cell 5: 331-44.

Makrantonaki, E., K. Vogel, S. Fimmel, M. Oeff, H. Seltmann, C.C. Zouboulis. 2008. Interplay of IGF-I and 17beta-estradiol at age-specific levels in human sebocytes and fibroblasts in vitro. Exp Gerontol 43: 939-46.

Makrantonaki, E., P. Schonknecht, A.M. Hossini, E. Kaiser, M.M. Katsouli, J. Adjaye, et al. 2010. Skin and brain age together: the role of hormones in the ageing process. Exp Gerontol 45: 801-13.

Makrantonaki, E., V. Bekou and C.C. Zouboulis. 2012a. Genetics and skin aging. Dermatoendocrinol 4: 280-4.

Makrantonaki, E., T.C. Brink, V. Zampeli, R.M. Elewa, B. Mlody, A.M. Hossini, et al. 2012b. Identification of biomarkers of human skin ageing in both genders. Wnt signalling – a label of skin ageing? PLoS One 7: e50393.

Makrantonaki, E., A.I. Liakou, R. Eckardt, M. Zens, E. Steinhagen-Thiessen and C.C. Zouboulis. 2012c. Skin diseases in geriatric patients. Epidemiologic data. Hautarzt 63: 938-46.

Makrantonaki, E., M. Vogel, K. Scharffetter-Kochanek and C.C. Zouboulis. 2015. Skin aging: Molecular understanding of extrinsic and intrinsic processes. Hautarzt 66: 730-7.

Mancini, M., A.M. Lena, G. Saintigny, C. Mahe, N. Di Daniele, G. Melino, et al. 2014. MicroRNAs in human skin ageing. Ageing Res Rev 17: 9-15.

McClintock, D., D. Ratner, M. Lokuge, D.M. Owens, L.B. Gordon, F.S. Collins, et al. 2007. The mutant form of lamin A that causes Hutchinson-Gilford progeria is a biomarker of cellular aging in human skin. PLoS One 2: e1269.

Medvedev, Z.A. 1990. An attempt at a rational classification of theories of ageing. Biol Rev Camb Philos Soc 65: 375-98.

Merideth, M.A., L.B. Gordon, S. Clauss, V. Sachdev, A.C. Smith, M.B. Perry, et al. 2008. Phenotype and course of Hutchinson-Gilford progeria syndrome. N Engl J Med 358: 592-604.

Meyer, L.J. and R. Stern. 1994. Age-dependent changes of hyaluronan in human skin. J Invest Dermatol 102: 385-9.

Michikawa, Y., F. Mazzucchelli, N. Bresolin, G. Scarlato and G. Attardi. 1999. Aging-dependent large accumulation of point mutations in the human mtDNA control region for replication. Science 286: 774-9.

Mitchell, R.E. 1967. Chronic solar dermatosis: a light and electron microscopic study of the dermis. J Invest Dermatol 48: 203-20.

Mizutari, K., T. Ono, K. Ikeda, K. Kayashima and S. Horiuchi. 1997. Photo-enhanced modification of human skin elastin in actinic elastosis by N (epsilon)– (carboxymethyl) lysine, one of the glycoxidation products of the Maillard reaction. J Invest Dermatol 108: 797-802.

Model, D. 1985 Smoker's face: an underrated clinical sign? Br Med J (Clin Res Ed) 291: 1760-2.

Monami, M., C. Lamanna, F. Gori, F. Bartalucci, N. Marchionni and E. Mannucci. 2008. Skin autofluorescence in type 2 diabetes: beyond blood glucose. Diabetes Res Clin Pract 79: 56-60.

Moragas, A., C. Castells and M. Sans. 1993. Mathematical morphologic analysis of aging-related epidermal changes. Anal Quant Cytol Histol 15: 75-82.

Mukherjee, A. and S. Swarnakar. 2015. Implication of matrix metalloproteinases in regulating neuronal disorder. Mol Biol Rep 42: 1-11.

Na, C.R., S. Wang, R.S. Kirsner and D.G. Federman. 2012. Elderly adults and skin disorders: common problems for nondermatologists. South Med J 105: 600-6.

Naylor, E.C., R.E. Watson and M.J. Sherratt. 2011. Molecular aspects of skin ageing. Maturitas 69: 249-56.

Nicolaides, A.N., C. Allegra, J. Bergan, A. Bradbury, M. Cairols, P. Carpentier, et al. 2008. Management of chronic venous disorders of the lower limbs: guidelines according to scientific evidence. Int Angiol 27: 1-59.

Nikolakis, G., E. Makrantonaki and C.C. Zouboulis. 2013. Skin mirrors human aging. Horm Mol Biol Clin Investig 16: 13-28.

Nikolakis, G., H. Seltmann, A.M. Hossini, E. Makrantonaki, J. Knolle and C.C. Zouboulis. 2015. Ex vivo human skin and SZ95 sebocytes exhibit a homoeostatic interaction in a novel coculture contact model. Exp Dermatol 24: 497-502.

Nouveau-Richard, S., Z. Yang, S. Mac-Mary, L. Li, P. Bastien, I. Tardy, et al. 2005. Skin ageing: a comparison between Chinese and European populations. A pilot study. J Dermatol Sci 40: 187-93.

Papakonstantinou, E., M. Roth and G. Karakiulakis. 2012. Hyaluronic acid: a key molecule in skin aging. Dermatoendocrinol 4: 253-8.

Paris, M., M. Rouleau, M. Puceat and D. Aberdam. 2012. Regulation of skin aging and heart development by TAp63. Cell Death Differ 19: 186-93.

Park, H.Y., J.H. Kim, M. Jung, C.H. Chung, R. Hasham, C.S. Park, et al. 2011. A long-standing hyperglycaemic condition impairs skin barrier by accelerating skin ageing process. Exp Dermatol 20: 969-74.

Paul, R.G. and A.J. Bailey. 1996. Glycation of collagen: the basis of its central role in the late complications of ageing and diabetes. Int J Biochem Cell Biol 28: 1297-310.

Pennacchi, P.C., M.E. Almeida, O.L. Gomes, F. Faiao-Flores, M.C. Crepaldi, M.F. Dos Santos, et al. 2015. Glycated reconstructed human skin as a platform to study pathogenesis of skin aging. Tissue Eng Part A 1: 1.

Perrotta, R.E., M. Giordano and M. Malaguarnera. 2011. Non-melanoma skin cancers in elderly patients. Crit Rev Oncol Hematol 80: 474-80.

Peters, E.M., D. Imfeld and R. Graub. 2011. Graying of the human hair follicle. J Cosmet Sci 62: 121-5.

Petrofsky, J., H. Lee, M. Trivedi, A.N. Hudlikar, C.H. Yang, N. Goraksh, et al. 2010. The influence of aging and diabetes on heat transfer characteristics of the skin to a rapidly applied heat source. Diabetes Technol Ther 12: 1003-10.

Petrofsky, J.S., K. McLellan, G.S. Bains, M. Prowse, G. Ethiraju, S. Lee, et al. 2008. Skin heat dissipation: the influence of diabetes, skin thickness and subcutaneous fat thickness. Diabetes Technol Ther 10: 487-93.

Plackett, T.P., E.D. Boehmer, D.E. Faunce and E.J. Kovacs. 2004. Aging and innate immune cells. J Leukoc Biol 76: 291-9.

Plowden, J., M. Renshaw-Hoelscher, C. Engleman, J. Katz and S. Sambhara. 2004. Innate immunity in aging: impact on macrophage function. Aging Cell 3: 161-7.

Pochi, P.E., J.S. Strauss and D.T. Downing. 1979. Age-related changes in sebaceous gland activity. J Invest Dermatol 73: 108-11.

Potten, C.S. 1974. The epidermal proliferative unit: the possible role of the central basal cell. Cell Tissue Kinet 7: 77-88.

Poundarik, A.A., P.C. Wu, Z. Evis, G.E. Sroga, A. Ural, M. Rubin, et al. 2015. A direct role of collagen glycation in bone fracture. J Mech Behav Biomed Mater 50: 82-92.

Rabe, E., J.J. Guex, A. Puskas, A. Scuderi and F. Fernandez Quesada. 2012. Epidemiology of chronic venous disorders in geographically diverse populations: results from the Vein Consult Program. Int Angiol 31: 105-15.

Racila, D. and J.R. Bickenbach. 2009. Are epidermal stem cells unique with respect to aging? Aging (Albany NY) 1: 746-50.

Ravelojaona, V., A.M. Robert and L. Robert. 2009. Expression of senescence-associated beta-galactosidase (SA-beta-Gal) by human skin fibroblasts, effect of advanced glycation end-products and fucose or rhamnose-rich polysaccharides. Arch Gerontol Geriatr 48: 151-4.

Rawlings, A.V. 2006. Ethnic skin types: are there differences in skin structure and function? Int J Cosmet Sci 28: 79-93.

Ressler, S., J. Bartkova, H. Niederegger, J. Bartek, K. Scharffetter-Kochanek, P. Jansen-Durr, et al. 2006. p16INK4A is a robust in vivo biomarker of cellular aging in human skin. Aging Cell 5: 379-89.

Robinson, M.K., R.L. Binder and C.E. Griffiths. 2009. Genomic-driven insights into changes in aging skin. J Drugs Dermatol 8: s8-11.

Rock, K., J. Tigges, S. Sass, A. Schutze, A.M. Florea, A.C. Fender, et al. 2015. miR-23a-3p causes cellular senescence by targeting hyaluronan synthase 2: possible implication for skin aging. J Invest Dermatol 135: 369-77.

Rosengardten, Y., T. McKenna, D. Grochova and M. Eriksson. 2011. Stem cell depletion in Hutchinson-Gilford progeria syndrome. Aging Cell 10: 1011-20.

Ruzankina, Y., C. Pinzon-Guzman, A. Asare, T. Ong, L. Pontano, G. Cotsarelis, et al. 2007. Deletion of the developmentally essential gene ATR in adult mice leads to age-related phenotypes and stem cell loss. Cell Stem Cell 1: 113-26.

Sakai, S., K. Kikuchi, J. Satoh, H. Tagami and S. Inoue. 2005. Functional properties of the stratum corneum in patients with diabetes mellitus: similarities to senile xerosis. Br J Dermatol 153: 319-23.

Samarasinghe, V. and V. Madan. 2012. Nonmelanoma skin cancer. J Cutan Aesthet Surg 5: 3-10.

Scaffidi, P. and T. Misteli. 2008. Lamin A-dependent misregulation of adult stem cells associated with accelerated ageing. Nat Cell Biol 10: 452-9.

Schmidt, E. and D. Zillikens. 2009. Diagnosis and clinical severity markers of bullous pemphigoid. F1000 Med Rep 1: 15.

Schmitt, J.V. and H.A. Miot. 2012. Actinic keratosis: a clinical and epidemiological revision. An Bras Dermatol 87: 425-34.

Schuler, N. and C.E. Rube. 2013. Accumulation of DNA damage-induced chromatin alterations in tissue-specific stem cells: the driving force of aging? PLoS One 8: e63932.

Seiberg, M. 2013. Age-induced hair greying – the multiple effects of oxidative stress. Int J Cosmet Sci 35: 532-8.

Sejersen, H. and S.I. Rattan. 2009. Dicarbonyl-induced accelerated aging in vitro in human skin fibroblasts. Biogerontology 10: 203-11.

Sell, D.R., E.C. Carlson and V.M. Monnier. 1993. Differential effects of type 2 (non-insulin-dependent) diabetes mellitus on pentosidine formation in skin and glomerular basement membrane. Diabetologia 36: 936-41.

Sestier, B. 2015. Hematopoietic stem cell exhaustion and advanced glycation end-products in the unexplained anemia of the elderly. Rev Esp Geriatr Gerontol 50: 223-231.

Shapiro, S.D. 1998. Matrix metalloproteinase degradation of extracellular matrix: biological consequences. Curr Opin Cell Biol 10: 602-8.

Sharpless, N.E. and R.A. DePinho. 2007. How stem cells age and why this makes us grow old. Nat Rev Mol Cell Biol 8: 703-13.

Stern, M.M. and J.R. Bickenbach. 2007. Epidermal stem cells are resistant to cellular aging. Aging Cell 6: 439-52.

Stitt, A.W. 2001. Advanced glycation: an important pathological event in diabetic and age related ocular disease. Br J Ophthalmol 85: 746-53.

Su, X. and E.R. Flores. 2009. TAp63: The fountain of youth. Aging (Albany NY) 1: 866-9.

Sugimoto, M., R. Yamashita and M. Ueda. 2006. Telomere length of the skin in association with chronological aging and photoaging. J Dermatol Sci 43: 43-7.

Sunderkotter, C., H. Kalden and T.A. Luger. 1997. Aging and the skin immune system. Arch Dermatol 133: 1256-62.

Swetter, S.M., A.C. Geller and J.M. Kirkwood. 2004. Melanoma in the older person. Oncology (Williston Park) 18: 1187-96; discussion 96-7.

Theisen, S., A. Drabik and S. Stock. 2012. Pressure ulcers in older hospitalised patients and its impact on length of stay: a retrospective observational study. J Clin Nurs 21: 380-7.

Thijssen, D.H., S.E. Carter and D.J. Green. 2015. Arterial structure and function in vascular ageing: "Are you as old as your arteries?". *J Physiol* [Epub ahead of print].

Thomson, J.A., J. Itskovitz-Eldor, S.S. Shapiro, M.A. Waknitz, J.J. Swiergiel, V.S. Marshall, et al. 1998. Embryonic stem cell lines derived from human blastocysts. Science 282: 1145-7.

Tomlinson, J.W., N. Holden, R.K. Hills, K. Wheatley, R.N. Clayton, A.S. Bates, et al. 2001. Association between premature mortality and hypopituitarism. The Lancet 357: 425-31.

Toole, B.P. 1997. Hyaluronan in morphogenesis. J Intern Med 242: 35-40.

Traianou, A., M. Ulrich, Z. Apalla, E. De Vries, D. Bakirtzi, D. Kalabalikis, et al. 2012. Risk factors for actinic keratosis in eight European centres: a case-control study. Br J Dermatol 167 Suppl 2: 36-42.

Tsai, S., C. Balch and J. Lange. 2010. Epidemiology and treatment of melanoma in elderly patients. Nat Rev Clin Oncol 7: 148-52.

Tsukahara, K., T. Fujimura, Y. Yoshida, T. Kitahara, M. Hotta, S. Moriwaki, et al. 2004. Comparison of age-related changes in wrinkling and sagging of the skin in Caucasian females and in Japanese females. J Cosmet Sci 55: 351-71.

Tsutsumi, M. and M. Denda. 2007. Paradoxical effects of beta-estradiol on epidermal permeability barrier homeostasis. Br J Dermatol 157: 776-9.

Tzellos, T.G., I. Klagas, K. Vahtsevanos, S. Triaridis, A. Printza, A. Kyrgidis, et al. 2009. Extrinsic ageing in the human skin is associated with alterations in the expression of hyaluronic acid and its metabolizing enzymes. Exp Dermatol 18: 1028-35.

Tzellos, T.G., X. Sinopidis, A. Kyrgidis, K. Vahtsevanos, S. Triaridis, A. Printza, et al. 2011. Differential hyaluronan homeostasis and expression of proteoglycans in juvenile and adult human skin. J Dermatol Sci 61: 69-72.

Valet, F., K. Ezzedine, D. Malvy, J.Y. Mary and C. Guinot. 2009. Assessing the reliability of four severity scales depicting skin ageing features. Br J Dermatol 161: 153-8.

Vina, J., C. Borras and J. Miquel. 2007. Theories of ageing. IUBMB Life 59: 249-54.

Vlassara, H., W. Cai, J. Crandall, T. Goldberg, R. Oberstein, V. Dardaine, et al. 2002. Inflammatory mediators are induced by dietary glycotoxins, a major risk factor for diabetic angiopathy. Proc Natl Acad Sci USA 99: 15596-601.

Waldera Lupa, D.M., F. Kalfalah, K. Safferling, P. Boukamp, G. Poschmann, E. Volpi, et al. 2015. Characterization of skin aging-associated secreted proteins (SAASP) produced by dermal fibroblasts isolated from intrinsically aged human skin. J Invest Dermatol 135: 1954-68.

Wang, Y., S. Zeinali-Davarani, E.C. Davis and Y. Zhang. 2015. Effect of glucose on the biomechanical function of arterial elastin. J Mech Behav Biomed Mater 49: 244-54.

Wenzel, V., D. Roedl, D. Gabriel, L.B. Gordon, M. Herlyn, R. Schneider, et al. 2012. Naive adult stem cells from patients with Hutchinson-Gilford progeria syndrome express low levels of progerin in vivo. Biol Open 1: 516-26.

Winkelspecht, K., V. Mahler and F. Kiesewetter. 1997. Metageria–clinical manifestations of a premature aging syndrome. Hautarzt 48: 657-61.

Wu, X. and V.M. Monnier. 2003. Enzymatic deglycation of proteins. Arch Biochem Biophys 419: 16-24.

Xue, M., N. Rabbani and P.J. Thornalley. 2011. Glyoxalase in ageing. Semin Cell Dev Biol 22: 293-301.

Yaar, M., Gilchrest B.A. 1997. Human melanocytes as a model system for studies of Alzheimer disease. Arch Dermatol 133: 1287-91.

Yamagishi, S., K. Fukami and T. Matsui. 2015. Evaluation of tissue accumulation levels of advanced glycation end products by skin autofluorescence: A novel marker of vascular complications in high-risk patients for cardiovascular disease. Int J Cardiol 185: 263-8.

Yang, Y.C., H.C. Fu, C.Y. Wu, K.T. Wei, K.E. Huang and H.Y. Kang. 2013. Androgen receptor accelerates premature senescence of human dermal papilla cells in association with DNA damage. PLoS One 8: e79434.

Yang, Y.I., H.I. Kim, M.Y. Choi, S.H. Son, M.J. Seo, J.Y. Seo, et al. 2010. Ex vivo organ culture of adipose tissue for in situ mobilization of adipose-derived stem cells and defining the stem cell niche. J Cell Physiol 224: 807-16.

Ye, J., A. Garg, C. Calhoun, K.R. Feingold, P.M. Elias and R. Ghadially. 2002. Alterations in cytokine regulation in aged epidermis: implications for permeability barrier homeostasis and inflammation. I. IL-1 gene family. Exp Dermatol 11: 209-16.

Yin, L., A. Morita and T. Tsuji. 2001. Skin aging induced by ultraviolet exposure and tobacco smoking: evidence from epidemiological and molecular studies. Photodermatol Photoimmunol Photomed 17: 178-83.

Zhu, P., C. Yang, L.H. Chen, M. Ren, G.J. Lao and L. Yan. 2011. Impairment of human keratinocyte mobility and proliferation by advanced glycation end products-modified BSA. Arch Dermatol Res 303: 339-50.

Zolla, V., I.T. Nizamutdinova, B. Scharf, C.C. Clement, D. Maejima, T. Akl, et al. 2015. Aging-related anatomical and biochemical changes in lymphatic collectors impair lymph transport, fluid homeostasis and pathogen clearance. Aging Cell 14: 582-94.

Zouboulis, C.C. and A. Boschnakow. 2001. Chronological ageing and photoageing of the human sebaceous gland. Clin Exp Dermatol 26: 600-7.

Zouboulis, C.C. and E. Makrantonaki. 2011. Clinical aspects and molecular diagnostics of skin aging. Clin Dermatol 29: 3-14.

Zouboulis, C.C., W.C. Chen, M.J. Thornton, K. Qin, R. Rosenfield. 2007. Sexual hormones in human skin. Horm Metab Res 39: 85-95.

Zouboulis, C.C., J. Adjaye, H. Akamatsu, G. Moe-Behrens and C. Niemann. 2008. Human skin stem cells and the ageing process. Exp Gerontol 43: 986-97.

12

CHAPTER

Skin Aging with a Focus on the Cornified Envelope

Mark Rinnerthaler,[1,a] *Maria Karolin Streubel*[1,b] *and Klaus Richter*[1,*]

❏ Introduction

The skin providing the protective barrier is the largest organ of the human body and confronted with the harshest conditions as it has to fend off a wide variety of insults from the environment. The skin is a complex organ consisting of 3 different layers and a series of different cell types. The innermost layer, the subcutis built up by fat tissue serves as an energy storage and provides insulation and protective padding.

The next layer is the dermis consisting predominantly of dermal fibroblasts which produce collagens, proteoglycans and elastic fibers forming an extensive extracellular matrix (ECM) (Ritz-Timme et al. 2003; Shapiro et al. 1991).

Elastic fibers are composed of fibrillin-rich microfibrils, elastins, glycoproteins and some other proteins (Kielty et al. 2002). They are connected to each other and to hyaluronic acid forming an extensive dermal network into which long fibrils of collagen I and III are interwoven (Naylor et al. 2011). This ECM gives the skin its physical strength and elasticity. During aging the ECM gets partially degraded by matrix metalloproteases (MMPs) (Birkedal-Hansen et al. 1993). Besides the most abundant fibroblasts a number of different immune cells (macrophages, dermal dentritic cells, mast cells, neutrophils and T-cells) and adipocytes are present in the dermis.

[1] Department of Cell Biology, Division of Genetics, University of Salzburg, Salzburg 5020, Austria.

[a] E-mail: mark.rinnerthaler@sbg.ac.at

[b] E-mail: mariakarolin.streubel@stud.sbg.ac.at

[*] Corresponding author: klaus.richter@sbg.ac.at

The outermost layer of the skin is the epidermis which provides the protective barrier against the environment. Its main cell type is the keratinocyte (more than 95%) but there are also melanocytes, Langerhans cells and Merkel cells. The epidermis itself comprises 4 sublayers: *stratum basale, stratum spinosum, stratum granulosum* and *stratum corneum*. The epidermis and the dermis are connected via the basal lamina a special kind of ECM. Cells of the *stratum basale* directly attach to the basal lamina. These are stem cells and undifferentiated proliferative keratinocytes (Hsu et al. 2014). Upon leaving the basal layer cells stop proliferating and start the differentiation program.

Finally the outermost layer the *stratum corneum* consists of terminally differentiated and dead corneocytes providing the barrier function of the skin.

During aging both the dermis and the epidermis are becoming thinner and the dermo-epidermal junction flattens. In the dermis the most dramatic changes during aging are the fragmentation and reduction of the extracellular matrix which leads to the formation of wrinkles the most obvious appearance of aged skin. In the epidermis the proliferation rate of keratinocytes slows down but the most dramatic effect is the change in the protein composition of the cornified envelope (Rinnerthaler et al. 2013).

❑ Composition of the Epidermis and the Cornified Envelope

The epidermis itself shows a thickness of 100 – 150 μm with remarkable histological changes from the basal lamina to the outside leading to the designation of the 4 sublayers *stratum basale, stratum spinosum, stratum granulosum* and *stratum corneum*. The cells of the *stratum basale,* the innermost layer are stem cells as well as undifferentiated proliferating progenitors so called transit amplifying cells which are characterized by the expression of keratins K5 and K14. As cells migrate into the spinous and granular layers they stop proliferating and start differentiating. On the contrary to the outermost layer, the *stratum corneum,* the cells in these two layers are still transcriptionally active. In the *stratum corneum* the terminally differentiated keratinocytes have changed their morphology to a flattened appearance; they are already dead and are now called corneocytes. In the *stratum spinosum* keratins K1 and K10 are expressed as well as 3 important proteins for the formation of the cornified envelope: involucrin, envoplakin and periplakin. Involucrin forms a complex together with envoplakin and periplakin (DiColandrea et al. 2000) which is the first scaffold in the formation of the cornified envelope to whom many more proteins are subsequently crosslinked (Sevilla et al. 2007).

In addition to this protein scaffold lamellar bodies are produced by the Golgi apparatus of keratinocytes in the *stratum spinosum* and *stratum granulosum* (Grayson et al. 1985; Chapman and Walsh 1989). These lamellar bodies are granulescomprising polar lipids like glucosylceramides, sphingomyelins, phospholipids and cholesterol (Raymond et al. 2008). But they also contain lipid processing enzymes, antimicrobial peptides proteases and protease inhibitors and corneodesmosin (Braff et al. 2005; Raymond et al. 2008; Galliano et al. 2006; Madison et al. 1998; Serre et al. 1991).

The lamellar bodies are of crucial importance for the formation of the cornified envelope. They fuse with the plasma membrane replacing phospholipids of the lipid bilayer by ω-OH-ceramids which are further on crosslinked to the periplakin-envoplakin-involucrin scaffold by transglutaminase 1 (Kalinin et al. 2001). Transglutaminase 1 is calcium dependent and together with transglutaminase 3 it is responsible to incorporate loricrin into the cornified envelope. Loricrin is the main component of the cornified envelope and its expression peaks in the *stratum granulosum* (Kalinin et al. 2001). Due to its poor solubility it is also packed into the lamellar bodies and crosslinked with members of the small proline rich repeat (SPRR) protein family. Finally the loricrin-SPRR complex is linked to the periplakin-envoplakin-involucrin scaffold. The cornified envelope is not yet finished at this stage however. Various other proteins still need to be incorporated. Filaggrin is one of them, it is bundling keratins in particular keratin 1 and 10 into macrofibrils with the result that corneocytes obtain their characteristic flattened shape (Proksch et al. 2008). Furthermore members of the S100 protein family are attached to the cornified envelope (Robinson et al. 1997). Finally the late cornified envelope proteins (LCE) are incorporated (Marshall et al. 2001) and now the cornified envelope has a mega-protein-lipid skeleton that occupies most of the corneocytes volume and is responsible for the barrier function of the skin. The corneocyte itself has degraded its nucleus, mitochondria and other organelles and is eventually shed off the surface as dead squama.

❑ Composition of the Cornified Envelope in Dependence of Age

During aging the turnover rate of keratinocytes in the epidermis slows down considerably. Whereas in young skin it takes about 28 days for a keratinocyte from leaving the basal layer until it scales off as a dead corneocyte in older individuals the same process takes place within 40 – 60 days (Grove and Kligman 1983). Even more dramatic are changes affecting the composition of the cornified envelope. The first scaffold upon which the cornified envelope is constructed comprises envoplakin, periplakin and involucrin. The expression pattern of these genes does not change during aging (Rinnerthaler et al. 2013). The expression of transglutaminase 1 responsible for crosslinking of envoplakin, periplakin and involucrin slightly increases during aging whereas the expression of transglutaminase 3 responsible for the crosslinking of loricrin and the SPRRs is almost unaffected. The most abundant protein in the CE is loricrin it is considerably down-regulated (2.7-fold) in old skin (Rinnerthaler et al. 2013).

On the contrary to loricrin the partner proteins which are predominantly crosslinked to loricrin, the SPRRs are upregulated. All SPRRs with the only exception of SPRR2G are dramatically upregulated which in the case of SPRR2F is more than 100 fold. This increase in SPRR expression might on the one hand be a compensation for the reduced expression of loricrin and on the other hand an increase of the anti-oxidative capacities of the epidermis. The epidermis is confronted with a high burden of ROS which is even increasing during aging. For this reason the CE itself shows anti-oxidative capabilities and a major role to accomplish this task is played by the SPRR2 subfamily. The composition of SPRRs is characterized by a high content of proline and cysteine the later having a pronounced anti-oxidative function. Pointing to the anti-oxidative function of SPRRs is also the fact that SPRRs are upregulated after tissue injury and burns (Vermeij et al. 2011; Rinnerthaler et al. 2015a). Furthermore SPRR genes are direct targets of the transcription factor Nrf2 and Nrf2 links anti-oxidative defense with epidermal barrier function via the up-regulation of SPRR2D and SPRR2H. Nrf2 is a major regulator of keratinocyte redox signaling and plays an important role in skin homeostasis, repair and disease (reviewed in (Schafer and Werner 2015)).

Filaggrin like loricrin a major component of the cornified envelope is also down-regulated considerably during aging (3.3 fold) (Rinnerthaler et al. 2013). It is bundling keratins which leads to the flattening of the corneocytes giving them their characteristic shape. An additional function of filaggrin is influencing the hydration state of the epidermis. During the maturation process of the corneoytes filaggrin undergoes a degradation process releasing hygroscopic amino acids which influence the water binding capacity of the skin (Tagami 2008).

Further components of the CE being incorporated at the late stage of cornification are the late cornified envelope proteins (LCEs). These proteins can be divided into 3 subfamilies. During aging the subfamilies 1 and 2 are down-regulated but subfamily 3 is upregulated. Remarkably, the subfamily 2 LCEs are up-regulated in keratinocyte cell culture experiments upon the addition of calcium whereas the expression of the 2 other subfamilies remains completely unaffected. Another family of which some members are incorporated by transglutaminases into the CE comprises the S100 proteins. The S100 proteins have been identified originally in bovine brain and have been characterized as a family of small calcium binding proteins. Their physiological functions cover a wide spectrum including the regulation of oxidative stress, wound healing, proliferation, differentiation, cell migration, membrane and vesicular trafficking and calcium homeostasis. S100A11 is involved in the differentiation of keratinocytes. Also during the differentiation process S100A10 is thought to play a role in remodeling of the cell membrane. S100A8 is thought to be protective against oxidative stress in skin and after external stresses like tape stripping it is up-regulated. S100A7 was identified as an amplifier of inflammation in psoriatic lesions. S100A9 is involved in wound healing and together with S100A8 it is up-regulated after injury. (fora review on S100 proteins see (Halawi et al. 2014)).

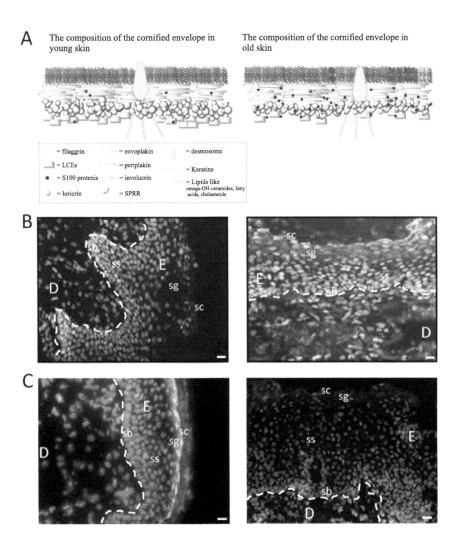

FIG. 1 Change in the composition of the cornified envelope during the aging process.
In (A) a schematic drawing of the changes in the composition of the cornified envelope is shown. The levels of lorcirin and filaggrin are decreasing whereas the levels of all SPRRs are dramatically increasing. Another highlight is the increase of many S100 proteins and a decrease of the group one and two of the LCE family. The protein content of involucrin, periplakin and envoplakin remains unchanged. In (B) immunohistochemistry of SPRR2A and in (C) immunohistochemistry of loricrin is presented (green colour). The distribution of nuclei is shown with Hoechst 33258 (blue). In each case on the left hand side the situation in young individuals and on the right hand side the situation in old individuals is shown. An increase in SPRR2A levels and a decrease of loricrin levels with age is very obvious. The following abbrevations are used: Stratum basale (sb), stratum granulosum (sg), stratum spinosum (ss) and stratum corneum (sc), epidermis (E) and (D) dermis. The dashed line should represent the basal membrane that separates the dermis from the epidermis. (Scale bar: 10 μm).

The expression of all these S100 proteinsis up-regulated during aging which is modest in the case of S100A10 (two-fold) and quite strong in the case of S100A9 (five–fold) (Rinnerthaler et al. 2013). A schematic drawing of all the CE changes summarized above is presented in Fig. 1A. The increase in SPRR2A levels and the decrease in loricrin levels are shown with the help of immunohistochemistry in Fig. 1B and Fig. 1C respectively.

❑ Epidermal Calcium Gradient and its Breakdown

Calcium is of utmost importance for the differentiation of keratinocytes and the formation of the CE as has been already demonstrated by Hennings & Holbrook 1983 (Hennings and Holbrook 1983). Although the differentiation/cornification continues without further cell divisions calcium itself initiates the differentiation process but does not stop cell proliferation. It has been demonstrated that keratinocytes are able to proliferate even at concentrations exceeding 1.8 mM calcium. Only when cells get into contact with each other upon reaching confluency the cell cycle inhibitors p21^{WAF1} and p27^{KIP1} are activated and cell division ceases (Kolly et al. 2005).

In the *stratum basale* the calcium concentration is very low (around 0.1 mM) which is necessary to keep keratinocytes in a proliferating and undifferentiated state. As keratinocytes migrate to the *stratum spinosum* they stop dividing and start differentiating with the expression of keratins 1 and 10, envoplakin, periplakin, involucrin, desmoplakin, corneodesmosin, desmoglein 1 and transglutaminase 1 (Streubel et al. 2015, in press) . For the expression of these proteins higher calcium concentrations are necessary with the exception of TG1 but this enzyme needs calcium for its activity. In the *stratum granulosum* calcium reaches the highest concentration in the epidermis as could be demonstrated with Molecular Probes™ Calcium Green™-1, AM, Cell Permeant (Rinnerthaler et al. 2013). Here the expression of filaggrin, transglutaminase 3 and loricrin the most abundant protein of the CE is activated (Kalinin et al. 2001).

In the *stratum corneum* the expression of the SPRRs, LCEs and S100 proteins takes place together with the concomitant final assembly of the CE. In the *stratum corneum* the calcium concentration is already remarkably reduced compared with the stratum granulosum. Previously it has been assumed that the calcium gradient in the epidermis is built up by using extracellular calcium. But recently it has been shown that intracellular calcium stores are providing the calcium for this gradient (Celli et al. 2010).

For the intracellular calcium stores the calcium sensing receptor CaSR is of crucial importance. It is localized in the plasma membrane of keratinocytes and belongs to the super family of G-protein coupled receptors (GPCRs) class C (Brown and MacLeod 2001). This receptor is essential for establishing the epidermal calcium gradient necessary for the differentiation of keratinocytes and the formation of the permeability barrier as has been demonstrated in keratinocyte-specific CaSR knock out mice (Tu et al. 2012). Upon binding of extracellular calcium the CaS- receptor activates phospholipase C gamma 1 which hydrolyses phosphatidyl inositol 4, 5-bisphosphate (PIP2) to diacylglycerol (DAG) and inositol 1, 4, 5 trisphosphate (IP3). DAG activates proteinkinase C which stimulates the expression, phosphorylation and activation of c-Fos and c-Jun both are dimerizing to AP-1 transcription factors. For AP-1 TFs it has been demonstrated that they are involved in the expression of a number of keratins (K1, K3, K4, K5, K12, K14, K15, K18) (Blumenberg 2006) as wells as the expression of TG 1, involucrin and loricrin (DiSepio et al. 1999; Maccarrone et al. 2003; Rossi et al. 2000). Like CaSR also localized in the plasma membrane are the calcium channel ORAI1, the ion channel transient receptor potential channel 1 (TRPC1) and TRPV5 which are responsible for the import of calcium into the cytosol of keratinocytes.

A rise in intracellular calcium results in the occupation of four calcium binding sites in the protein calmodulin which in turn causes the activation of many enzymes among them calcineurin a serine phosphatase which dephosphorylates the four members of the NFAT family of transcription factors. The dephosphorylated NFATs shuttle from the cytosol into the nucleus. Here they interact with the AP-1 transcription factors starting the differentiation process by activating the transcription of CE proteins like involucrin, filaggrin and later on loricrin (Tu and Bikle 2013).

The transport of calcium from the cytosol into the ER and Golgi is mediated by the P-type sarco/endoplasmic reticulum Ca2+ −ATPases (ATP2A1, ATP2A2, ATP2A3) with the result that the calcium stores are filled up (Brini et al. 2012). Celli et al. demonstrated that the release of calcium from the ER into the cytosol taking place in the *stratum granulosum* is a key event for the terminal differentiation of keratinocytes (Celli et al. 2011).

In fact using calcium specific staining on histological sections of human skin it can be demonstrated that there is a peak of calcium concentration in the *stratum granulosum* (Rinnerthaler et al. 2013). This peak in calcium concentration is present during childhood and also in young adults but disappears in aging skin. This is even more surprising as neither the expression of genes involved in calcium metabolism mentioned in this chapter does change significantly during aging nor does the overall concentration of calcium in the epidermis (117 µg calcium per gram epidermis in young adults versus 109 µg calcium per gram epidermis in old individuals) (Rinnerthaler et al. 2013).

❑ Calcium and Skin Diseases

Calcium homeostasis is not only disturbed during aging but also in some skin diseases. Mutations in the gene ATP2A2/SERCA2 encoding a calcium pump of the P-type ATPase family which transports calcium from the cytosol into the ER are causing Darier disease (Sakuntabhai et al. 1999). In total 130 mutations in the ATP2A2 gene are known that cause Darier disease and they all lead to a failure of the calcium transport and a depletion of calcium from the ER (Savignac et al. 2011).

A direct effect of these mutations is an increase of the calcium concentration in the cytosol, causing an impaired transport of desmoplakins to the periphery and therefore desmosomes cannot form properly.

As a consequence keratinocytes lose cell-cell adhesions produce an abnormal keratinization pattern and not the typical flattened but a rounded shape. At the clinical level Darier disease shows itchy malodorous keratotic papules which are very susceptible to infections (Savignac et al. 2011).

Mutations in the gene ATP2C1 are causing Hailey-Hailey disease. ATP2C1 belongs to the family of P-type cation transport ATPases. Its function is to transport calcium into the Golgi (Hu et al. 2000; Alfonso-Prieto et al. 2009) and mutations in ATP2C1 result in higher levels of free calcium in the cytoplasmconcomitant with the failure to respond to extracellular calcium. In these patients the calcium gradient is also affected similar to the aging phenotype. Due to reduced adhesion of keratinocytes, the clinical phenotype shows epidermal vesiculation or clefting which leads to painful erosions scaly plaques and vesicopustules (Sudbrak et al. 2000).

In contrary to Darier disease and Hailey-Hailey disease psoriasis is not caused by a single mutation but is a chronic inflammatory disease affecting up to 1% of children and 3% of adults (Parisi et al. 2013) caused by T helper cells (Belge et al. 2014) combined with an infiltration of the dermis and epidermis with immune cells. Characteristic for this disease is an enormously increased proliferation rate and turnover of keratinocytes from normally 28 days to 3-4 days in psoriasis. This leads to dry red lesions of the skin which are covered with silvery scales. Comparing normal with psoriatic skin using gene expression profiling identified differentially expressed genes involved in calcium binding, apoptosis, keratinization, lipid transportation and homeostasis in addition to the immune processes (Sudharsana et al. 2015). Of the calcium binding proteins in particular S100A7 and S100A15 are up-regulated which are responsible for an exaggerated inflammatory response (Wolf et al. 2010). It was also demonstrated that in psoriatic skin the calcium gradient is disturbed similar to aged skin (Menon and Elias 1991). Furthermore an altered calcium metabolism leads to a defective calcium-mediated cell signaling (Karvonen et al. 2000) and it was shown that reduced TRPC channel expression causes impaired differentiation and enhanced proliferation (Leuner et al. 2011).

Like Psoriasis atopic dermatitis is a chronic inflammatory skin disease originating from a complex interplay between keratinocytes and immune cells. This results in a dry and scaly skin showing red raised lesions that often weep and crack (Thomsen 2014). A characteristic feature of atopic dermatitis is a disturbed epidermal barrier function (Cork et al. 2009) as well as a disturbed epidermal calcium gradient (Forslind et al. 1999). Associated with this are reduced levels of S100 proteins, filaggrin, hornerin and filaggrin 2 in the epidermis of atopic dermatitis patients (Pellerin et al. 2013). Furthermore it was demonstrated that calmodulin-like skin protein (CLSP) is increased in the differentiated layers of the atopic dermatitis-epidermis. It is speculated that it helps to restore the calcium gradient and regulates the calcium dependent proteins which are forming the epidermal barrier (Donovan et al. 2013).

❑ Recovery of the Aged Cornified Envelope by Calcitriol, Sulforaphane, Hyperforin, UVB, Niclosamide and Several Lipids

The age-dependent change in the composition of the cornified envelope results in an altered barrier function of the epidermis, leading to an increased TWEL, increased thickness of the *stratum corneum*, a reduced recovery rate after physical damage of the epidermis, an increased sensitivity against tape stripping and a decreased resistance against an aceton treatment (Celli et al. 2011). Therefore it is of utmost importance to compensate for the loss of the epidermal calcium gradient and induce the formation of the cornified envelope. A substance that could fulfill this task is Vitamin D_3 or its biological active metabolite 1, 25-dihydroxyvitamin D_3. In a first step 7-Dehydrocholesterol is synthesized by the body and under the influence of UVB irradiation in the epidermis previtamin D_3 is formed. In a next step previtamin D_3 is metabolized in the liver to 25-hydroxyvitaminD [25(OH)D] by the mitochondrial localized cytochrome P450 enzyme CYP27A1. Finally 25-hydroxyvitaminD [25(OH)D] is converted by the renal cytochrome p450 enzyme CYP27B1 to 1,25-dihydroxyvitamin D_3, better known as calcitriol (Reichrath 2007). Calcitriol has a strong effect on the proliferation as well as differentiation of keratinocytes. The cellular target of calcitriol is the vitamin D receptor (VDR), a member of the nuclear receptor family of transcription factors. Activation of VDR by calcitriol promotes heterodimerization with the retinoid-X receptor. This heterodimer binds to genomic hormone response elements that are called vitamin D response elements (VDRE) resulting in a transcription of target sites. Activation of the VDR in human keratinocytes leads to both induction of proliferation and differentiation (Hu et al. 2014; Haussler et al. 1998). This discrepancy can be explained by the fact that VDR can recruit several coactivators (Bollag 2007). Similar to calcium these vitamin D interacting coactivators are organized in a gradual way. In the *stratum basale* the D receptor interacting protein (DRIP) complex is localized that is constantly declining towards the *stratum granulosum*. In contrast to this the steroid receptor coactivator (SRC) complexes (of which only SRC2 and SRC3 are expressed in human keratinocytes) are highly abundant in the *stratum granulosum* and are not detectable in the *stratum basale* (Bikle 2012; Oda et al. 2003). The combination of VDR with DRIP in the *stratum basale* interacts with the Wnt/β-catenin signaling pathway and induces the expression of such proteins as the cell cycle regulator cyclin D1, oncogene glioma-associated oncogene homolog (Gli1) and, peptidyl arginine deiminase 1 (PADI1). The promotor of these genes harbor VDRE as well as TCF/Lef response elements (target sites for β-catenine). Especially cyclin D1 and Gli1 promote the proliferation of the keratinocyte stem cells (Talwar et al. 1995; Grigoryan et al. 2008). The opposing effect is achieved by the combination of VDR with SRC2/3. This results in a recruitment of the CREB-binding protein, histone acetyltransferases and methltransferases. Typical target genes that are expressed are K1, K10, filaggrin, loricrin, catheldicidin and ABCA12 (Bikle 2012; Christakos et al. 2003). All these genes are involved in the terminal differentiation process of keratinocytes. Of special interest is the VDR target gene CaR because it reflects the gradual action of the VDR as well as the epidermal calcium gradient. The calcium-sensing receptor CaSR is expressed under the influence of calcitriol in the suprabasal keratinocyte layers. In this skin section CaSR is needed most, because calcium peaks in the *stratum basale* where this small ion renders to be a main driving force for keratinocyte differentiation. The combination of calcium and calcitriol induces the expression of several phosphoinositide phospholipase C family members, transgluatminases and involucrin (Ratnam et al. 1999; Bikle 2012). A topical treatment of skin with calcitriol should therefore greatly improve the skin barrier function in the elderly. A positive effect of vitamin D on the skin was already shown for the skin disorder *psoriasis* (Fogh and Kragballe 2004) . As we have discussed elsewhere psoriasis in many cases resembles aged human skin (Rinnerthaler et al. 2015b).

The already mentioned transcription factor Nrf2 could also be a suitable target to restore the composition of the cornified envelope. It was demonstrated that an activation of Nrf2 via sulforaphane led to a transcriptional upregulation of Sprr2d and Sprr2h and in this way had a positive effect on the barrier formation in loricrin deficient mice (Schafer and Werner 2015). A good way to improve the barrier function of the skin seems to be an enforced increase in the cytoplasmatic calcium levels. Members of the Transient receptor potential cation channel, subfamily C encode non-selective calcium-permeable cation channels that could have the capacity to increase intracellular calcium levels. Especially, TRPC4, TRPC6 and TRPC7 seem to be involved in the differentiation process of keratinocytes. Addition of hyperforin leads to an activiation of TRPC6 accompanied with a calcium influx and this results in an immediate inhibition of keratinocyte proliferation and induction of keratinocyte differentiation (HaCat cells as well as primary keratinocytes) (Muller et al. 2008; Leuner et al. 2011). By interfering downstream of calcium in the differentiation process the necessity for this small ion should be no more essential. A good target for this approach is the transcription factor activatorprotein 1 (AP-1). AP-1 after activation forms a heterodimeric protein that consists in various combinations of members of the c-FOS, c-JUN, ATF and JDP family. Depending on the cell type AP-1 has a broad variety of effects. In human keratinocytes that transcription factor is a central element in the epidermal differentiation process acting downstream of calcium. The big opponent of AP-1 is the signal transducer and activator of transcription 3 (STAT3) pathway that inhibits AP-1 expression. Therefore STAT3 inhibition leads to premature differentiation of keratinocytes (Saeki et al. 2012). This task can be fulfilled pharmaceutically by a treatment with niclosamide that rendered to be an inhibitor of the STAT3 pathway (Ren et al. 2010).

The effect of UVB irradiation on the epidermal barrier is ambivalent. It was demonstrated that high doses of UVB disrupt the epidermal barrier. In contrast to this results it was shown that low doses of UVB as well as suberythermal doses of UVB for three days greatly improved the epidermal barrier (Permatasari et al. 2013).

An improvement of the epidermal barrier can not only be achieved on the protein level (cornified envelope) but can also be obtained on the lipid level. It was demonstrated that several lipids that are externally applied can penetrate the *stratum corneum*, are taken up by keratinocytes, are packed into lamellar bodies that are pinching off from the ER, are then secreted and contribute to the epidermal barrier by forming lamellar bilayers. An optimal improvement could be achieved by administration of an equimolar ratio between ceramides, cholesterols and free fatty acids (Man et al. 1996; Valdman-Grinshpoun et al. 2012). In sum twelve ceramide sublasses have been identified to contribute to the epidermal barrier (Hon et al. 2013). But the best effect in improving the *stratum corneum* was achieved by synthetic ceramids such as N-ethyl dihydrogenphosphate-2-hexyl-3-oxo-decanamide (Kang et al. 2008) or pseudoceramide-5 [N-(2-hydroxyhexadecanoyl) sphinganin] (Del Rosso 2011) that are rebuilt into endogenous ceramides.

An improvement of the epidermal barrier was also achieved:

- by urea that strengthened the *stratum corneum* and induced the expression of antimicrobial peptides such as LL-37 and β-defensin-2 (Grether-Beck et al. 2012; Hon et al. 2013)
- by macrocarpal A, a component of an Eucalyptus extract that increased the levels of ceramides and the water holding capacity in the SC (Ishikawa et al. 2012)
- by N-acetyl-glucosamine that induced an upregulation of several differentiation markers such as keratin 10 and involucrin, (Mammone et al. 2009)
- by nicotinamide that induced an upregulation of the palmitoyl-transferase leading to an increased synthesis of ceramides (Tanno et al. 2000)
- by panthenol that increased the water binding capacity of the stratum corneum and at the same time reduced the transepidermal water loss (Gehring and Gloor 2000)

- by samples from Dead-Sea-Salts that are rich in magnesium and led to an increased skin hydration (Proksch et al. 2005)
- by Chinese herbal mixtures that induced both an increased synthesis of lipids and an increased expression of antimicrobial peptides (Man et al. 2011)

None of this substances and methods mentioned above was tested on aged skin, but they should have the potential to help to increase the epidermal barrier function in the elderly and are waiting for further investigation.

❑ Acknowledgments

We are grateful for financial support to the OeAD, project number (CZ 10/2014) (to Mark Rinnerthaler). We want to thank Prof. Johann Bauer (Head of dermatology, SALK/The Paracelsus Medical University, Salzburg), Prof. Dr. med. Nikolaus Schmeller (head of urology, The Hospital of the Brothers of St. John of God in Salzburg) and Prof. Dr. med. Gottfried Wechselberger (head of plastic surgery, The Hospital of the Brothers of St. John of God in Salzburg) for continuing support and fruitful discussions.

❑ References

Alfonso-Prieto, M., X. Biarnes, P. Vidossich and C. Rovira. 2009. The molecular mechanism of the catalase reaction. J Am Chem Soc 131: 11751-11761.

Belge, K., J. Bruck and K. Ghoreschi. 2014. Advances in treating psoriasis. F1000Prime Rep 6: 4.

Bikle, D.D. 2012. Vitamin D and the skin: physiology and pathophysiology. Rev Endocr Metab Dis 13: 3-19.

Birkedal-Hansen, H., W.G. Moore, M.K. Bodden, L.J. Windsor, B. Birkedal-Hansen, A. DeCarlo, et al. 1993. Matrix metalloproteinases: a review. Crit Rev Oral Biol Med 4: 197-250.

Blumenberg, M. 2006. Transcriptional regulation of keratin gene expression. Intermediate Filaments. Springer/Landes Bioschience, USA: 93-109.

Bollag, W.B. 2007. Differentiation of human keratinocytes requires the vitamin D receptor and its coactivators. J Invest Dermatol 127: 748-750.

Braff, M.H., A. Di Nardo and R.L. Gallo. 2005. Keratinocytes store the antimicrobial peptide cathelicidin in lamellar bodies. J Invest Dermatol 124: 394-400.

Brini, M., T. Cali, D. Ottolini and E. Carafoli. 2012. Calcium pumps: why so many? Compr Physiol 2: 1045-1060.

Brown, E.M. and R.J. MacLeod. 2001. Extracellular calcium sensing and extracellular calcium signaling. Physiol Rev 81: 239-297.

Celli, A., S. Sanchez, M. Behne, T. Hazlett, E. Gratton and T. Mauro. 2010. The epidermal Ca2+ gradient: measurement using the phasor representation of fluorescent lifetime imaging. Biophys J 98: 911-921.

Celli, A., D.S. Mackenzie, D.S. Crumrine, C.L. Tu, M. Hupe, D.D. Bikle, et al. 2011. Endoplasmic reticulum Ca2+ depletion activates XBP1 and controls terminal differentiation in keratinocytes and epidermis. Brit J Dermatol 164: 16-25.

Chapman, S.J. and A. Walsh. 1989. Membrane-coating granules are acidic organelles which possess proton pumps. J Invest Dermatol 93: 466-470.

Christakos, S., P. Dhawan, Y. Liu, X.R. Peng and A. Porta. 2003. New insights into the mechanisms of vitamin D action. J Cell Biochem 88: 695-705.

Cork, M.J., S.G. Danby, Y. Vasilopoulos, J. Hadgraft, M.E. Lane, M. Moustafa, et al. 2009. Epidermal barrier dysfunction in atopic dermatitis. J Invest Dermatol 129: 1892-1908.

Del Rosso, J.Q. 2011. Repair and maintenance of the epidermal barrier in patients diagnosed with atopic dermatitis: an evaluation of the components of a body wash-moisturizer skin care regimen directed at management of atopic skin. J Clin Aesthet Dermatol 4: 45-55.

DiColandrea, T., T. Karashima, A. Maatta and F.M. Watt. 2000. Subcellular distribution of envoplakin and periplakin: insights into their role as precursors of the epidermal cornified envelope. J Cell Biol 151: 573-585.

DiSepio, D., J.R. Bickenbach, M.A. Longley, D.S. Bundman, J.A. Rothnagel and D.R. Roop. 1999. Characterization of loricrin regulation in vitro and in transgenic mice. Differentiation 64: 225-235.

Donovan, M., A. Ambach, A. Thomas-Collignon, C. Prado, D. Bernard, O. Jammayrac, et al. 2013. Calmodulin-like skin protein level increases in the differentiated epidermal layers in atopic dermatitis. Exp Dermatol 22: 836-837.

Fogh, K. and K. Kragballe. 2004. New vitamin D analogs in psoriasis. Curr. Drug Targets Inflamm. Allergy 3: 199-204.

Forslind, B., Y. Werner-Linde, M. Lindberg and J. Pallon. 1999. Elemental analysis mirrors epidermal differentiation. Acta Derm Venereol 79: 12-17.

Galliano, M.F., E. Toulza, H. Gallinaro, N. Jonca, A. Ishida-Yamamoto, G. Serre, et al. 2006. A novel protease inhibitor of the alpha2-macroglobulin family expressed in the human epidermis. J Biol Chem 281: 5780-5789.

Gehring, W. and M. Gloor. 2000. Effect of topically applied dexpanthenol on epidermal barrier function and stratum corneum hydration. Results of a human in vivo study. Arzneimittelforschung 50: 659-663.

Grayson, S., A.D. Johnsonwinegar, B.U. Wintroub, E.H. Epstein, R.R. Isseroff and P.M. Elias. 1985. Lamellar Bodies from Neonatal Mouse Epidermis – Functional Implications of Lipid and Enzyme Content. Clin Res 33: A155-A155.

Grether-Beck, S., I. Felsner, H. Brenden, Z. Kohne, M. Majora, A. Marini, et al. 2012. Urea uptake enhances barrier function and antimicrobial defense in humans by regulating epidermal gene expression. J Invest Dermatol 132: 1561-1572.

Grigoryan, T., P. Wend, A. Klaus and W. Birchmeier. 2008. Deciphering the function of canonical Wnt signals in development and disease: conditional loss- and gain-of-function mutations of alpha-catenin in mice. Genes Dev 22: 2308-2341.

Grove, G.L. and A.M. Kligman. 1983. Age-associated changes in human epidermal cell renewal. J Gerontol 38: 137-142.

Halawi, A., O. Abbas and M. Mahalingam. 2014. S100 proteins and the skin: a review. J Eur Acad Dermatol 28: 405-414.

Haussler, M.R., G.K. Whitfield, C.A. Haussler, J.C. Hsieh, P.D. Thompson, S.H. Selznick, et al. 1998. The nuclear vitamin D receptor: biological and molecular regulatory properties revealed. J Bone Miner Res 13: 325-349.

Hennings, H. and K.A. Holbrook. 1983. Calcium regulation of cell-cell contact and differentiation of epidermal cells in culture. An ultrastructural study. Exp Cell Res 143: 127-142.

Hon, K.L., A.K. Leung and B. Barankin. 2013. Barrier repair therapy in atopic dermatitis: an overview. Am J Clin Dermatol 14: 389-399.

Hsu, Y.C., L.S. Li and E. Fuchs. 2014. Emerging interactions between skin stem cells and their niches. Nat Med 20: 847-856.

Hu, L.Z., D.D. Bikle and Y. Oda. 2014. Reciprocal role of vitamin D receptor on beta-catenin regulated keratinocyte proliferation and differentiation. J Steroid Biochem 144: 237-241.

Hu, Z., J.M. Bonifas, J. Beech, G. Bench, T. Shigihara, H. Ogawa, S. Ikeda, et al. 2000. Mutations in ATP2C1, encoding a calcium pump, cause Hailey-Hailey disease. Nat Genet 24: 61-65.

Ishikawa, J., Y. Shimotoyodome, S. Chen, K. Ohkubo, Y. Takagi, T. Fujimura, et al. 2012. Eucalyptus increases ceramide levels in keratinocytes and improves stratum corneum function. Int J Cosmet Sci 34: 17-22.

Kalinin, A., L.N. Marekov and P.M. Steinert. 2001. Assembly of the epidermal cornified cell envelope. J Cell Sci 114: 3069-3070.

Kang, J.S., W.K. Yoon, J.K. Youm, S.K. Jeong, B.D. Park, M.H. Han, et al. 2008. Inhibition of atopic dermatitis-like skin lesions by topical application of a novel ceramide derivative, K6PC-9p, in NC/Nga mice. Exp Dermatol 17: 958-964.

Karvonen, S.L., T. Korkiamaki, H. Yla-Outinen, M. Nissinen, H. Teerikangas, K. Pummi, et al. 2000. Psoriasis and altered calcium metabolism: downregulated capacitative calcium influx and defective calcium-mediated cell signaling in cultured psoriatic keratinocytes. J Invest Dermatol 114: 693-700.

Kielty, C.M., M.J. Sherratt and C.A. Shuttleworth. 2002. Elastic fibres. J Cell Sci 115: 2817-2828.

Kolly, C., M.M. Suter and E.J. Muller. 2005. Proliferation, cell cycle exit and onset of terminal differentiation in cultured keratinocytes: pre-programmed pathways in control of C-Myc and Notch1 prevail over extracellular calcium signals. J Invest Dermatol 124: 1014-1025.

Leuner, K., M. Kraus, U. Woelfle, H. Beschmann, C. Harteneck, W.H. Boehncke, et al. 2011. Reduced TRPC channel expression in psoriatic keratinocytes is associated with impaired differentiation and enhanced proliferation. PLoS One 6: e14716.

Maccarrone, M., M. Di Rienzo, N. Battista, V. Gasperi, P. Guerrieri, A. Rossi, et al. 2003. The endocannabinoid system in human keratinocytes. Evidence that anandamide inhibits epidermal differentiation through CB1 receptor-dependent inhibition of protein kinase C, activation protein-1 and transglutaminase. J Biol Chem 278: 33896-33903.

Madison, K.C., G.N. Sando, E.J. Howard, C.A. True, D. Gilbert, D.C. Swartzendruber, et al. 1998. Lamellar granule biogenesis: a role for ceramide glucosyltransferase, lysosomal enzyme transport and the Golgi. J Investig Dermatol Symp Proc 3: 80-86.

Mammone, T., D. Gan, C. Fthenakis and K. Marenus. 2009. The effect of N-acetylglucosamine on stratum corneum desquamation and water content in human skin. J Cosmet Sci 60: 423-428.

Man, M., M. Hupe, D. Mackenzie, H. Kim, Y. Oda, D. Crumrine, et al. 2011. A topical Chinese herbal mixture improves epidermal permeability barrier function in normal murine skin. Exp Dermatol 20: 285-288.

Man, Mq M., K.R. Feingold, C.R. Thornfeldt and P.M. Elias. 1996. Optimization of physiological lipid mixtures for barrier repair. J Invest Dermatol 106: 1096-1101.

Marshall, D., M.J. Hardman, K.M. Nield and C. Byrne. 2001. Differentially expressed late constituents of the epidermal cornified envelope. Proc Natl Acad Sci USA 98: 13031-13036.

Menon, G.K. and P.M. Elias. 1991. Ultrastructural-localization of calcium in psoriatic and normal human epidermis. Arch Dermatol 127: 57-63.

Muller, M., K. Essin, K. Hill, H. Beschmann, S. Rubant, C.M. Schempp, et al. 2008. Specific TRPC6 channel activation, a novel approach to stimulate keratinocyte differentiation. J Biol Chem 283: 33942-33954.

Naylor, E.C., R.E.B. Watson and M.J. Sherratt. 2011. Molecular aspects of skin ageing. Maturitas 69: 249-256.

Oda, Y., C. Sihlbom, R.J. Chalkley, L. Huang, C. Rachez, C.P.B. Chang, et al. 2003. Two distinct coactivators, DRIP/mediator and SRC/p160, are differentially involved in vitamin D receptor transactivation during keratinocyte differentiation. Mol Endocrinol 17: 2329-2339.

Parisi, R., D.P. Symmons, C.E. Griffiths and D.M. Ashcroft. 2013. Global epidemiology of psoriasis: a systematic review of incidence and prevalence. J Invest Dermatol 133: 377-385.

Pellerin, L., J. Henry, C.Y. Hsu, S. Balica, C. Jean-Decoster, M.C. Mechin, et al. 2013. Defects of filaggrin-like proteins in both lesional and nonlesional atopic skin. J Allergy Clin Immunol 131: 1094-1102.

Permatasari, F., B. Zhou and D. Luo. 2013. Epidermal barrier: Adverse and beneficial changes induced by ultraviolet B irradiation depending on the exposure dose and time (Review). Exp Ther Med 6: 287-292.

Proksch, E., H.P. Nissen, M. Bremgartner and C. Urquhart. 2005. Bathing in a magnesium-rich Dead Sea salt solution improves skin barrier function, enhances skin hydration and reduces inflammation in atopic dry skin. Int J Dermatol 44: 151-157.

Proksch, E., J.M. Brandner and J.M. Jensen. 2008. The skin: an indispensable barrier. Exp Dermatol 17: 1063-1072.

Ratnam, A.V., D.D. Bikle and J.K. Cho. 1999. 1, 25 dihydroxyvitamin D3 enhances the calcium response of keratinocytes. J Cell Physiol 178: 188-196.

Raymond, A.A., A. Gonzalez de Peredo, A. Stella, A. Ishida-Yamamoto, D. Bouyssie, G. Serre, et al. 2008. Lamellar bodies of human epidermis: proteomics characterization by high throughput mass spectrometry and possible involvement of CLIP-170 in their trafficking/secretion. Mol Cell Proteomics 7: 2151-2175.

Reichrath, J. 2007. Vitamin D and the skin: an ancient friend, revisited. Exp Dermatol 16: 618-625.

Ren, X.M., L. Duan, Q.A. He, Z. Zhang, Y. Zhou, D.H. Wu, et al. 2010. Identification of niclosamide as a new small-molecule inhibitor of the STAT3 signaling pathway. Acs Med Chem Lett 1: 454-459.

Rinnerthaler, M., J. Duschl, P. Steinbacher, M. Salzmann, J. Bischof, M. Schuller, et al. 2013. Age-related changes in the composition of the cornified envelope in human skin. Exp Dermatol 22: 329-335.

Rinnerthaler, M., J. Bischof, M.K. Streubel, A. Trost and K. Richter. 2015a. Oxidative stress in aging human skin. Biomolecules 5: 545-589.

Rinnerthaler, M., M.K. Streubel, J. Bischof and K. Richter, 2015b. Skin aging, gene expression and calcium. Exp Gerontol 68: 59-65.

Ritz-Timme, S., I. Laumeier and M.J. Collins. 2003. Aspartic acid racemization: evidence for marked longevity of elastin in human skin. Brit J Dermatol 149: 951-959.

Robinson, N.A., S. Lapic, J.F. Welter and R.L. Eckert. 1997. S100A11, S100A10, annexin I, desmosomal proteins, small proline-rich proteins, plasminogen activator inhibitor-2 and involucrin are components of the cornified envelope of cultured human epidermal keratinocytes. J Biol Chem 272: 12035-12046.

Rossi, A., M.V. Catani, E. Candi, F. Bernassola, P. Puddu and G. Melino. 2000. Nitric oxide inhibits cornified envelope formation in human keratinocytes by inactivating transglutaminases and activating protein 1. J Invest Dermatol 115: 731-739.

Saeki, Y., T. Nagashima, S. Kimura and M. Okada-Hatakeyama. 2012. An ErbB receptor-mediated AP-1 regulatory network is modulated by STAT3 and c-MYC during calcium-dependent keratinocyte differentiation. Exp Dermatol 21: 293-298.

Sakuntabhai, A., V. Ruiz-Perez, S. Carter, N. Jacobsen, S. Burge, S. Monk, et al. 1999. Mutations in ATP2A2, encoding a Ca2+ pump, cause Darier disease. Nat Genet 21: 271-277.

Savignac, M., A. Edir, M. Simon and A. Hovnanian. 2011. Darier disease: a disease model of impaired calcium homeostasis in the skin. Biochim. Biophys. Acta 1813: 1111-1117.

Schafer, M. and S. Werner. 2015. Nrf2-A regulator of keratinocyte redox signaling. Free Radic Biol Med 88b: 243-252.

Serre, G., V. Mils, M. Haftek, C. Vincent, F. Croute, A. Reano, et al. 1991. Identification of late differentiation antigens of human cornified epithelia, expressed in re-organized desmosomes and bound to cross-linked envelope. J Invest Dermatol 97: 1061-1072.

Sevilla, L.M., R. Nachat, K.R. Groot, J.F. Klement, J. Uitto, P. Djian, et al. 2007. Mice deficient in involucrin, envoplakin and periplakin have a defective epidermal barrier. J Cell Biol 179: 1599-1612.

Shapiro, S.D., E.J. Campbell, H.G. Welgus and R.M. Senior. 1991. Elastin degradation by mononuclear phagocytes. Ann Ny Acad Sci 624: 69-80.

Streubel, M.K., M. Rinnerthaler, J. Bischof, K. Richter. 2015. Changes in the composition of the cornified envelope during skin aging: A calcium centric point of view. Tb aging skin. Springer (in press).

Sudbrak, R., J. Brown, C. Dobson-Stone, S. Carter, J. Ramser, J. White, et al. 2000. Hailey-Hailey disease is caused by mutations in ATP2C1 encoding a novel Ca(2+) pump. Hum Mol Genet 9: 1131-1140.

Sudharsana, S., L. Sajitha and A. Mohanapriya. 2015. Insights into protein interaction networks reveal non-receptor kinases as significant druggable targets for psoriasis. Gene 566: 138-147.

Tagami, H. 2008. Functional characteristics of the stratum corneum in photoaged skin in comparison with those found in intrinsic aging. Arch Dermatol Res 300: S1-S6.

Talwar, H.S., C.E. Griffiths, G.J. Fisher, T.A. Hamilton and J.J. Voorhees. 1995. Reduced type I and type III procollagens in photodamaged adult human skin. J Invest Dermatol 105: 285-290.

Tanno, O., Y. Ota, N. Kitamura, T. Katsube and S. Inoue. 2000. Nicotinamide increases biosynthesis of ceramides as well as other stratum corneum lipids to improve the epidermal permeability barrier. Brit J Dermatol 143: 524-531.

Thomsen, S.F. 2014. Atopic dermatitis: natural history, diagnosis and treatment. ISRN Allergy 2014: 354250.

Tu, C.L. and D.D. Bikle. 2013. Role of the calcium-sensing receptor in calcium regulation of epidermal differentiation and function. Best Pract Res Clin Endocrinol Metab 27: 415-427.

Tu, C.L., D.A. Crumrine, M.Q. Man, W. Chang, H. Elalieh, M. You, et al. 2012. Ablation of the calcium-sensing receptor in keratinocytes impairs epidermal differentiation and barrier function. J Invest Dermatol 132: 2350-2359.

Valdman-Grinshpoun, Y., D. Ben-Amitai and A. Zvulunov. 2012. Barrier-restoring therapies in atopic dermatitis: current approaches and future perspectives. Dermatol Res Pract 2012: 923134.

Vermeij, W.P., A. Alia and C. Backendorf. 2011. ROS quenching potential of the epidermal cornified cell envelope. J Invest Dermatol 131: 1435-1441.

Wolf, R., F. Mascia, A. Dharamsi, O.M.Z. Howard, C. Cataisson, V. Bliskovski, et al. 2010. Gene from a Psoriasis Susceptibility Locus Primes the Skin for Inflammation. Sci Transl Med 2: 61ra90.

Index

T - #0412 - 071024 - C264 - 234/156/12 - PB - 9780367783006 - Gloss Lamination